Neurologic Localization and Diagnosis

T0073862

Neurologic Localization and Diagnosis

Differential Diagnosis by Complaint-Based Approach

ELI E. ZIMMERMAN, MD

Associate Professor
Neurology
Vanderbilt University Medical Center
Nashville, Tennessee, United States

MARTIN A. SAMUELS, MD

Miriam Sydney Joseph Distinguished Professor of Neurology
Harvard Medical School
Founding Chair
Department of Neurology
Brigham and Women's Hospital
Boston, Massachusetts, United States

HOWARD S. KIRSHNER, MD

Professor and Vice Chairman
Neurology
Vanderbilt University Medical Center
Nashville, Tennessee, United States

KARL E. MISULIS, MD, PhD

Professor and Director of Neurohospitalist Service
Neurology
Professor
Biomedical Informatics
Vanderbilt University School of Medicine
Nashville, Tennessee, United States

ELSEVIER

Elsevier
1600 John F. Kennedy Blvd.
Ste 1800
Philadelphia, PA 19103-2899

NEUROLOGIC LOCALIZATION AND DIAGNOSIS: ISBN: 978-0-323-81280-1
DIFFERENTIAL DIAGNOSIS BY COMPLAINT-BASED APPROACH

Content Strategist: Melanie Tucker/Mary Hegeler
Senior Content Development Manager: Somodatta Roy Choudhury
Senior Content Development Specialist: Malvika Shah
Publishing Services Manager: Shereen Jameel
Project Manager: Vishnu T. Jiji
Design Direction: Brian Salisbury

Printed in India

Last digit is the print number: 9 8 7 6 5 4 3 2 1

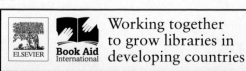

We are pleased to bring you *Neurologic Localization and Diagnosis*. It has been 25 years since the original book of the same name was published. In this new book, we have expanded the text and covered substantial new ground. We have also engaged new authors who are experienced educators and clinicians at Vanderbilt University Medical Center and Harvard Medical School.

We begin Part 1 with an overview of neurologic diagnosis, then progress to the details of taking a neurologic history and examination.

Part 2 explores clinical neuroscience, with anatomy and physiology as they pertain to neurologic diagnosis.

Part 3 is localization by anatomy, where we cover syndromes and disorders affecting the central and peripheral nervous systems.

Part 4 focuses on localization by dysfunction, helping to guide differential diagnosis of specific clinical presentations.

Part 5 considers the diagnosis of some suspected disorders for which localization is particularly helpful for diagnosis.

It is a pleasure to bring this text to another generation of clinicians in training. We hope this book will be helpful not only for those planning careers in neurology and neurosurgery but also in other specialties, because neurologic disorders are omnipresent in the practice of medicine.

CONTENTS

PART 1

Approach to Neurologic Diagnosis

PART OUTLINE

Overview of Neurologic Diagnosis

Howard S. Kirshner, Martin A. Samuels, Eli E. Zimmerman, and Karl E. Misulis

First Localize

This book has a principal focus on the use of history and examination to localize lesions affecting the nervous system and to guide diagnosis of many conditions. We presume the reader has a foundation in basic neuroanatomy and neurophysiology as would be covered early in medical training, though we will review critical details. Beginning with that foundation, the first task of the neurologist is to localize the patient's presenting complaints to a specific area of the nervous system. In taking a history from a patient, the neurologist listens carefully for symptoms that localize the problem to a specific area of the nervous system: brain, spinal cord, cranial and peripheral nerves, neuromuscular junction, or muscle. Then the examination demonstrates findings that suggest one or more specific locations for a neurologic disorder. Hence, a history and an examination go most of the way to establishing a diagnosis (or, at least, a differential diagnosis).

The history begins with the chief complaint, which is usually the reason for the encounter, although sometimes the patient and the referring provider have different reasons in mind. Neurology is concerned not only with the neurologic complaint but also with other medical issues that might be related, because many neurologic disorders are manifestations of systemic processes.

The history is not limited to the timing of the onset of the symptoms. It also includes the patient's past medical history, family history, and social history, which serve to identify risk factors for the problem at hand. The onset and time course of the symptoms give major clues to both the localization and the cause of the problem. For example, stroke might be the obvious diagnosis in a patient who presents with sudden onset of right-sided weakness and aphasia, based on the timing of onset and the neurologic deficit. On the other hand, a patient with several months of progressive right hemiparesis and aphasia is more likely to have a tumor.

Further details of the history can lead to a more specific diagnosis. For example, the patient might have a history of transient ischemic attacks involving speech difficulty plus right-sided weakness. This would suggest that the problem originates from atherosclerotic disease of the left internal carotid artery. A history of risk factors of stroke, such as hypertension, diabetes, dyslipidemia and smoking, would make atherosclerotic carotid disease even more likely. A family history of stroke might also increase the likelihood of this diagnosis. On the other hand, a patient with ongoing intravenous drug abuse and new fever may raise a clinical suspicion of endocarditis as causation. A history of recent neck injury in a patient without significant vascular risk factors would raise concern for carotid artery dissection.

Objective information for localizing a lesion can be gained from details of the neurologic examination. If a patient presents with right hemiplegia from a presumed stroke, the proposed localization of the lesion is very different depending on whether they have aphasia or not. Elements of aphasia are evidence of cortical involvement, whereas if a patient has severe right hemiparesis without language deficit, a subcortical lesion is more likely.

In neurology perhaps more than any other medical specialty, the time course in which symptoms develop often leads to the specific etiologic diagnosis. Strokes, as in the example above, begin suddenly, but space-occupying lesions such as brain tumors produce symptoms in an insidious,

3

slowly developing fashion. A patient with a brain tumor and a patient with a stroke may have nearly identical examinations, but their histories will provide the clues to the diagnosis. The timing and evolution of the symptoms thus aid the clinician in reaching a specific diagnosis.

Then Diagnose

Once the neurologist localizes the neurologic lesion and analyzes the history, they then obtain confirmation from laboratory and imaging studies. In our stroke example, a magnetic resonance imaging (MRI) scan will show the acute infarction in the brain, and specific sequences will identify the age of the stroke. Computer tomography (CT) angiography can show the obstruction in the carotid artery.

If the stroke does not appear related to a lesion in the carotid artery, the neurologist would also look at the heart as a possible source of embolism, and studies such as echocardiography and cardiac monitoring would be appropriate. The neurologist would also look to laboratory studies such as fasting lipid profile and hemoglobin A1c.

In the patient with an apparent brain tumor, MRI will again be helpful in identifying the lesion. The neurologist might then go to studies as CT scan of the chest, abdomen, and pelvis to look for a primary tumor that might have metastasized to the brain. In a case of infection, such as meningitis, encephalitis, or brain abscess, brain imaging might localize the lesion, but a lumbar puncture or brain biopsy might be needed to confirm the infectious organism. This process of neurologic diagnosis depends critically on an accurate history and physical and neurologic examination.

Pitfalls in Localization and Diagnosis

History, examination, and subsequent localization are key to accurate diagnosis, but our human execution of these techniques is not perfect. The multitude of interconnections and associative processing occurring in the clinician's mind is both an asset and a liability to diagnosis.

Workflow for optimal care is commonly some variation on the following sequence:
- Identify the patient.
- Identify the reason for the encounter.
- Obtain the patient's medical history.
- Perform a physical examination.
- Develop a differential diagnosis.
- Gather additional data to narrow the differential diagnosis, which can be done by obtaining additional historical or examination data from the patient, obtaining information from family or medical records.
- Arrive at a most likely diagnosis with a short list of differential diagnoses.
- Decide on an action, which could either be acquiring more information or initiating management of the provisionally diagnosed condition.

At some subsequent point, usually during a follow-up encounter, response to management and other additional data is acquired, and the provisional diagnosis is confirmed, refuted, or reclassified.

The pitfalls in diagnosis include:
- Anchoring,
- Bias, and
- Incorrect knowledge-base.

Anchoring is the tendency to cling to a thought or diagnosis despite evidence to the contrary. Clinicians sometimes have a hard time admitting that they are wrong about their conclusions.

Perhaps replace strikeout with "An example would be a provider seeing a young patient with spells which sound convincing for epileptic seizures. EEG was normal but there were no events captured during the EEG. The provider diagnoses epilepsy on clinical grounds and treats. Some time later, the patient presents to the emergency department with clinical seizures and EEG shows no abnormalities during the events. The diagnosis of nonepileptic events is made in the ED, but the first provider rejects the new diagnosis and continues to treat for epilepsy." The clinician is anchored in their thought process.

Bias is giving preferential consideration based on data that are not relevant to a specific patient. When a neuroimmunologist who does research on autoimmune encephalitis covers the emergency department, they think of that diagnosis every time they see a patient with unexplained encephalopathy. The diagnosis is probably not autoimmune encephalitis, and so the clinician needs to look harder for a diagnosis (or, commonly, multiple diagnoses).

Incorrect knowledge-base will happen to all clinicians. It is impossible to keep up with all medical literature. During our careers, we have noticed swings in treatment recommendations that are not trivial. Not having the most current information can place patients at risk.

How can these pitfalls be avoided? First, recognize them and try to avoid anchoring and bias in patient encounters. A patient with untreated HIV may have a headache due to a migraine rather than to toxoplasmosis. Second, keep up with literature as best you can, and consult literature and other information sources when needed. Third, discuss a complex patient's situation directly with colleagues, including others on the treatment team and your specialist team.

Taking a History

Howard S. Kirshner and Martin A. Samuels

Chief Complaint

The chief complaint is the reason for the encounter. The encounter always has a defined purpose, even if the visit is for a medical screening of an individual with no known medical complaints or issues. This should be documented prominently in the encounter note so that the purpose of the visit is clear.

History of Present Illness

In taking a history, the neurologist asks the patient to give an account of the symptoms, how they began, and how they evolved over time. This is the History of Present Illness (HPI). The neurologist should always identify sources of information: Did the information come from direct interview of the patient or from secondhand reports? History taking often requires the neurologist to redirect the patient. For example, some patients use vague terms to describe their symptoms, and the examiner must be sure that they understand what the patient means. For example, patients may use the word "weakness" when they mean sensory disturbance. A host of symptoms can be encoded in the term "dizzy"; for example, some patients mean a spinning sensation of the room or of themselves, which is called vertigo, whereas others mean lightheadedness or a sensation of impending syncope. The precise sequence and timing of how the symptoms developed give key clues to the diagnosis. Another example of misleading history is when patients relate what diagnoses other clinicians have made, rather than what symptoms they experienced.

Past Medical History

In neurology, as in other areas of medicine, a complete history also includes past medical history (PMH), family history, social history, and review of systems. The PMH contains clues based on prior medical problems or risk factors. For example, in a patient with abrupt onset of right-sided weakness, a history of atrial fibrillation or a prosthetic heart valve would be clues to an embolic stroke. A history of severe hypertension would raise the concern of a cerebral hemorrhage or thrombotic stroke. A history of head trauma would make the provider suspect a subdural hematoma or perhaps a carotid dissection. A history of systemic cancer would bring up a metastatic tumor as a possibility, and a history of immunosuppression from chemotherapy or HIV infection might raise suspicion of an abscess or meningitis. History of surgical procedures, medications, and allergies complete the PMH.

Family History

Family history can also provide clues, especially in the case of genetic diseases. There are many inherited neurologic diseases, including hereditary peripheral neuropathies or myopathies or neurodegenerative diseases such as Alzheimer disease, Parkinson disease, or Huntington disease.

Even seemingly sporadic diseases such as stroke have genetically inherited risk factors including diabetes mellitus, heart disease, and clotting disorders.

Social History

The social history contains clues about risk factors such as smoking or the use of alcohol or illicit drugs. Toxic exposures might also be relevant. The patient's level of education and highest vocational attainments are important for understanding the significance of lost functions in acquired neurologic diseases.

Review of Systems

The Review of Systems (ROS) can reveal clues to the effects of the disease process on other organ systems. A frequent notation in History and Physical (H&P) examination notes is "a complete ROS was negative, except as in the HPI." This statement is almost never true. Even healthy patients have occasional headaches, nasal congestion, cough, refractive visual deficits requiring corrective lenses, hearing loss, joint pain, or fatigue. Almost everyone suffers periods of depressed mood, frustration, and disappointment. Stress-induced insomnia is nearly universal in our society. The review of systems should provide a general picture of the health and emotional status of the individual.

Combining the Data

History is often taken in some variation of the order of chief complaint, history of present illness, PMH, family history, social history, and review of systems. The information should be gathered in a systematic method, so that there are no gaps. This is not only important for accuracy of documentation but also for ensuring that the documentation meets criteria for clinical practice and for billing. Omitting even a single section may make the charge on the encounters at a much lower level than expected.

Once the neurologist has all of the historical data, they can tailor the examination so that problems are evaluated thoroughly. It is impossible to complete a total examination or even a total neurologic examination on every patient. Basic requirements must be met, so the examination has a focus derived from the synthesis of the historical information.

The Neurologic Examination

Karl E. Misulis and Martin A. Samuels

Mental Status

Mental status examination consists of evaluating level of consciousness, cognitive function, and language. The neurologist obtains a great deal of information regarding mental status as they take a history. Questions may be answered clearly or not, the historical details may be remembered in chronological order or not, patients may lose focus, or forget details that they would be expected to remember such as children's names. Patients sometimes provide contradicting information during their examination. Part of the neurologist's task is to determine whether this is a cognitive disturbance or an intent to deceive. After taking the patient's history, the neurologist has a fairly good, although not complete, assessment of mental status.

LEVEL OF CONSCIOUSNESS

Level of consciousness (LOC) assessment begins with observation of the patient. The approach differs depending on the setting. On entry into the examination room, the examiner immediately surveys the appearance, attention, demeanor, and social graces of the patient. Of course, the patient and others are assessing the same in the examiner.

In the emergency department or intensive care unit (ICU), the assessment may begin with a brief observation of the patient through the glass doors, watching for spontaneous movements and interactions with family or medical staff already in the room. This survey must be short, otherwise it can seem inappropriate.

We discuss the approach to cognitive and language function assessment first, and then we discuss some of the formal assessment tools used for delirium and dementia.

COGNITIVE FUNCTION

Cognitive function is assessed by casual encounter, informal examination, and by observation during performance of the rest of the neurologic examination. As the examiner greets the patient, they assess the mood and attention of the patient.

Cognition is assessed in part by observing task completion. Patients with cognitive impairments may have difficulty following verbal commands (e.g., "Touch your left ear with your right thumb"), or they may have difficulty with some task instructions (e.g., they are shown how to do a task with the right arm, and then they are asked to do the same task with their other arm).

Language comprehension can be a challenge in our increasingly global society, so assessment of cognitive deficits should ideally be performed by an examiner who is fluent in the language of the patient. A few cognitive assessment screening tools are available in multiple languages, although some degree of fluency is needed to interpret the responses.

Close observation during history and assessment of cognitive function during conversation can also give clues to some other portions of the examination. For example, the patient might have no difficulty using limbs to express emotion and punctuate speech during casual conversation, yet the patient might demonstrate inability to use a limb during formal examination. This discrepancy would suggest a psychogenic (functional) process rather than an organic process.

Orientation

Formal examination often begins with assessment of orientation. Many clinicians prefer to perform the motor examination first, so the patient is more relaxed with the history and physical examination (H&P) process and is more likely to give a consistent (and often better) performance on mental status testing.

A common script is "Alert and oriented × 3." This generally means person (states full name), place (specific hospital or office), and time (year, month, day). "A&O × 4" includes the addition of another element, which is usually the purpose of the visit. This can be obtained before the formal examination by asking the patient at the beginning of the encounter the purpose of the visit. For example, "What is your understanding of why Dr. X wanted you to see me?" An inaccurate response might not indicate orientation deficit but rather suboptimal communication between referring provider and patient, so this response is not analyzed in isolation.

Short-Term Memory

The examiner usually gives the patient three objects to remember. They are stated clearly and slowly enough to facilitate the patient's registration and recall. For example, "I am going to give you three words to remember, and I will ask you repeat them in a few minutes." Common elements are "ball, flag, and tree." Many examiners use at least one element that is a word the patient cannot visualize in their mind's eye, such as "theory."

The patient repeats the words; if the patient needs a second chance, it is given. After the patient successfully registers the three words, the examination continues with other tasks. Five minutes after registration, the patient is asked to recite the words. Many examiners give the patient hints if elements are missed to determine whether the patient can make a connection with the stored item.

Long-Term Memory

The examiner often assesses long-term memory by asking the patient to recall items from the distant past; typically the examiner asks the patient some details about their youth. However, these responses are usually not verifiable by the examiner. If a family member is present and contradicts the patient's recollection, this is often sufficiently disconcerting to the patient to affect adversely-subsequent performance. Many examiners use historical information that is commonly known. For example, "Who was the president when you were in high school?" Knowing the patient's age will allow the examiner to pose a question that the patient has a good chance answering correctly.

Concentration

Tests of concentration usually involve either serial 7s or backward spelling. In serial 7s, the examiner will tell the patient to start from 100 and count backwards by 7s. If the patient does not seem to understand, then the examiner can provide further detail such as, "Start from 100, take 7 away from that, and then 7 from what's left." In backward spelling, the examiner can instruct the patient to spell the word "world." After the patient has done that, the examiner instructs them to spell it backwards. If the patient does not understand, the examiner can rephrase the request as "give me the letters in reverse order." This is not a test of spelling per se but rather a test of attending to the task.

Construction

Construction is usually tested by asking a patient to copy a figure, such as a three-dimensional box. The critical elements are the angles and connections, with an emphasis on capturing the three-dimensional character rather than just copying a two-dimensional diagram.

LANGUAGE

Language is primarily tested during the history taking and mental status examination. More detailed language testing is indicated in patients who have a chief complaint of speech or comprehension difficulty or if there are abnormalities in language detected during mental status examination. Components of language assessment include casual speech during history taking, naming, reading, writing, and repetition.

Speech is assessed while the patient is answering questions or giving historical details or even during casual conversation. Does the patient struggle to find words? Do they make word substitutions? Paraphasic errors? Paraphasic errors can be sound substitutions (e.g., wrong phoneme such as "hat" for "pat"), word substitutions that can be in the same category (e.g., wrong daughter's name), or rarely substitution with neologism. Inability to express oneself is expressive aphasia or anterior aphasia. Inability to understand spoken words is receptive aphasia or posterior aphasia. Deficits in both is global aphasia.

Naming is usually tested by asking the patient to name objects in the room and objects not immediately in sight. The examiner can point to their watch and ask, "What is this called?" Then they might ask, "What is the hard center of a peach called?" If deficits are detected, the examiner performs additional testing with naming of objects in and out of the patient's sight and with naming of words that are independent of visual imagery. Inability to name objects is anomia.

Reading is tested by asking the patient to read a short passage aloud. The educational level of the text should be appropriate. Some patients with incipient dementia report the ability to read but have impaired registration of the meaning of the passage; however, this is usually tested only with detailed speech and language assessments. Inability to read is alexia.

Writing is tested by having the patient write a brief sentence; this should generally be spontaneous rather than dictated so that word usage and grammar errors can be better seen. Spelling is not generally considered. Inability to write is agraphia.

Repetition is tested by having the patient repeat a brief phrase. A common example is "No ifs, ands, or buts'." Deficit in repetition that is out of proportion to comprehension difficulty is typical of a conduction aphasia.

Details of these and other forms of language deficits are discussed in Chapter 5.2.

MENTAL STATUS TOOLS

Dementia

There are a variety of tools for assessment of mental status in the setting of potential dementia. These include:

- Mini-Mental State Examination (MMSE),
- Montreal Cognitive Assessment (MoCA),
- Mini-Cog, and
- ACE-III (Addenbrooke's Cognitive Examination) and Mini-Ace (Mini-Mini-Addenbrooke's Cognitive Examination)

Details of performance and interpretations are discussed in the websites of these copyrighted tools. Some of these are also discussed in more detail in Chapter 4.1. A brief summary follows:

Mini-Mental State Examination. The MMSE tool is often used in the ambulatory patient to screen for cognitive disturbance. It has a 30-point scale assessing memory, orientation, reading, writing, constructions, attention, and language. It takes about 10 minutes to perform. Some training is required for the tool to be useful.

Montreal Cognitive Assessment. The MoCA is a sensitive screen for dementia. It is not an intelligence test, and it does not identify individuals who are intellectually gifted. Training is needed to administer the test, and certification is recommended for valid results. It is free for use in medical care. The MoCA cannot distinguish between dementia and confusional (inattentive) states, so this and most other tools should be used mainly in the outpatient setting. The MoCA tests orientation, memory, construction, abstraction, executive function, and reading.

Mini-Cog. This is a very brief screen for patients with cognitive deficit. There are only three elements, and they test memory and constructions. Some patients with cognitive deficit can score well, but in general this is well-validated and quite sensitive.

ACE-III and Mini-ACE. These are fairly complex and powerful assessments. The Mini-ACE is a briefer version that can be performed in just a few minutes. These test memory, attention, fluency, and constructions.

Delirium and Encephalopathy

There are multiple tools used for assessment of delirium and encephalopathy, principally in the emergency and inpatient areas. The predominant one in importance is the Glasgow Coma Scale (GCS), which we will discuss in some detail. Other scales will be introduced only briefly.

Glasgow Coma Scale. The GCS is an assessment of LOC routinely used for patients, especially in the acute care setting. An aggregate score is reached with assessment of eye opening, verbal response, and motor response. A score of 3 indicates no function; a score of 15 indicates full function. The elements of the GCS are as follows:
- Eye opening is tested by initially observing the patient for spontaneous eye opening. If there is none, then a verbal command is given to the patient to open their eyes. If there is no response to that command, then a noxious stimulation is delivered to the body (e.g., shoulder, extremity). Responses are graded according to level of response:
  - Spontaneous eye opening = 4 points
  - Opening to verbal command or speech = 3 points
  - Opening to pain (but not on the face) = 2 points
  - No response = 1 point
- Verbal response is tested by observing for spontaneous speech. If there is none, then the examiner speaks to the patient, asks questions, and gives commands to determine whether language of any kind can be elicited. Responses are graded on the basis of the speech output:
  - Speaking and oriented = 5 points
  - Responds to questions and commands but is confused = 4 points
  - Responds only with inappropriate words = 3 points
  - Speech is incomprehensible = 2 points
  - No verbal response = 1 point
- Motor response is observed for spontaneous movement, movement to command, and reflexive movement. Responses are graded as follows:
  - Moves to command appropriately = 6 points
  - Makes purposeful movement to noxious stimuli = 5 points
  - Withdraws to pain = 4 points
  - Flexion to noxious stimuli (decorticate posturing) = 3 points
  - Extension to noxious stimuli (decerebrate posturing) = 2 points
  - No response to command or noxious stimuli = 1 point
- Interpretation of the responses is generally as follows:
  - Mild deficit = GCS 13 or better
  - Moderate deficit = GCS 9-12
  - Severe deficit = GCS 8 or less

Sedation-Agitation Assessments. There are multiple sedation-agitation assessment scales. The most commonly used scale is the Richmond Agitation-Sedation Scale (RASS); it is often a field of entry in many electronic health record (EHR) programs. Other scales are the Confusion Assessment Method for the ICU (CAM-ICU); the Riker Sedation-Agitation Scale (SAS); and the Ramsay Sedation Scale.

The RASS is commonly used in ICUs with patients on mechanical ventilation. It is a component of the CAM-ICU. RASS is especially useful as ventilatory and sedation needs are considered in critically ill patients.

The scoring is based on observation of the patient in the ICU.

+4 = *Combative*. Overtly agitated or combative, potentially violent. A risk to staff.

+3 = *Very agitated*. Often pulling lines, aggressive. Difficult for staff to work with.

+2 = *Agitated*. Often significant extremity or truncal movement. Often irregular respirations on vent.

+1 = *Anxious* but without aggressive movements.

0 = Alert and calm.

−1 = *Drowsy* but makes eye contact with examiner to voice.

−2 = *Light sedation*. Briefly makes eye contact to voice.

−3 = *Moderate sedation*. Moves to voice but no eye contact.

−4 = *Deep sedation*. Moves to physical stimulation but not to voice.

−5 = *Unarousable*. No response to voice or physical stimulation.

Performance of the assessment begins with observation of the patient. Testing response begins with verbal commands and questions and then moves to physical stimulation if needed.

INTERPRETATION OF MENTAL STATUS TESTING

Deficits in many of these tests may occur for protean reasons, from dementia to intoxication to delirium to psychiatric disorders. With diffuse disorders, such as dementia, most modalities will be affected. However, there are some focal structural lesions that can produce more isolated clinical findings.

Short-term memory deficit is usually a diffuse disorder, but frontal or medial temporal lesions can produce this. Naming and word-finding deficits are most suggestive of left temporal and posterior frontal lesions. Calculation errors along with problems with reading and writing are most suggestive of a left parietal lesion. Construction deficits are seen in patients with right centroparietal lesions and in patients with degenerative dementia. In patients with Alzheimer disease, construction deficit can be seen quite early.

Cranial Nerves

The cranial nerves (CN) exit the brainstem segmentally, making their assessment useful for diagnosing disorders that affect these structures. Cranial nerves can be thought of in clusters: smell, eyes, face, auditory/vestibular function, swallowing and speech, and head turning/shoulder shrugging. Details of each cranial nerve follows and in Chapter 3.4.

During the clinical examination, a rapid survey of all cranial nerves can be performed in just a few minutes, except for olfaction. This survey should be performed with a focused additional detailed examination depending on clinical findings and the clinical question under consideration.

CN I OLFACTORY

Olfaction should be assessed when there is concern about pathology that is in the region of the cribriform plate or inferior frontal region, such as an anterior cerebral artery distribution stroke, meningioma, or hydrocephalus, and when neurodegenerative disorders (such as Alzheimer and Parkinson disease) are suspected.

Testing is performed by asking the patient to identify some common odor. Coffee and chocolate, which can be kept in powder form in small containers, are often used. Mint and ammonia are not used because they are trigeminal stimulants.

Abnormalities in olfaction indicate the possibility of a conductive deficit rather than a sensorineural deficit, that is, the chemicals might not be getting to the receptors because of sinus disease. Therefore, the differential diagnosis should include sinus deficit.

CN II OPTIC

Examination of optic nerve function includes assessment of eye function. Some disorders of the eye or optic nerve can be difficult to differentiate.

Examination begins with assessment of visual fields and acuity. Visual acuity of each eye is tested with a Snellen eye chart or similar device. Visual fields are often then tested by asking patients to count fingers in the visual fields in four quadrants: right, left, superior, and inferior. Abnormalities are classified as monocular versus binocular, superior and/or inferior quadrant.

Fundus examination should be performed on all patients. However, the neurologist using a pocket ophthalmoscope can miss subtle papilledema and other significant abnormalities, so it is recommended that an ophthalmologist be consulted if there is any question.

Pupil responses are tested individually and collectively. Ambient lighting is dimmed, and a focused light is used to illuminate one eye to look for ipsilateral and contralateral pupillary constriction. Normal examination is for the pupils to be equal in diameter and both respond to stimulation of each eye. If there is a CN III palsy, the pupil on the affected side will have a reduced response. If there is CN II dysfunction, both pupils will not respond as well to illumination of the affected eye. This is an afferent pupillary defect (APD).

- Monocular visual loss suggests a lesion in the eye or optic nerve before the chiasm.
- Binocular homonymous hemianopia suggests lesion of the contralateral optic radiation after the chiasm or of the visual cortex.
- Binocular homonymous superior quadrantanopia suggests a lesion on the contralateral optic radiations after the chiasm extending into the temporal region or inferior aspect of the occipital visual cortex.
- Binocular homonymous inferior quadrantanopia suggests a lesion of the contralateral optic radiations or upper aspect of the occipital cortex. A contralateral parietal lesion can produce a quadrant defect, but occipital lesions are much more likely as a cause.

Optic nerve lesions usually produce monocular visual loss, and subacute deficits may not be initially noticed by the patient. Careful testing may reveal reduced visual acuity that cannot be improved by correcting for refractive error by having the patient look through a pin hole, which helps to focus light on the retina. Color vision is often impaired. If a focal portion of the optic nerve is compressed or otherwise damaged, there may be a monocular abnormality in visual fields. Fig. 1.3.1 shows changes in visual fields with lesions of the optic nerves, chiasm, and tracts.

OCULAR MOVEMENTS: CN III, IV, VI

Ocular movements test CN III, CN IV, and CN VI together. The lesions are then localized to one or more cranial nerves or to a brain lesion causing a constellation of findings. Fig. 1.3.2 shows neural control over eye movements.

CN III Oculomotor

Superior, inferior, and medial rectus muscles are innervated by CN III along with the levator palpebrae superioris. These muscles have a host of effects, so their function is most easily noted when considering lesions of the nerve.

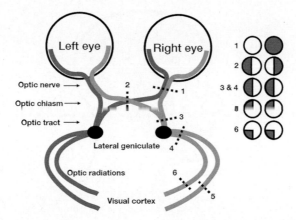

Fig. 1.3.1 Visual field pathways and abnormalities. Visual pathways with regions for common neurologic lesions. Visual field defects that are expected from the indicated lesions are shown on the right. Note that the lesions and associated visual field defects are usually not precise and complete.

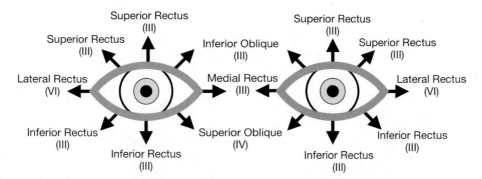

Fig. 1.3.2 Eye movements. Eye movements with responsible muscle and cranial nerves indicated in parentheses.

CN III palsy can have varying severity, but it typically produces diplopia with lateral deviation of the eye associated with ptosis and sometimes mydriasis if the parasympathetic fibers accompanying the nerve are damaged. The eye is sometimes referred to as "down-and-out" because of unopposed abduction by the lateral rectus and depression by the superior oblique, along with some rotation.

A variety of lesions can affect CN III function, including aneurysmal compression, microvascular disease, increased intracranial pressure from almost any cause, trauma, and inflammatory and infectious disorders affecting the orbit, cavernous sinus, meninges, and cerebrospinal fluid (CSF).

CN IV Trochlear

CN IV innervates the superior oblique and is responsible for depression of the eye especially when adducted and intorsion of the eye especially when abducted.

Lesions of CN IV produce diplopia due to loss of the depression from the superior oblique and loss of intorsion, resulting in head tilt to the opposite side.

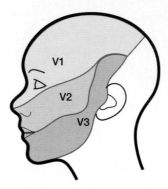

Fig. 1.3.3 Trigeminal nerve distribution. The trigeminal nerve innervation is shown with the three divisions as indicated. *V1*, Ophthalmic division; *V2*, maxillary division; *V3*, mandibular division.

Note that while intorsion of the eye is often spoken of as a particular effect of the superior oblique and CN IV, all of the extraocular muscles may have a torsional effect on the eye that varies depending on direction of gaze.

CN VI Abducens

Lateral rectus is innervated by CN VI, and it is responsible for abduction of the eye during lateral gaze. Lesions produce horizontal diplopia due to unopposed adduction of the eye.

Lesions of CN VI are common and often microvascular; they are seen particularly in people with diabetes. Damage can also occur in the cavernous sinus or on the clivus as the nerve ascends from the pontine-medullary junction to join CN III and IV to enter the cavernous sinus and then orbit.

CN V Trigeminal

CN V supplies motor innervation to muscles of mastication, but the predominant innervation of clinical concern is sensory to the face. Three branches are ophthalmic (V1), maxillary (V2), and mandibular (V3) (Fig. 1.3.3).

Testing of the trigeminal nerve varies depending on the clinical question. Testing light touch of each division takes seconds and can screen for deficits. If the clinical question clinically involves a potential lesion of the trigeminal nerve, then sharp and dull sensation in all three divisions is recommended.

Motor function of the trigeminal nerve is not routinely tested. If there is specific concern, it can be tested by asking the patient to forcibly close the jaw and feeling for tightness of the masseter muscle on both sides. Forced opening of the jaw against resistance results in jaw deviation to the side of the weak pterygoid muscle.

Lesions of CN V branches can occur anywhere from the brainstem to the face. Common lesions are in the cavernous sinus, often with V1 and sometimes V2 distribution of sensory loss. Pain in the trigeminal distribution is distinct from sensory loss; when present, specifics of involvement of branches of the trigeminal nerve should be documented.

CN VII FACIAL

CN VII supplies motor innervation to the face, and special sensory function (taste) to the soft palate and anterior two-thirds of the tongue.

Examination of the facial nerve is usually best conducted by watching facial expression during history taking. Spontaneous movements are often more revealing than forced movements during formal testing. During examination, the function of the upper and lower facial muscles are assessed. Weakness may be subtle, including only mild flattening of the nasolabial fold.

Subtle asymmetries in facial movement can be preexisting, and family members might not have noticed. Asking to see pictures of the patient can be helpful. Most people have a driver's license that has a photo taken previously. In addition, many people have pictures of various ages on their phones.

Lesions of CN VII produce weakness of the ipsilateral face involving upper and lower segments as opposed to upper motor neuron lesions that affect mainly the lower face. Distinguishing features suggesting a CN VII lower motor neuron lesion include impaired eye closure and loss of wrinkling of the forehead with upgaze.

Common causes of CN VII dysfunction include Bell palsy, other inflammatory conditions (e.g., Lyme disease, sarcoidosis), and lesions at the cerebellopontine angle (CPA).

CN VIII VESTIBULOCOCHLEAR

CN VIII serves hearing and vestibular function, including position in space, and linear and angular acceleration. Function is tested by assessing hearing in both ears, often by a soft sound that would not be detected bilaterally.

Weber test is performed by placing a tuning fork on the patient's forehead and assessing whether there is lateralization of sound perception. Rinne test is performed by placing a tuning fork on the mastoid. When the sound decays to undetectable, the fork is moved so that the vibrating end is adjacent to the external ear; this indicates whether air conduction is better than bone conduction, which is a normal response.

Depending on the chief complaint, vestibular maneuvers may also be performed such as the Barany maneuver. This is performed with the patient sitting upright with head straight; then the patient is laid back so that the head can hang off the bed at about a 30-degree angle. The maneuver is first performed with the patient's head turned to the right, and then the movement is repeated with the head turned to the left. A positive response is the generation of nystagmus with a rotatory movement in the down eye and a vertical movement in the up eye.

Another useful test of vestibular function is the Halmagy horizontal head thrust maneuver, which is a test of the vestibuloocular reflex. The examiner asks the patient to fix their gaze on the examiner's eyes, and the examiner passively moves the patient's head to one side and then the other. Normally the patient's eyes stay fixed on the examiner's eyes. If the vestibular system is defective on one side, the eyes will move with the head and then be seen to jerk back to retain fixation on the examiner's eyes. A positive horizontal head thrust maneuver is a sensitive and specific sign of a peripheral vestibular disorder in one ear (such as vestibular neuritis). The examiner can alternatively cover one eye while the patient fixes their gaze on the examiner. Any vertical readjustments of the eyes indicate a central nervous system disorder. Bidirectional nystagmus in a single position of the eyes also indicates a central nervous system etiology.

Newman-Toker has devised an acronym, HINTS, that means head impulse (HI), nystagmus (N), and tests of skew (TS) as a mnemonic for this three-part simple test. This test is highly sensitive for discriminating a central from a peripheral cause of vertigo; it is a very useful technique for assessing a patient with acute vertigo in emergency department. The HINTS test is not designed to examine patients with dizziness other than vertigo, such as gait instability, near faint, or anxiety.

Lesions of CN VIII can include CPA, vestibular schwannoma, and toxins including some antibiotics and some chemotherapies. In performing an evaluation, note that most hearing loss is not due to a CN VIII lesion but rather is due to ear pathology, with infection being the most common.

OROPHARYNGEAL EXAMINATION: CN IX, CN X, AND CN XII

CN IX, X, and XII are often examined together as part of the oropharyngeal examination. CN IX sensory function is tested by gag, and the efferent side is CN X. CN XII function is tested by tongue protrusion.

Lesions of these cranial nerves can be oropharyngeal mass lesions, but the spectrum of disorders is broad. Usually, multiple lower cranial nerves are affected.

CN XI ACCESSORY

CN XI supplies motor innervation to the sternocleidomastoid and trapezius muscle and some laryngeal muscles.

Testing of CN XI involves examination of activation and power of the sternocleidomastoid muscle with head turning and the trapezius by shoulder shrug. Other innervated muscles are not practically testable.

Lesion of CN XI is most commonly seen after neck surgery, especially neck dissection for cancer.

Motor

Tone is tested through passive movement of the extremities, usually at least one movement per limb. Increased tone can indicate nonacute corticospinal tract dysfunction. Reduced tone can occur in acute corticospinal tract dysfunction and cerebellar ataxia, but it is most commonly seen in lower motor neuron, peripheral nerve, and some muscle disorders.

Strength is tested by examining representative muscles of each limb, with a focused examination based on the patient's complaint. Examination of the right arm of a patient complaining of arm weakness will be much more extensive than in a patient with report of headaches. When weakness is detected, individual muscles are selected for examination in the affected limb(s) and other limbs to utilize knowledge of neuroanatomy to localize the lesion.

For a screening examination, proximal and distal muscles in each limb are often tested. One combination for the arm may be shoulder abduction, elbow flexion and extension, wrist flexion and extension, and finger abduction. One combination for the leg may be hip flexion and extension, knee flexion and extension, dorsiflexion and plantarflexion, and foot inversion and eversion.

Sensory

Sensory examination is tailored to the patient's complaint and to motor findings. Because the sensory examination is generally subjective, there is inherent variability and even frank inconsistency in sensory reporting. With different modalities and with duration of the examination, the patient can become fatigued and give responses they otherwise might not, especially if the sensory examination produces a long series of monotonous responses.

A screening examination for sensory deficits can include light touch of each side of the face and then of a distal aspect of the arm and leg, such as back of the hand and top of the foot. More detailed sensory examination is warranted if there are motor or other sensory deficits or a sensory component to the presenting condition.

Light touch is tested with the pad of the examiner's finger. A tool such as a brush can be used, but this is not usually necessarily.

Sharp sensation is not always necessary. Reusable safety pins or sharp part of medical equipment are not recommended because of the risk of infection, skin breakage, especially in older patients.

Vibration is tested if neuropathy or a posterior column spinal lesion is suspected.

Temperature is tested most commonly by touching the metal of the tuning fork or reflex hammer to the patient's skin and asking whether they can feel the coolness. This response often fatigues especially as with multiple uses as the metal begins to warm.

Proprioception is tested by moving the patient's finger or toe up or down while holding onto the lateral aspects of the digit. In the absence of lesion, even small movement is perceived. The Romberg test is a useful method for assessing proprioception (discussed later).

Coordination

Coordination is tested by several maneuvers. Although these are predominantly considered to be tests of cerebellar function, performance relies on the entirety of the motor system.

In finger-nose-finger (FNF), the examiner asks the patient to alternately touch the examiner's finger and then their own nose. Alternatively, the examiner may ask the patient to touch their own chin, as masks are prevalent. Emphasis is on accuracy rather than speed.

For heel-knee-shin (HKS), the examiner asks the seated patient to run their heel down the front of their shin. Emphasis is on accuracy and not speed.

Rapid alternative movements are tested by the examiner asking the patient to alternately tap the front and back of their hand on their thigh.

For finger tapping, the patient is asked to tap the index finger to the thumb as fast as they can do so accurately. Alternatively, the patient is asked to touch each finger in turn with the thumb going from index to little finger.

Orbiting or the forearm rolling test is when the patient's arms are held in front and the patient is asked to roll the forearms around each other. Patients with mild corticospinal tract dysfunction will tend to hold the affected arm relatively still while the unaffected arm makes the greater component of the movements. This can reveal corticospinal deficits when frank weakness or other signs are absent.

Gait

Gait assessment includes stance, normal gait, and tandem gait. Stance and gait are often best observed by watching the patient walk outside of the examination room in the hall.

Stance is tested by asking the patient to stand. If the initial stance is broad-based, then the examiner asks the patient to stand on a narrow base and watches for wavering. The examiner often asks the patient to close their eyes to see whether wavering of stance worsens. This is often a prelude to the Romberg test.

Casual gait is observed. Although this can be done in the examination room, it is best performed in the hall where there is ample room for the patient to accelerate to the normal speed of natural gait. Multiple abnormalities can be observed, including steppage gait (e.g., foot drop), circumduction (often corticospinal dysfunction), short-step or shuffling gait (e.g., parkinsonism), and stiff-straight leg (often mechanical). This observation is key to recognizing the gait abnormalities seen with hemiparesis, cerebellar ataxia, and parkinsonism.

Tandem gait is tested by observing the patient walking with one toe in front of the other, as if on a tightrope or in a field sobriety test. This gets more difficult with advanced age under normal circumstances. If this gait is significantly abnormal in the absence of other major deficits, sidesteps suggest truncal ataxia and often indicate cerebellar disorder, but this is far from specific.

Romberg test is not a test of cerebellar function but rather it reveals a proprioceptive disorder either in the peripheral (e.g., neuropathy) or central (posterior columns) nervous system.

Reflex

TENDON

Tendon reflexes are tested with the patient's limb in a position that the distal tendon of the studied muscle can be tapped to transiently lengthen the muscle.

Commonly tested proprioceptive reflexes include the following, with their associated innervation:

- Biceps: C6 root, musculocutaneous nerve
- Triceps: C7 root, radial nerve
- Brachioradialis: C6 root, radial nerve
- Patellar: L2-4 roots, femoral nerve
- Achilles: S1 root, sciatic nerve

Depressed reflexes usually indicate a peripheral lesion, such as neuropathy.

Enhanced reflexes usually indicate a corticospinal lesion, although the level of the lesion cannot be determined from a single reflex.

PLANTAR

Plantar reflex is produced by stroking the bottom of the foot from the lateral midsole across the base of the toes.

Normal response is for the great toe to go down (flex). An abnormal response is for the great toe to go up (extend). An abnormal response indicates a corticospinal tract lesion.

Stimulation can produce a false-positive response if a painful stimulus results in withdrawal of the foot.

There is confusion about terminology. The Babinski reflex is sometimes used to indicate the test; the Babinski response or Babinski sign is often used to indicate the abnormal result. The interpretation of upgoing toes and other features of the response suggesting corticospinal tract dysfunction depends on age, with the Babinski sign being present in newborns. We recommend using the term "plantar reflex," with the response being upgoing, downgoing, or neutral. The term "Babinski sign" is most helpful for those who like eponyms.

RELEASE SIGNS

Release signs are reflexes that are pathologic when identified. The most common are presented here. These are sought predominantly when there is concern for frontal or global cerebral dysfunction, such as dementia, frontal lobe injury, hydrocephalus, or bihemispheric ischemia.

The examiner elicits the glabellar response by tapping the patient between the eyebrows, ensuring their hand is out of the patient's line of sight. Normal response is no blink or perhaps a subtle blink or two. An abnormal response is an eye blink that the patient cannot suppress despite being told to keep their eyes open. Glabellar is abnormal in Parkinson disease and in frontal lobe dysfunction.

Snout is elicited by the examiner tapping the patient's skin above the midline of the upper lip. A normal response is no response. An abnormal response is pursing of the lips, a finding that can be mild. Snout is abnormal in patients with dementia and in others with frontal lobe dysfunction from a variety of causes.

Palmomental reflex is elicited by the examiner stroking the patient across the palm of their hand and watching for ipsilateral depression of the corner of the mouth. Normal response is no depression of the mouth. Abnormal response is transient depression of the corner of the mouth.

Grasp reflex is elicited by the examiner brushing their fingers down the palm of the patient's hand to the base of the fingers. Normal response is none. Abnormal response is curling of the fingers as if a mild attempt to close grasp. Grasp reflex is abnormal in some patients with dementia and frontal lobe lesions.

Putting It Together

The examination as presented here is comprehensive and reasonably detailed. However, there are other portions of the examination that can be performed to focus in on a localization. For example, in the initial examination, the examiner might test one representative muscle of each nerve and nerve root; if they detect weakness, they often will have to examine more muscles and nerves to determine whether the deficit is due to nerve, plexus, or nerve root dysfunction. Hence, elements of the examination are not performed in isolation.

At the conclusion of the examination, the neurologist considers the findings together and determines the localization of the lesion(s). Then they create a differential diagnosis based on the history and clinical findings on examination. As they synthesize the localization and diagnosis, they often have to ask more questions or check for additional examination findings.

Medical Examination in Neurologic Patients

Karl E. Misulis, Martin A. Samuels, and Howard S. Kirshner

Many specialists, including neurologists, are first trained in general medicine. As such, they interpret their findings in the context of the entire body. For this reason, they must remain facile in performance and interpretation of the general medical examination. However, they do not perform the entire examination on every patient but rather select specific portions for focus that are appropriate to their study. For example, if a neurologist is seeing a stroke patient in the emergency department, the general medical examination segment of greatest interest is cardiovascular. However, if they are examining a patient in the clinic with worsening myasthenia gravis, they may pay special attention to the pulmonary examination with concern for respiratory drive and the possibility of aspiration.

Therefore, this chapter will consider both the basic general medical examination that might be performed on most patients and the focused examination that is indicated for specific entities.

Basic Medical Examination

The basic medical examination usually includes cardiac, pulmonary, musculoskeletal, and vascular examinations. These are the most important for correlation with neurologic conditions, especially in the acute care environment.

Cardiac examination is probably the most important. This is where the return on investment of the time of examination is the greatest. The examination might reveal a heart murmur or an irregularity that would have implications, especially in a patient in whom cardiovascular or cerebrovascular disease is considered.

Vascular examination goes hand in hand with the cardiac examination. Carotid bruits can be reflective of previously undetected disease. In addition, peripheral pulses are important because their absence or association with other findings suggesting vascular disease can indicate the possibility of nonvascular pathology.

Musculoskeletal examination is performed largely by observation during history taking. However, when gait is tested as part of the neurologic examination, the examiner watches the patient walk and observes how the limbs and body move. Abnormalities can be manifested that may suggest spinal pathology, peripheral nerve pathology, or myopathy.

Skin examination is mainly for rash or edema. Rash is a rare accompaniment to several diseases involving the nervous system, such as dermatomyositis, but edema is quite important, as it can be a sign of peripheral vascular disease, renal disease, or cardiac disease. Any of these may be important contributors to the neurologic presentation.

Focused Medical Examination

In select instances, there is a focused examination that is specific to the problem under consideration. We will discuss some general guidelines and then some specific scenarios.

GENERAL PRINCIPLES OF THE FOCUSED EXAMINATION

Direct signs of specific neurologic disorders are occasionally visible. The most obvious would be signs of stroke with spastic posture of a hemiplegia. It is quite rare that the examiner will see some of the other signs of disease on casual inspection, but some of those include:

- Bilateral ptosis suggesting myasthenia.
- Bilateral facial weakness suggesting myotonic dystrophy.
- Dysmorphic features suggesting Down syndrome.
- Presence of mobility device and interaction with the environment suggesting significant corticospinal or other motor deficit.

Cardiovascular

Elements of the cardiovascular examination can provide clues as to whether the patient is at increased risk for stroke. Signs of peripheral edema, peripheral ischemia indicating peripheral vascular disease, or scars from cardiac or vascular surgery can indicate elevated stroke risk. If the patient is seen in the hospital where they are on telemetry, then the examiner may see arrhythmias, significant tachycardia, or bradycardias. Clinicians listen to the carotid arteries and the heart on every patient, but they listen especially closely on those with suspected cerebrovascular disease.

Pulmonary

Pulmonary examination is especially important for patients with vascular disease because often they will have cardiorespiratory and cerebrovascular manifestations. Patients who are critically ill may have chest injuries separate from their neurologic injuries. Additionally, it is important to listen to the lungs in patients with significant neuromuscular weakness, such as amyotrophic lateral sclerosis (ALS) or myasthenia, to ensure that there are no early signs of aspiration or consolidation.

Skin

Skin examination is especially important in acute care medicine to identify the signs of peripheral emboli that may suggest a cardiac source or skin changes that suggest thrombocytopenia or other coagulopathy. For example, one of our emergency department patients was found unresponsive, and we had no medical history or observer to offer additional information. It was evident from his skin examination that he was anticoagulated or had other coagulopathy or thrombocytopenia on the basis of significant cutaneous bleeding on exposed surfaces. He turned out to have intracranial hemorrhage as the cause of his neurologic presentation.

Eye

Clinicians look at the eyes of every patient. This is an integral part of the neurologic examination as the eye is considered to be an extension of the brain; this is indeed true of the optic nerve. Special attention to the eye is necessary in a broad spectrum of patient presentations. Among these are headache, any visual loss, double vision, and subacute cognitive disturbance that might suggest increased intracranial pressure.

Ear

Detailed inspection of the external ear is important, especially for patients who have a report of hearing loss. It is also important for patients who might be at risk for Ramsay Hunt syndrome, including those with suspected Bell palsy.

Recommended Examination Elements

Our recommendation is to perform a complete neurologic examination, with the only exception being very acute cases in which only a focused neurologic assessment is performed. Regarding general medical examination, we recommend eyes, skin, heart, vascular, and pulmonary.

Focused examination should be applicable to the presentation and initial differential diagnosis. Some specific scenarios include:

- Generalized weakness—pulmonary and cardiac examinations;
- Stroke—cardiac and vascular examinations;
- Seizure—oral (for tongue laceration), pulmonary (for aspiration), and musculoskeletal survey (for injury); and
- Coma or trauma without history—skin examination (to assess for scars and other signs of medical problems or injury).

Synthesis of the Assessment and Plan

Karl E. Misulis, Martin A. Samuels, and Eli E. Zimmerman

Synthesis of assessment and plan includes methods to determine the information we want to convey as well as the method for presenting the information. We will consider these separately.

Development of the Assessment and Plan

Assessment is formulated by considering the information that has been obtained from the history and physical examination (H&P) within the context of the reason the patient as being seen. The assessment of a general practitioner performing a yearly checkup will be different from that of specialist addressing a specific condition. This chapter will focus on the specialist assessment and plan.

To develop the assessment, the neurologist formulates an opinion using algorithmic and syndromic approaches.

In the algorithmic approach, the neurologist considers the information they have obtained and then localizes the lesions by their knowledge of neuroanatomy and neuropathology. Can the presentation be explained by a single lesion in one location? If so, where? What types of pathology could produce that focal deficit? If not one lesion, might there be multiple discrete lesions? Is the presentation explained by a diffuse process affecting a range of neuronal types and loci? What systems other than neurologic are affected, and is that because of the direct relation to the neurologic diagnosis or to a concurrent unrelated condition?

When the neurologist has localized the lesion, they then consider what pathologies can produce the presentation. They identify tests or additional H&P findings that need to be explored to further narrow the differential diagnosis.

In the syndromic approach, we take the data that we have obtained through the standard H&P and determine whether the clinical presentation fits into one or more syndromes. If so, that becomes the foundation of the differential diagnosis. The neurologist then leverages further H&P or study data to narrow the differential diagnosis. An example includes a patient with parkinsonism, where a constellation of neurologic findings indicates the clinical diagnosis but none of them in isolation would define the diagnosis.

There are merits to both the algorithmic and the syndromic approach. The algorithmic approach should be used extensively by people early in training when they are establishing their skills at evaluation, diagnostic thought processes, and approaches to diagnostic confirmation. The algorithmic approach is more time-intensive, but it is less likely to be derailed by anchoring on the part of the provider.

The syndromic approach is used by many neurologists in practice. In an emergent situation, this is often the first approach that the neurologist uses. When seconds count, the algorithmic approach is often too slow. If the syndromic approach is not working well, the neurologist stabilizes the patient, initiates essential studies and treatments, and then takes a little more time to think though the case with an algorithmic approach. This is often the method of action when the first couple of considered diagnoses are not correct.

When there is a proposed diagnosis, there must always be a differential diagnosis. This is essential, because it is not uncommon for a confident conclusion to be incorrect. In that case, the neurologist starts the process again, often repeating portions of the examination and exploring new avenues to get additional history.

Plan can be an action that the neurologist takes directly, as when they are seeing a patient in the emergency department or in clinic. Alternatively, if the neurologist is a consultant giving a report to a referring provider, they are not expected to execute the plan directly. In that case, they write recommendations. It is a recommendation rather than a plan for the referring provider, because the provider may have information or an insight into the case that might make some of the neurologist's recommendations inappropriate, or the patient or other decision makers may decide against the recommendations. If the neurologist does not directly execute the plan, they do not want to commit the referring provider to the wrong course or action.

There are multiple methods of documenting assessments and plans. The problem-based approach is common for primary care, internal medicine, general pediatrics, and admitting services where each diagnosis is given a brief assessment and plan. This works for neurologists also when they are the principal provider in the inpatient or outpatient arena. However, neurologists are commonly consultants, so that they confine their assessments and recommendations to the neurologic issues.

We generally provide an assessment that is a short paragraph, summarizing the essential facts of the case, our reasoning, and the journey to the diagnosis. One useful approach is to have a bulleted or numbered list of diagnoses, beginning with the one(s) we feel is most applicable to our specialty. We do not list all of the diagnoses for that patient, but we do list the nonneurologic diagnoses that pertain to the neurologic presentation or diagnosis.

The plan or recommendation section should likewise be a list that is either bulleted or numbered. The plan should be granular. If medications are recommended, the neurologist should suggest specific doses, because not every provider is savvy to medication dose adjustments for organ insufficiency or concurrent medications. Tests also should be specific, so that the referring provider does not have to wonder whether the neurologist wanted that scan with contrast or not.

Long discussions typical of a textbook are not helpful; most providers do not have the time to work through that. For example, for a patient with a transient ischemic attack (TIA), the provider does not need to be instructed on an ABCD2 score for diagnosis. Instead, the neurologist should perform the calculation and place their specific recommendations based on that and other data.

Occasionally there is some nonneurologic issue that the requesting provider might not have seen or considered. This should be mentioned as appropriate to the neurologic presentation and report, but it should done with sensitivity and should not place other providers in a situation where they could become defensive or even targeted for critique. If there is an issue in this arena, the neurologist should talk with the provider directly.

Below are two sample Assessment and Recommendation sections for hypothetical clinical scenarios.

SAMPLE 1

Assessment

57M referred by Dr. Alpha for imbalance. He has had progressive slowness and stiffness of gait for 2 years. Associated symptoms are resting tremor, left more than right. Exam shows stooped posture, increased tone, and resting tremor. Intellect is normal. The most likely diagnosis is Parkinson disease, with the differential diagnosis including vascular parkinsonism, less likely drug-induced parkinsonism.

Diagnosis

Parkinsonism, most likely Parkinson disease
DDx includes vascular parkinsonism and other degenerative Parkinson disease conditions
No predisposing factors identified

Recommend

MRI brain without contrast
Trial of immediate-release carbidopa-levodopa 25-100 TID
Physical therapy followed by a sustained program of exercise

SAMPLE 2

Assessment

42F presenting to the ED with acute right hemiparesis and aphasia, most consistent with acute ischemic stroke. NIH Stroke Scale was 10 for right-sided weakness and aphasia. She met clinical criteria for tPA, and this is being administered. CTA head and neck shows left M1 thrombus, so she is being considered for endovascular therapy (EVT).

Diagnosis

Acute onset of right hemiparesis and aphasia
Left M1 occlusion d/t thrombus
Acute ischemia stroke
IV tPA candidate, and being administered
Risk factors include DM2, HTN, smoking

Recommend

Complete IV tPA
EVT is under consideration
Post-tPA care including BP parameters per protocol
Will need MRI stroke protocol but after stability assured following TPA administration and immediate observation period
Completion of stroke work-up with lipid panel, A1c, TTE-bubble study, and cardiac monitoring
Admit Neuro ICU

Documenting and Presenting Findings

Karl E. Misulis and Eli E. Zimmerman

Purpose

The principal reason for documenting the history and examination findings is communication, whether with other providers, with patients, or with themselves when they see the patient again in a future encounter. These different communications used to have different content—a letter to a referring provider, clinic notes for the examiner, and layperson level notes for patients. Now, there is usually a single document to meet all communication and billing requirements; patients and all connected providers have access to it. Even so, the documentation often does not meet all of the communication needs well. Hence when these documents are generated, they have to be carefully constructed and worded to inform but not offend all parties.

Documentation must meet the needs of the recipients. As such, the most important sections are assessment and recommendations. These must be concise yet complete, and the recommendations must be granular. They must include contingencies that anticipate some of the possible courses the case may take. Discussion of the presentation of these and samples are presented in Chapter 1.5.

Text Documentation

PROSE VERSUS TEMPLATED ENTRY

Two methods for entering data into the record are prose entry where the user types or uses speech recognition to enter the text and templated entry where a complex series of taps or clicks generates the entry. The latter is commonly used in acute care settings, such as emergency department and urgent care facilities, and in procedural areas where there are many standard aspects to documentation.

Templated entry is efficient, but some information and context are lost compared with prose entry. However, use of the template can reduce the chance that key elements will be missed, especially those that are part of required documentation. For example, the checklist before a procedure or thrombolytic administration needs to be standardized and complete to optimize patient safety.

For the history of present illness (HPI), prose entry is recommended. For many other elements of the neurologic history and examination, templated entry is acceptable.

METHOD OF ENTRY

Common methods of data entry are typing, voice recognition, and scribe. Typing is essential for some portion of the entry, and this can be done in the presence of the patient and family. Voice recognition is widely used. It can be awkward in the presence of patient and family, especially when items with a negative connotation are entered, such as "morbid obesity," a term that is specifically looked for when coding comorbid conditions.

Entry by the provider while they are looking at their screen has disadvantages for the encounter. The time looking at the screen results in loss of nonverbal communication. With the lack of sustained eye contact, the provider can miss observational components of the examination, including facial expression, spontaneous movements, and gestures. The computer becomes a barrier between the provider and patient, even if they are both looking at the screen; this is better than the alternative but is still suboptimal. Direct entry into the electronic health record (EHR) also results in the provider having less intellectual bandwidth to apply to the patient, having to wrestle with the user interface, making corrections, and having to look through the tabs of the chart during the discussion.

Scribes are in widespread use except in many academic medical centers. They can free the provider to be hands-on and to look at the patient. Some limited data indicate that quality of care may be enhanced by the addition of another teammate. In a multicenter study, scribes reduced emergency department length of stay and improved the number of patients seen by the provider per hour by 25.6%. A University of Chicago study in the primary care setting showed improved provider satisfaction, with more than 50% reduction in postclinic documentation time, with no decline in patient satisfaction; in fact there were some improvements.

Outline of the Elements

DEMOGRAPHICS AND ENCOUNTER DETAILS

Name, date of birth, and medical record number should be prominent; these elements should be on every page if the document is a PDF or is printed. Encounter details include date of encounter, institution, location, specialty, and provider.

CHIEF COMPLAINT

Chief complaint, or the reason for the encounter, is entered even if the patient is not able to express one. If the patient is able to communicate, then their impression of the reason for the encounter should be documented in addition to a reason that was indicated at the time of the encounter request, whether it was requested by the family, patient, or provider. Wording such as "here for neurology appointment" is not useful and should not be used. "Referred by Dr. X for Y problem, but the patient and daughter report they are here for Z problem" is a more appropriate documentation.

HISTORY OF PRESENT ILLNESS

HPI includes the story of the events and observations leading up to the encounter. This includes items directly pertaining to the chief complaint and other events that may be important.

For inpatient evaluation, the HPI should include the relevant hospital course to the time of the encounter. For many presentations, it is appropriate to documente future plans for the patient's hospitalization. For example, "Patient is referred for consideration of anticoagulation for atrial fibrillation depending on the risk of CNS bleeding." The assessment and plan depend on this information.

PAST MEDICAL AND SURGICAL HISTORY

Past medical history (PMH) and surgical history can be sourced from the data already entered in the EHR, from the patient directly, and/or from family and other caregivers. Review of the EHR documentation is essential, but it is recommended that the provider ask questions about this history independently to verify accuracy of the prior documentation and ensure that nothing has been missed.

SOCIAL HISTORY

Social history (SH) includes the patient's living situation, marital status, and substance use, including tobacco products, ethanol, and other drugs. This is often prepopulated in the EHR, but it should be verified.

REVIEW OF SYSTEMS

The standard review of systems (ROS) covers most of the organ systems, and there are various formats. This is a standard ROS statement that is sometimes used: "ROS: The following systems were reviewed with pertinent positives and negatives documented in the HPI: Constitutional, Eyes, HEENT, CV, Respiratory, GI, GU, Skin, Neurologic, Psychiatric, Musculoskeletal, and Sleep."

For documentation of the ROS, an alternative and more classic method is to have each positive and negative documented in this section. For busy clinicians, this is not valuable; it is better for them to place positive and pertinent negatives in the HPI.

FAMILY HISTORY

Family history (FH) includes the medical histories of family members that are relevant and possibly relevant. If a patient is being seen for cancer, FH of a similar diagnosis is appropriate. If a patient is being seen for stroke, FH of stroke or cardiovascular disease is important to note. This is especially true for inherited diseases such as Huntington disease.

MEDICATIONS

Accurate knowledge of prescribed medications, compliance, and administration is key when considering assessment and plans. The provider cannot rely on EHR-generated lists to be complete and accurate and to reflect compliance. Database queries can determine what medications have been filled at many pharmacies, but they do not include data from all pharmacies.

The medication record needs to include vitamins and nutritional supplements.

ALLERGIES, SENSITIVITIES, AND ADVERSE REACTIONS

Documentation of allergies, sensitivities, and adverse reactions includes not only pharmaceuticals but also contrast agents, biological exposures, and other elements. If the patient has reacted to medical agents, these details are important. The decision about the type of premedication depends on the patient's previous reaction.

EXAMINATION

All elements of the examination are documented. It is recommended that abnormal or key normal elements are highlighted. In a long list of body systems, important findings might not be noticed. Many clinicians bold or otherwise highlight key findings. Sometimes, key findings are placed at the beginning of the examination documentation to emphasize them.

The specific components of the examination are determined by the patient's clinical presentation and also by requirements for documentation of the encounter at a particular level of service.

These guidelines are changing, but at the time of this writing, Centers for Medicare & Medicaid Services (CMS) specifies which components of which organ systems are required to be examined and the results documented to meet criteria for billing at a specific level of service.

ASSESSMENT

Assessment is a statement of the provider's impression of the clinical presentation in the context of the medical background of the patient. As such, the HPI and PMH should not be restated. For an assessment to be read and to be helpful to other clinicians, it must be concise and targeted. The assessment may be written in prose or as a list.

This example of an assessment is presented in the wrong order: "77M with CAD, s/p CABG, Afib on warfarin, COPD, SCLC, 50-pack smoking history, here with CHF exacerbation now with right sided weakness." The reader wants to know the reason for the encounter before all of the background information. Better wording would be, "77M with right-sided weakness in the setting of CHF exacerbation."

The assessment should indicate the differential diagnosis, beginning with the most likely diagnosis. In the previous example, it would be stated as, "Right-sided weakness is most likely due to ischemic stroke, with the differential diagnosis including intracerebral hemorrhage or brain metastasis." Not every possibility needs to be listed. Brain abscess in this patient might be mentioned in the differential diagnosis because the patient may be predisposed to bacterial endocarditis.

It is important to answer the question that prompted the encounter. If this is a consult where the request was "rule out neuromuscular causes of weakness," then the assessment would include, "No evidence of primary neuromuscular disease; the identified weakness conforms to a vascular distribution and is most likely cerebrovascular."

Always have a differential diagnosis. Unless the provider arrives in the trauma bay and sees a pole sticking out of a patient's head, there is always more than one possibility for the clinical presentation, although one diagnosis might seem more obvious than others.

Be concise in the assessment. Studies have shown that the longer an assessment is, the less likely a provider is to read it. Do not put the HPI into the assessment. The assessment can be a paragraph or bullet points, and many providers use a combination of both, such as a short assessment paragraph followed by a diagnosis list that is then followed by a plan or recommendation list.

PLAN OR RECOMMENDATIONS

The label of "plan" or "recommendations" depends on whether the encounter is a consultation. If it is, then the plan for patient care is a recommendation for the providers who ordered the consult. There may be a relationship where the consulting provider is expected to execute the plan, but this should be understood by both parties.

Recommendations should be granular. "Recommend workup for TIA" is unacceptable unless the statement is followed by a list of elements that the clinician recommends in the TIA workup.

Consult recommendations should generally be confined to the consultant's specialty and reason for the consultation. A neurologist should not give recommendations on antibiotic management to an infectious disease provider unless they were specifically requested to. If there are issues of concern outside the consultant's sphere, they should be raised verbally with the requesting provider.

Verbal Presentation

Throughout their careers, neurologists and all other providers deliver verbal presentations. The content and presentation format differ markedly depending on the context and stage of the provider's career. A second-year medical student is expected to give a comprehensive presentation, a neurology resident is expected to give a concise presentation, and colleagues at the resident and attending level give each other handoff presentations. In addition, there are bedside presentations to the patient and family.

COMPREHENSIVE PRESENTATION

Comprehensive presentation does not mean completely replaying the script of the encounter. There is not time or attention for that. It means an organized presentation starting with the reason for the encounter followed by the HPI with the often disorganized data acquisition sculpted into a coherent patient story. PMH is complete for active problems and inactive ones that pertain to the presentation. Similarly, FH and SH are pertinent to the presentation. ROS is often not part of the verbal presentation; if something of importance was identified in the ROS, it should be in the patient story that was already presented. It is part of the role of the presenter to organize the data.

Examination elements can be presented in a variety of ways. For a comprehensive verbal presentation, it is appropriate to list each system examined along with abnormal findings or indication of normal findings. Elements that could not be examined should be mentioned, for example, "unable to visualize fundi due to corneal scarring."

Assessment and plan are concise and focused, even in a comprehensive presentation. The HPI is not repeated; most people are able to recall it.

In all presentations and writings, the clinician must remember that their audience has a limited attention span and are able to incorporate a limited amount of data in one sitting.

CONCISE PRESENTATION

Concise presentation includes all of the elements in a comprehensive presentation, but only positives and pertinent negatives are presented. PMH is woven into the HPI; key elements are incorporated into the presentation of the condition under consideration and other elements mentioned at the end of the HPI presentation. FH is not presented at all unless during case discussion someone offers a differential diagnosis for which FH would be relevant.

Assessment and plan are presented together. A differential diagnosis is always included with an estimate of likelihood. For example, "Acute onset of right hemiparesis and aphasia is most likely due to stroke, likely ischemic. Differential diagnosis includes hemorrhage but absence of headache and alteration of consciousness makes this less likely. Seizure is possible but less likely."

BEDSIDE PRESENTATION

Bedside presentation should be concise, so the amount of information is not overwhelming. Elements of the presentation that are sensitive should be discussed appropriately.

The patient and family should be invited to enter the discussion. This can be by a statement such as, "Did I summarize correctly?" or "Anything else we need to know?"

COLLEAGUE BRIEFING

Discussion between colleagues who are sharing care of a patient is often called a handoff. This is just a few sentences to summarize the clinical situation, to give concise assessment and plan, and to highlight any issues that are likely to arise. A hypothetical example for a patient with possible seizures would be: "This is a 24-year-old female with clinical seizures that are likely psychogenic nonepileptic events. She has 24-hour video-EEG on for spell capture. If she has an event, the nurse will message you, so please check the EEG. If epileptic, then order levetiracetam load and maintenance. If not, let them know I will be back in the morning to go over the situation. Any questions?"

An example for a patient with myasthenia gravis would be: "This is a 74-year old male with seropositive myasthenia gravis who has more weakness and now cannot swallow. I changed him to IV steroids and pyridostigmine and asked for frequent pulmonary assessments. If he deteriorates, have a low threshold for intubation and increase his methylprednisolone. I will start plasma exchange in the morning."

Colleague briefings, as well as all recommendations and plans, must have granular recommendations and contingencies.

Clinical Neuroscience

Overview of a Systems-Based Approach

Eli E. Zimmerman and Karl E. Misulis

Neuroanatomy is an enormous field, with textbooks devoted solely to the subject. In this book, we presume the reader has a foundation in basic neuroanatomy and neurophysiology. Here we will take the clinical approach to neuroanatomy. We will organize by locations but also by functional systems. Subsequent chapters cover the individual segments of the nervous system.

General Principles

SYMMETRY

With few exceptions, the nervous system is symmetric across the midsagittal plane. This is from a structural standpoint, not completely a functional one. For example, each cerebral hemisphere serves motor function to the contralateral body. Many structures of the brain have principal responsibility for the opposite side of the body.

Lateralization

There are exceptions to this symmetry. The cerebellum has predominantly ipsilateral responsibility to the body on motor control. There are function-specific lateralizations, such as left hemisphere for speech and right hemisphere for attention and some visuospatial functions.

In neuroanatomical terms, there is extensive lateralization among symmetric and asymmetric functions, and these lateralizations are complex and incompletely understood.

PATHWAYS AND RELAYS

For connections between central centers to happen, long pathways must decussate (that is cross the midsagittal plane) to end up at their targets. As we will discuss, these decussations occur at different points across the neuraxis for each pathway. Along the way, there are relays from one neuron to another, but this is usually more than a simple handoff; there is almost always, if not always, processing at the point of relay.

CENTRAL AND PERIPHERAL NERVOUS SYSTEMS

All neurologists are familiar with the distinction between central nervous system (CNS) and peripheral nervous system (PNS). Some of the elements of this classification, however, are complex. For example, the cell bodies of motor neurons are in the spinal cord for appendicular and axial muscles, and they are in the brain for voluntary muscles innervated by the cranial nerves. So are these CNS or PNS? The neuron cell bodies are considered to be in the CNS, but the axons are in the PNS; so whether motor neurons are affected in the central or peripheral arena depends on the etiology of the damage.

GRAY MATTER VERSUS WHITE MATTER

Gray matter contains primarily neuron cell bodies, hence its color, and it forms the cortex, ganglia, and nuclei. White matter, from lipid-rich myelin, forms the tracts connecting regions of the brain and spinal cord.

Systems

Details of the systems are discussed in the following chapters, but some of the key neurologic systems are:

- Motor system,
- Sensory system,
- Visual system, and
- Language system (speech and hearing).

All of the systems have intertwined and interdependent activity. Although it is helpful to silo these systems, they are all connected. For example, motor activity in the sensory system is essential for feedback on success of movement, but the cerebellum depends on sensory input to determine how to adjust motor function.

The systems are considered individually and collectively in the chapters that follow.

Cerebral Hemispheres

Eli E. Zimmerman and Howard S. Kirshner

Introduction

The cerebral hemispheres contain the very essence of our being. They allow us to speak, form complex thought, interact with the world, have interpersonal relationships, understand humor, and more. They accomplish this through complex organization and specificity. A theme throughout the organization of the nervous system is that everything is arranged in a highly organized and predictable manner. Nothing in the nervous system is an accident.

Structural Organization

The major landmarks of the cerebral hemisphere are shown in Fig. 2.2.1. During the explosive development of the central nervous system, the cortex develops gyri (folds of brain tissue) and sulci (the spaces between them) to increase surface area. Several deeper sulci are the fissures. The interhemispheric fissure separates the left and right halves of the brain. On each side, the central sulcus separates the frontal and the parietal lobes, and the deeper Sylvian fissure separates the frontal and parietal lobes from the temporal lobe. The parietooccipital sulcus, only visible on the medial aspect of the cortex, separates the parietal lobe from the occipital lobe. The gyrus just rostral (anterior) to the central sulcus is the precentral gyrus, and the gyrus just caudal (posterior) to it is the postcentral gyrus. A key in the structural arrangement of the cortex is that the brain is typically relatively symmetric; this is structural symmetry rather than functional symmetry. In most people, the left hemisphere is the dominant hemisphere. It is identified as such because of its role in language.

Functional Organization

FRONTAL LOBES

Starting with the caudal aspect of the frontal lobes, there is the precentral gyrus, which is bordered rostrally by the precentral sulcus and caudally by the central sulcus. This strip of cortex is the primary motor cortex—the area of the cortex responsible for the initiation of voluntary movement. The arrangement of the motor cortex (Fig. 2.2.1) follows a pattern of the homunculus, with the leg represented medially, the face represented laterally, and the arm and trunk superiorly. Anterior to the primary motor cortex are the premotor and supplementary motor cortices, which assist in the planning of movement. The frontal eye field is anterior to these and is responsible for the initiation of volitional gaze to the contralateral side. Most rostrally is the prefrontal cortex, which is responsible for executive function, including personality and inhibition. In the inferior frontal gyrus lies Broca area (in the dominant hemisphere), which is responsible for the productive elements of speech. This area lies adjacent to the motor portion of the cortex responsible for movement of the face and mouth.

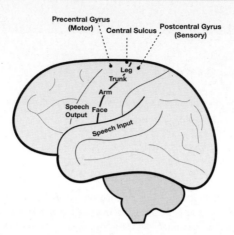

Fig. 2.2.1 Cerebral hemisphere anatomy. Left cerebral hemisphere is shown with important functional regions indicated.

PARIETAL LOBES

Starting with the rostral aspect of the parietal lobe, there is the postcentral gyrus, which is bordered rostrally by the central sulcus and caudally by the postcentral sulcus. Just as the primary motor cortex resides in the frontal lobe with its characteristic organization, this is the primary somatosensory cortex, and it is responsible for the reception of somatosensory information from the body. Its arrangement mirrors the primary motor cortex. More caudally in the parietal lobe lie the supramarginal and angular gyri, responsible for written language and reading.

TEMPORAL LOBES

Within the posterior aspect of the superior temporal gyrus lies Wernicke area, the cortical area in the dominant hemisphere responsible for language comprehension. This, unsurprisingly, lies adjacent to the primary auditory cortex, where sounds are first perceived.

OCCIPITAL LOBES

The main function of the occipital lobes is vision. The primary visual cortex lies at the very posterior aspect of the occipital lobe, with each hemisphere responsible for vision from the contralateral visual field. Information is then sent anteriorly for processing (interpretation of color, figure, faces, etc.).

Basal Ganglia and Thalamus

Eli E. Zimmerman and Karl E. Misulis

Basal Ganglia

The basal ganglia are composed of the following deep nuclei, which have complex interrelationships:

- Globus pallidus
- Putamen
- Caudate nucleus
- Subthalamic nucleus
- Claustrum
- Substantia nigra

The neostriatum consists of the putamen and caudate nucleus. The lentiform nucleus consists of the globus pallidus and putamen; it is called "lentiform" because its geometry is similar to that of an optical lens.

The basal ganglia are mainly involved in control of movement, especially the automatic components of locomotion and posture. Fine movements are initiated in the cortex, whereas the basal ganglia are involved in feedback control of movements.

Major inputs to the basal ganglia are from the cerebral cortex, thalamus, and brainstem. Major outputs from the brainstem are from the globus pallidus to the ventral anterior (VA) and ventrolateral (VL) nuclei of the thalamus; the thalamus projects back to the cerebral cortex as well.

Interconnections between the nuclei in the basal ganglia are plentiful. The following are some of the most important:

- From the substantia nigra to the striatum
- Between the substantia nigra and globus pallidus in both directions
- From the striatum to the globus pallidus
- Between the subthalamic nucleus and globus pallidus in both directions

With these afferent, efferent, and associative connections, there are complex and interwoven circuits, the details of which are outside the scope of this text. Lesions often affect multiple elements in these circuits. Some important circuits involve the following:

- Cerebral cortex → striatum → thalamus → cerebral cortex
- Neostriatum → globus pallidus + substantia nigra → neostriatum
- Globus pallidus → subthalamic nucleus and back

Circuits in the basal ganglia are probably involved in execution of patterned movements and error checking. The motor system can be thought of as a hierarchical network of controls. At the top is the cortex, which determines the focus and intent of the movement at this level. The movement may be a concept of an action rather than an action of individual muscles and muscle groups. Output from the cortex projects to the basal ganglia, brainstem, and spinal cord. The purpose of the brainstem and spinal cord is to decode the intent to move into individual muscle movements, activating specific motor neurons and receiving feedback on the success of the intended movements.

The cerebellum receives input on movement and provides information used to correct movement. The basal ganglia also receive input regarding success of movement; however, unlike the brainstem brainstem, cerebellarr, and spinal cerebellar and spinal centers, the basal ganglia have a major projection of their output ultimately back to the cortex, which, in turn, modifies its output in accordance with the information received.

The basal ganglia have multiple functions, including control of the speed of movement and automatic motor programs. Lesions of the basal ganglia can occur due to a variety of etiologies, including neurodegenerative (Parkinson disease), genetic (Huntington disease), metabolic (Wilson disease), toxic (carbon monoxide poisoning), and vascular (stroke) causes.

Lesions of these structures usually affect the speed of movement, either making it too fast or causing too much movement (hyperkinetic) or making it too slow or causing too little movement (bradykinetic). A key distinction between lesions of the corticospinal tract and disorders of the basal ganglia is the presence of rigidity. Compared to spasticity (which is a velocity-dependent increase in tone and is characteristic of upper motor neuron lesions), disorders of the basal ganglia cause rigidity, which is a velocity-independent increase in tone.

Thalamus

The thalamus has many functions, although its basic task is processing afferent information. The ventroposterior (VP) nuclear complex is the main somesthetic receiving area; it consists of the ventroposterolateral (VPL) and ventroposteromedial (VPM) nuclei. Ascending information from the head and face projects to the VPM nuclei, whereas input from the rest of the body projects to VPL nuclei. The VP complex projects mainly to the primary somatosensory region of the cortex on the postcentral gyrus (areas 3, 1, and 2).

An exception is taste, which ascends to VPM nuclei and projects to the ventral aspect of the precentral gyrus, adjacent to the insula.

The posterior nuclear group receives nociceptive input from the spinothalamic tracts and projects to the secondary somesthetic region on the inner aspect of the postcentral cortex, adjacent to the insula.

The VA nucleus receives input from the substantia nigra and globus pallidus and from other thalamic nuclei, brainstem reticular formation, and cerebral cortex. Projections are to the premotor area of the frontal lobe (area 6) and the supplementary motor area on the superior frontal gyrus (also area 6). The VA nucleus is probably involved in processing the information that causes alerting. Damage to this area results in decreased alertness and inattention, which can resemble frontal lobe deficits.

The VL nucleus receives input from the cerebellum, substantia nigra, and globus pallidus. In addition, it receives lesser input from the cerebral cortex, reticular formation, and other thalamic nuclei. The VL nucleus has projections to and from the primary motor cortex on the precentral gyrus (area 4). It is involved in control over movement, and it is an integral part of two control loops, as described below.

CONNECTIONS AND BLOOD SUPPLY

The control loops and Cerebellar Loop and Basal Ganglia loop:
- Cerebellar loop: cerebral cortex → pons → cerebellum → red nucleus → thalamus → cerebral cortex
- Basal ganglia loop: cerebral cortex → basal ganglia → thalamus → cerebral cortex

Damage to the cerebellar loop results in predominantly cerebellar ataxia. Damage to the basal ganglia loop results in extrapyramidal findings, including parkinsonism, dystonia, and dyskinesias.

The medial geniculate body receives auditory input from the brainstem, especially the inferior colliculus. Projections are to the auditory cortex in the superior temporal gyrus (area 41).

The lateral geniculate body receives visual input via the optic tracts. Because the lateral geniculate is central to the optic chiasm, the lateral geniculate conveys information from the contralateral visual hemifield. There are six layers, with each layer relaying information from only one eye; the ipsilateral eye fibers project to layers 2, 3, and 5, and the contralateral eye fibers project to layers 1, 4, and 6. Projections are via the optic radiations to the primary visual cortex (area 17) on the medial aspect of the occipital lobe.

ARTERIAL SUPPLY

The thalamus is supplied mainly by branches of the posterior cerebral artery, with some supply from posterior communicating arteries. The vessels enter the substance of the thalamus in a manner similar to that of the lenticulostriate vessels.

Brainstem, Cerebellum, and Cranial Nerves

Eli E. Zimmerman and Karl E. Misulis

Brainstem

Brainstem anatomy includes associated connections with the cerebellum, spinal cord, and hemispheres. In addition, cranial nerve anatomy and function are integral to brainstem anatomy. Clinical diagnosis of brainstem dysfunction requires an understanding of motor and sensory pathways through the brainstem and a working knowledge of segmental anatomy at different levels of the brainstem. Table 2.4.1 presents the localization and clinical features of some important brainstem syndromes.

OVERVIEW

Remembering the segmental anatomy of the brainstem is easier if sites of exit of the cranial nerves (CN) are thoroughly understood. Fig. 2.4.1 shows a ventral view of the brainstem with sites of exit of each cranial nerve, and Fig. 2.4.2 shows the vascular supply of the brainstem.

The oculomotor nerve exits the midbrain on the ventral surface between the cerebral peduncles. The trochlear nerve exits the midbrain near the inferior colliculus and wraps around the cerebral peduncle. The optic nerve only projects a small proportion of its fibers to the midbrain, but the optic tracts sit just above the oculomotor and trochlear nerves as they travel toward the orbit.

Immediately below the midbrain is the pons, which on ventral view appears to wrap around the brainstem and attach to the cerebellar hemispheres on either side. The trigeminal nerve exits the lateral aspect of the pons.

The abducens, facial, and vestibulocochlear nerves exit at the pontomedullary junction. The most medial is the abducens nerve, which has a long course past the pons to project to the orbit. The facial nerve exits laterally to the abducens and just adjacent to the vestibulocochlear nerve. The glossopharyngeal, vagus, and hypoglossal nerves exit the medulla, and the accessory nerve has fibers that exit both at the level of the medulla and at the upper cervical cord.

Localization of lesions affecting the brainstem is easier if a systematic approach is used. When faced with a difficult diagnostic problem, the neurologist should try to rely on this method rather than trying to fit the symptoms into one of the many syndrome descriptions. Important questions to answer include the following:

- Is the lesion intraaxial or extraaxial?
- What is the rostrocaudal location of the lesion?
- Is the intraaxial lesion unilateral or bilateral?
- What clinical conditions can produce damage in this localization?

Isolated single cranial nerve palsies are usually extraaxial, that is, not in the substance of the brainstem. Multiple cranial nerve palsies can still be due to extraaxial disease. An intraaxial lesion is suggested by the combination of cranial nerve palsies and signs of damage to ascending and descending tracts. For example, an isolated CN VI palsy, which causes impaired abduction

47

TABLE 2.4.1 ■ Brainstem Syndromes

Syndrome	Structures Involved	Features
Midbrain		
Parinaud	Dorsal midbrain; pretectal region; posterior commissure	Vertical gaze deficit, usually supranuclear; light-near dissociation of pupil response; convergence-retraction nystagmus; lid retraction; lid lag
Weber	CN III; ventral midbrain; CST	CN III palsy; contralateral hemiparesis
Benedikt	CN III; ventral midbrain; CST; red nucleus	CN III palsy; contralateral hemiparesis; intention tremor; cerebellar ataxia
Top of the basilar	Occipital lobes; midbrain ocular motor nuclei; cerebral peduncle; medial temporal lobe; thalamus	Cortical blindness; ocular motor deficits; CST signs; memory deficit; sensory deficit
Pons		
Millard-Gubler	CN VI, VII; ventral pons	CN VI, VII palsies; contralateral hemiparesis
Clumsy-hand dysarthria	CST; facial nerve	Hemiparesis; dysarthria; often facial weakness
Locked-in	CST; CN VI, VII	Quadriplegia; facial weakness; lateral gaze palsy
Pure motor hemiparesis	CST in ventral pons	Hemiparesis with CST signs
Ataxic hemiparesis	CST at basis pontis (or internal capsule)	Hemiparesis with impaired coordination
Foville	CN VII; ventral pons; PPRF	CN VII palsy; contralateral hemiparesis; gaze palsy to side of lesion
Medulla		
Lateral medullary	Inferior cerebellar peduncle; descending sympathetic tract; spinothalamic tract; trigeminal nucleus	Ipsilateral ataxia; Horner syndrome; vertigo; contralateral pain and temperature loss; ipsilateral facial sensory loss
Medial medullary	CST; medial lemniscus; hypoglossal nerve	Contralateral hemiparesis; loss of position and vibratory sensation; ipsilateral tongue paresis

CN, Cranial nerve; *CST,* corticospinal tract; *PPRF,* paramedian pontine reticular formation.

of the ipsilateral eye, is relatively common and can result from microvascular disease, trauma, and increased intracranial pressure; it is often idiopathic. In contrast, a CN VI palsy combined with damage to the medial longitudinal fasciculus (MLF), which causes internuclear ophthalmoplegia (INO), is due to a lesion in the pons.

Rostrocaudal localization is most easily identified by carefully determining which cranial nerves are affected. For example, an oculomotor lesion with signs of intraaxial damage suggests a midbrain lesion, whereas glossopharyngeal and vagus damage suggest a medullary lesion.

The determination of whether the lesion is unilateral or bilateral requires an understanding of which tracts are crossed and at which level. The descending corticospinal tracts cross in the medulla. Dorsal column axons, which serve touch, vibration, and position sense, ascend the cord uncrossed, synapse in the nucleus gracilis and nucleus cuneatus in the medulla, and cross as they

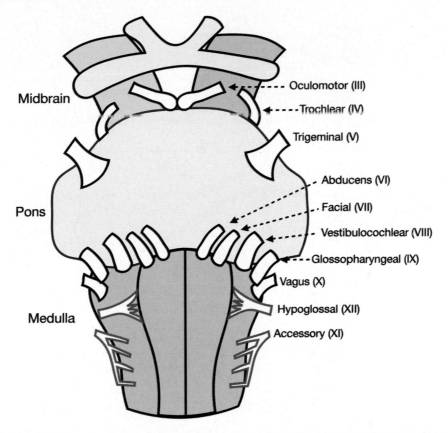

Fig. 2.4.1 Brainstem anatomy including cranial nerves. The sites of exit of the cranial nerves are seen. Knowledge of key anatomic relationships helps with localization of structural lesions.

ascend through the medulla, forming the medial lemniscus. The spinothalamic tract axons, which convey pain and temperature sensations, cross at the level of the spinal cord segment and ascend crossed in the cord. The spinothalamic tract stays lateral in the brainstem and ascends to the midbrain where it joins with the medial lemniscus to enter the thalamus.

When the lesion has been determined to be intraaxial and the rostrocaudal and unilateral or bilateral localization has been made, individual syndromes can be considered. Specific etiologies are suggested by associated symptoms; for instance, acute onset of a deficit suggests a stroke, sudden onset of headache and vomiting suggests a hemorrhage, and a slowly progressive deficit suggests an expanding mass lesion.

MIDBRAIN

Fig. 2.4.3 shows a cross section of the midbrain between the superior and inferior colliculi. Important landmarks are the cerebral peduncles, red nucleus, substantia nigra, aqueduct and surrounding periaqueductal gray matter, medial lemniscus, MLF, and midbrain tectum.

The cerebral peduncles carry descending information from the cerebral hemispheres to the brainstem and spinal cord. The red nucleus receives outflow from the contralateral cerebellum and

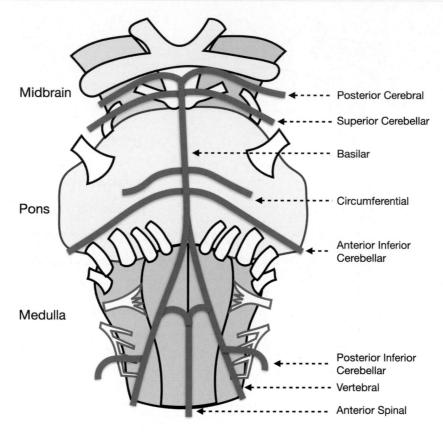

Fig. 2.4.2 Brainstem vascular supply. The major blood vessels are shown. These are the ones that can produce vascular ischemic syndromes.

sends efferents to the thalamus. The medial lemniscus carries ascending fibers from the nucleus gracilis and nucleus cuneatus in the medulla to the thalamus. The substantia nigra has extensive interconnections with other nuclei, but the most important are its reciprocal connections with the striatum.

The oculomotor nuclear complex is adjacent to the midline and ventral to the aqueduct. The trochlear nucleus is in a similar position, but it is caudal to the oculomotor nucleus although still within the midbrain. The MLF carries outflow from the contralateral paramedial pontine reticular formation, the center that governs lateral gaze, and projects to the oculomotor nuclear complex.

Blood supply to the midbrain is largely through the basilar artery, which lies on the ventral surface. The basilar artery sends several penetrating branches into the midbrain before bifurcating into the posterior cerebral arteries (PCAs), which wrap laterally around the midbrain. The PCAs also give off penetrating branches.

PONS

Fig. 2.4.4 shows a cross section of the pons. There are rostrocaudal differences in organization, so this figure is slightly stylized to show important structures. Important landmarks include the corticospinal tract, pontine nuclei, medial lemniscus, spinothalamic tract, lateral lemniscus, nuclei

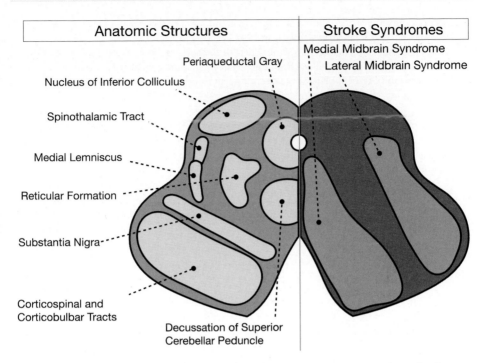

Fig. 2.4.3 Midbrain cross section. Cross section of the midbrain is shown. It is somewhat stylized because there is significant rostrocaudal change in nucleus and pathway localization. Left side of the figure highlights key structures. Right side shows approximate regions affected by ischemic syndromes.

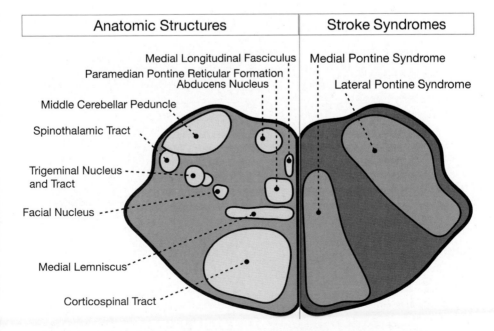

Fig. 2.4.4 Pons cross section. Cross section of the pons in a stylized format as for Fig. 2.4.3.

and intraaxial portions of the abducens, trigeminal and facial nerves, vestibular nucleus, paramedian pontine reticular formation (PPRF), and MLF.

The corticospinal tract lies in the ventral aspect of the pons, and it is still uncrossed at this level. The medial lemniscus, carrying fibers from the nuclei gracilis and cuneatus, is already crossed. The PPRF, which is important for lateral gaze, sends output to the abducens nucleus and through the MLF to the midbrain. The MLF is not dedicated solely to the PPRF; however, it also carries descending axons of the medial reticulospinal and vestibulospinal tracts and the tectospinal tract. The motor and sensory nuclei of the trigeminal nerves lie rostral to the abducens and facial nuclei, which lie in the caudal half of the pons. The facial nerve exits the facial nucleus and moves dorsally to loop around the abducens nucleus before moving ventrally and medially to exit the brainstem at the pontomedullary junction.

The vertebral arteries join to form the basilar artery near the pontomedullary junction, and the basilar artery ascends to the midbrain. There are major and minor circumferential branches as well as direct penetrating paramedial branches of the basilar artery. Major circumferential branches include the anterior inferior cerebellar artery (AICA) and superior cerebellar arteries. Transverse arteries have a variable projection bilaterally and send penetrating arteries into the pons.

MEDULLA

Fig. 2.4.5 shows a cross section of the medulla. There are rostrocaudal differences in organization, so the figure is slightly stylized. Important landmarks include the corticospinal tracts, olivary nucleus, medial lemniscus, MLF, vestibular nucleus, nucleus ambiguus, hypoglossal nucleus and

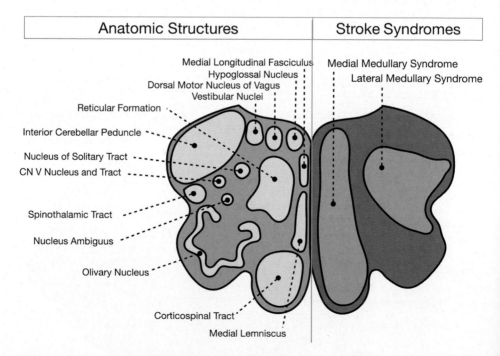

Fig. 2.4.5 Medulla cross section. Cross section of the medulla in a stylized format as for Figs. 2.4.3 and 2.4.4.

nerve, nucleus of the tractus solitarius, descending sympathetic tract, spinothalamic tract, and inferior cerebellar peduncle.

The blood supply to the medulla is from branches of the vertebral arteries because the basilar artery has not formed yet at this location. The major vessels are the posterior inferior cerebellar artery (PICA) and medial branches of the vertebral artery, which join to form the anterior spinal artery.

The corticospinal tract travels in the medullary pyramids. The corticospinal tract decussates in the medulla, with the arm axons crossing slightly rostral to the crossing of the leg axons. This arrangement allows a very localized lesion to produce corticospinal dysfunction affecting the ipsilateral arm and contralateral leg; although in practice, this combination is uncommon.

Underlying the olives are the olivary nuclei, which project somatosensory information to the contralateral cerebellum. Nucleus gracilis and nucleus cuneatus are in the most caudal section of the medulla, on the dorsal surface, in continuity with the dorsal columns. Outflow crosses the midline and forms the medial lemnisci. The spinothalamic tract is a continuation of the same tract in the spinal cord and stays lateral through its course in the medulla and into the pons. The nucleus ambiguus provides axons that control muscles of the pharynx and larynx via the glossopharyngeal, and vagus nerves. The solitary tract nucleus receives taste and visceral sensation input from the facial, glossopharyngeal, and vagus nerves. The descending sympathetic tract projects into the cervical cord. The MLF contains the medial vestibulospinal and reticulospinal tracts and the tectospinal tract. The restiform body forms the inferior cerebellar peduncle.

Cerebellum

ANATOMY

The cerebellum sits dorsal to the brainstem in the posterior fossa. All of its inputs and outputs pass through the brainstem. The cerebellum can be divided into several phylogenetic and physiologic divisions; in clinical practice, the most important distinction is between disorders affecting the vermis and those affecting the cerebellar hemispheres.

The cerebellum is divided into the anterior lobe, posterior lobe, and flocculonodular lobe. The anterior lobe is the section rostral to the primary fissure of the cerebellum. This lobe receives prominent input from the spinocerebellar pathways and is involved in gait and truncal coordination. The posterior lobe receives extensive input from the cerebral hemispheres and is concerned with coordination of individual limb movements. The flocculonodular lobe receives input from the vestibular nuclei and is concerned with proximal coordination.

Inputs to the cerebellum are largely through the middle and inferior cerebellar peduncles, although the ventral spinocerebellar tract and a few other minor afferent tracts pass through the superior cerebellar peduncle. Outflow from the cerebellum is through the superior cerebellar peduncle. Axons from the cerebellar cortex project to the deep nuclei, which in turn project axons through the superior cerebellar peduncle to the contralateral red nucleus, contralateral ventrolateral nucleus of the thalamus, reticular formation, and vestibular nuclei.

The cerebellum is involved in control of movement. The flocculonodular lobe, anterior lobe, and especially the vermis are involved in control of gait and truncal movement (Fig. 2.4.6). The posterior lobe, especially the hemispheres, is involved in coordinating movements of individual ipsilateral limbs.

FUNCTION

The cerebellum can be considered to have three major roles, which are:

- Maintenance of balance and posture,
- Moment-to-moment coordination of the trunk and limbs, and
- Higher order cognitive functions.

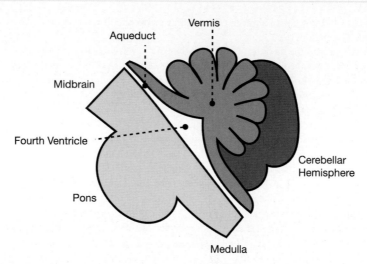

Fig. 2.4.6 Cerebellum. Sagittal and axial views of the cerebellum indicating regions of potential dysfunction. Vermis is more involved with gait and axial stability, whereas the cerebellar hemispheres are more involved with appendicular coordination.

Each of these regions has distinct inputs and outputs that allow their respective regions to serve these functions. These are divided functionally into the:

- Vestibulocerebellum (responsible for balance and posture),
- Spinocerebellum (responsible for moment-to-moment coordination), and
- Neocerebellum (responsible for higher order cognitive function).

With one exception (the vestibulocerebellum), cerebellar zones send output to the brainstem via the four (on each side) cerebellar nuclei. Each hemisphere of the cerebellum controls the ipsilateral side of the body.

In addition, three fiber bundles (the cerebellar peduncles) carry information in and/or out of the cerebellum. They are termed the superior, middle, and inferior cerebellar peduncles.

Vestibulocerebellum

This zone consists of the flocculonodular lobe. As this portion of the cerebellum developed with the vestibular system, it shares much in common. It receives inputs from vestibular system and sends outputs (without a relay through a deep cerebellar nucleus) to the vestibular system and reticular formation.

Spinocerebellum

This zone has within it a median zone (the vermis) and an intermediate zone. The median zone is responsible for corrections in posture and balance. It receives inputs from the vestibular system and the spinocerebellar tracts and sends outputs (via the fastigial nucleus) to the vestibular system and reticular formation. The intermediate zone is responsible for corrections in movement of the extremities. It receives information from the spinocerebellar tracts and sends outputs (via the globose and emboliform nuclei or the "interposed nuclei") to the red nucleus and to the ventroanterior (VA) and ventrolateral (VL) nuclei of the thalamus.

Neocerebellum

This zone, as its name suggests, is the most recently evolved portion of the cerebellum, responsible for planning and timing of complex movements, learned sequences, and higher order cognitive function. It receives input from the pontine gray nuclei and sends outputs (via the dentate nucleus) to the red nucleus and to the VA and VL nuclei of the thalamus.

Cerebellar Peduncles

The cerebellum communicates with the brainstem via three fiber bundles or peduncles.

Superior cerebellar peduncle mostly contains cerebellar output to the thalamus, the red nucleus, and the reticular formation and inputs from the ventral spinocerebellar tract.

Middle cerebellar peduncle, by far the largest, contains only input fibers into the cerebellum via the pontine grey nuclei.

Inferior cerebellar peduncle contains mostly input to the cerebellum (via the dorsal spinocerebellar tract and the cuneocerebellar tract, the vestibular nuclei, the reticular formation, and the inferior olive) and has output to the vestibular nuclei.

Cranial Nerves

The brainstem contains many nuclei related to cranial nerves, both for transmitting efferent (outgoing) motor information and for receiving afferent (incoming) sensory information. Each nucleus is responsible for either sensory or motor information but never both.

However, a single nucleus in the brainstem can send motor information via one or more cranial nerves. Similarly, a single nucleus in the brainstem can receive sensory information from one or more cranial nerves. For example, the nucleus ambiguus sends motor information out via CN IX and X. Another example is the spinal trigeminal nucleus, which is responsible for pain/temperature sensation for the face; it receives information via CN V, VII, IX, and X.

The converse is true as well: Cranial nerves carry efferent motor and afferent sensory information to and from multiple brainstem nuclei. For example, CN VII carries motor efferents to the muscles of facial expression and contains sensory afferents containing somatic sensation from the ear and visceral sensation (taste). Another example is CN III, which contains both motor efferents to several eye muscles but also parasympathetic efferents to pupillary constrictors.

OVERVIEW OF CRANIAL NERVE ANATOMY

The oculomotor nerve exits the midbrain on the ventral surface between the cerebral peduncles. The trochlear nerve exits the midbrain near the inferior colliculus and wraps around the cerebral peduncle. The optic nerve only projects a small proportion of its fibers to the midbrain, but the optic tracts sit just above the oculomotor and trochlear nerves as they travel toward the orbit.

Immediately below the midbrain is the pons, which on ventral view appears to wrap around the brainstem and attach to the cerebellar hemispheres on either side. The trigeminal nerve exits the lateral aspect of the pons.

The abducens, facial, and vestibulocochlear nerves exit at the pontomedullary junction. The most medial is the abducens nerve, which has a long course ascending ventral to the pons to project to the orbit. The facial nerve exits laterally to the abducens and just adjacent to the vestibulocochlear nerve. The glossopharyngeal, vagus, and hypoglossal nerves exit the medulla, and the accessory nerve has fibers that exit at both the level of the medulla and the upper cervical cord.

FUNCTIONAL CLASSIFICATION

There are six types of information contained within cranial nerves: three motor and three sensory. The cranial nerves will be discussed in detail in subsequent chapters.

Motor:

Somatic motor (CN III, IV, VI, XII): These are responsible for eye movements (CN III, IV, VI) and tongue muscles (CN XII).

Branchial motor, named because they are from the cranial nerves derived from branchial arches (CN V, VII, IX, X, XI): These are responsible for mastication (CN V), facial expression (CN VII), pharynx/larynx (CN IX, X), and sternocleidomastoid and trapezius (CN XI).

Parasympathetic (CN III, VII, IX, X): The parasympathetic nervous system originates in the brain and in the sacral portions of the spinal cord; these nuclei are responsible for parasympathetic innervation of the head/neck, the thorax, and the abdomen above the splenic flexure of the colon.

Sensory:

Somatic sensory (CN V, VII, IX, X): These are responsible for typical modalities of sensation (pain, temperature, vibration, etc.) of the face, sinuses, and even meninges (mainly CN V, but small components from CN VII, IX, X)8.

Visceral sensory (CN VII, IX, X): These are responsible for taste (CN VII, IX, X) and visceroception (CN IX, X).

Special sensory (CN VIII in brainstem): Special sensory includes smell, vision, hearing, and vestibular sensation; only CN VIII has brainstem nuclei.

OLFACTORY NERVE

The sensory receptors of the olfactory nerve are located at the superior aspect of the nasal cavity. Multiple small fiber bundles enter the cranial vault through the cribriform plate and then enter the olfactory bulb where they synapse on the second-order neurons.

The axons travel posteriorly through the olfactory tract beneath the frontal lobes. In the region of the optic chiasm, the olfactory tracts divide into medial and lateral striae; some of the former decussate in the anterior commissure. The lateral stria project to temporal lobe.

OPTIC NERVE

The optic nerve is formed from axons leaving the retina that gather in the optic disc and exit the eye. The nerve passes through the posterior aspect of the orbit and enters the skull through the optic canal. Nerve fibers serving the temporal field of each eye decussate at the optic chiasm. The optic tract exits the chiasm and projects to the lateral geniculate.

Optic nerve axons synapse in the lateral geniculate and project to the primary visual cortex. A small proportion of the fibers exit the lateral geniculate and project to the Edinger-Westphal nucleus in the midbrain to influence pupil diameter.

OCULAR MOTOR SYSTEM

CN III, IV, and VI are considered together in one discussion because of their cooperative role in eye movements.

The final pathway for eye movement begins in the brainstem with the midbrain and pontine nuclei, but voluntary control of eye movement originates in the cerebral hemispheres.

There are four basic types of eye movements:

- Pursuit movements
- Saccadic movements
- Vergence movements
- Corrective movements

Pursuit movements are synchronous movements of the eyes to follow a target that is moving relative to the head.

Saccades are quick synchronous movements to direct attention at a new target.

Vergence movements keep the target on the fovea of both eyes as it moves toward or away from the head.

Corrective movements are small movements of the eyes produced by motion of the head in space; they depend on the vestibular system and feedback from smooth pursuit mechanisms.

Supranuclear Control of Eye Movement

Pursuit mechanisms depend on input to the cortex about target location, direction of movement, and speed. Visual information from one hemifield is relayed to the contralateral visual cortex through subcortical pathways. Even though the pathways in humans are not completely known, visual information is believed to be relayed to the parietooccipital region for processing into the target parameters mentioned earlier. This information is then sent to the frontal eye fields for feedback on needed eye movements.

After the visual information is received and processed, the motor system acts to follow the target. Efferents from the frontal eye fields project to the pons and then to ocular motor nuclei. Efferents from visual processing areas also project to the pons, but output is relayed through the cerebellum, the medial vestibular nucleus, and then the ocular motor nuclei.

Pursuit eye movements are directed by the ipsilateral hemisphere, that is, pursuit to the left is directed by the left hemisphere. Pursuit therefore requires interaction between visual receiving areas in the occipital lobe, parietal and temporal association areas, and frontal eye fields. Commands to move are probably relayed via pontine nuclei to the ocular motor nuclei, bypassing the PPRF.

Saccadic eye movements are fast conjugate movements that cause the eyes to acquire a new target. Activation of the left frontal eye fields in area 8 of the frontal lobe, posterior on the second frontal gyrus, produces a saccade to the right. This is mediated by projections from the frontal lobe to the PPRF.

Saccadic eye movements can also be induced by novel visual stimuli at the periphery of vision. The superior colliculus directly receives input from optic nerve fibers representing the contralateral visual field; this input triggers a saccade in the direction of the novel stimulus.

Brainstem Control of Eye Movement

Pontine Gaze Centers. The PPRF is just lateral to the midline and adjacent to the sixth nerve nucleus. This region is responsible for lateral gaze. Descending input to the PPRF from the cerebral hemispheres directs gaze to the right or left. If right gaze is needed, the right PPRF is activated, and it in turn directs the ipsilateral sixth nerve (abducens) nucleus to activate the lateral rectus and abduct the right eye. Efferents from the PPRF cross to the contralateral side of the brainstem and ascend in the MLF to the midbrain where they direct the third nerve (oculomotor) nucleus to activate the medial rectus and adduct the left eye.

Lesion of the PPRF produces a lateral gaze palsy. Differentiation of a gaze palsy due to a cerebral lesion from one due to a brainstem lesion is aided by response to caloric stimulation, movement of the eyes in response to irrigation of the ear with cool water, and by associated weakness. With a frontal lobe lesion, the eyes can be forced across the midline by caloric testing or doll's eye maneuver; this finding points to a gaze preference rather than a gaze palsy. With a pontine lesion, the eyes cannot be forced across the midline, even with caloric testing, unless the lesion is incomplete. With both frontal and pontine lesions, weakness is contralateral; however, the gaze difficulty differs. With frontal lesions, the eyes look toward the side of the lesion, that is, away from the paralyzed side. With a pontine lesion, the eyes look away from the side of the lesion, that is, toward the side of the paralysis.

Lesion of the MLF produces INO. This is characterized by impaired adduction of the contralateral eye with gaze to one side. For example, with right gaze, the ipsilateral eye is abducted correctly, but the contralateral eye is not adducted. The patient perceives diplopia with lateral gaze when looking to the side opposite to the lesion because the MLF is crossed. Nystagmus of the right (abducting) eye is common: The right eye returns toward the midline in an attempt to correct the diplopia, but then the PPRF forces the eye to abduct again. Given the location of the MLF near the midline, bilateral INO is not uncommon. It presents with difficulty adducting either eye with lateral gaze. Occasionally, patients with INO are erroneously labeled as having sixth nerve palsies because of the diplopia with lateral gaze, but examination of the eye movements makes the distinction clear. The two most common causes of INO are multiple sclerosis and paramedian brainstem infarction.

Midbrain Centers. The midbrain contains the nuclei of CN III and CN IV, which form a complex network responsible for eye movement and also coordinates conjugate vertical movements, convergence, accommodation (change in lens shape for near focusing), and pupil diameter.

Input to the midbrain ascends and descends, as already discussed. Light reflex is caused by axons that project from the lateral geniculate to the Edinger-Westphal nucleus.

Vertical eye movements are mainly accomplished by activation of individual muscles innervated by CN III. Axons from the frontal lobes project to CN III nuclei to evoke vertical movement. Convergence is initiated by a neuronal group in the midline of the midbrain called the rostral interstitial nucleus of the MLF (riMLF) convergence causes activation of the medial recti, accommodation, and pupil constriction.

Pupil diameter is controlled by the combined action of constrictor and dilator muscles. Constrictor fibers are innervated by parasympathetic neurons that arise in the Edinger-Westphal nucleus and project to the eye via CN III. Dilator fibers are innervated by sympathetic neurons that arise in the hypothalamus and project through the brainstem and into the spinal cord; they descend to the level of T1, where the sympathetic fibers exit and join the cervical sympathetic chain. In the neck, the axons leave the chain and ascend into the skull with the carotid artery. Axons innervating the eyelid join CN III for its final course. Axons innervating the pupil join the nasociliary nerve, a branch of CN VI, and then extend to the pupil via the long ciliary nerve.

Eyelid elevation is controlled jointly by sympathetic and CN III axons. The sympathetic axons have the course already described, and the course of the CN III axons is described later. Damage to either CN III or the sympathetic pathway can produce ptosis. Eyelid closure is accomplished by the orbicularis oculi, which are innervated by CN VII.

Cranial Nerves Involved in Eye Movement

Oculomotor Nerve. The oculomotor nucleus lies medially in the midbrain, adjacent to the aqueduct of Sylvius at the level of the superior colliculus. The nucleus is a complex: The most anterior portion is the Edinger-Westphal nucleus, which controls pupillary constriction by the sphincter of the iris and accommodation by the ciliary muscle. The rest of the oculomotor nerve complex controls the other third nerve muscles. The nuclei for the two sides are separate except for the Edinger-Westphal nucleus and the portion of the complex controlling the superior rectus; therefore, localized nuclear lesions affecting one side affect the other as well. The axons exit the midbrain between the cerebral peduncles and then pass through the cavernous sinus and the superior orbital fissure. At the fissure, the nerve divides into superior and inferior rami; the superior ramus innervates the superior rectus and lid elevators, and the inferior ramus innervates the inferior rectus, inferior oblique, sphincter of the iris, and ciliary muscle.

Trochlear Nerve. The trochlear nucleus lies immediately caudal to the oculomotor nucleus at the level of the inferior colliculus. Axons cross the midline, then exit the midbrain on the dorsal surface near the inferior colliculus. The nerve turns around the brainstem to extend anteriorly, passing through the cavernous sinus and the superior orbital fissure. The superior oblique is the only muscle supplied by this nerve.

Abducens Nerve. The abducens nucleus is located in the caudal pons. Motor neurons give rise to axons that course rostrally and medial to the facial nerve and nucleus and then turn to exit lateral to the corticospinal tract fibers at the pontomedullary junction. The axons then ascend ventral to the pons, travel on the lateral wall of the cavernous sinus, and enter the orbit through the superior orbital fissure. Interneurons in the abducens nucleus cross the midline and ascend to the midbrain in the MLF.

Abducens palsy presents with impaired lateral rectus function and decreased eye abduction. There is no ptosis, so the diplopia is obvious, which is in contrast to third nerve palsy. Important causes of CN VI palsy are increased intracranial pressure and small vessel disease (diabetes, hypertension); some cases are idiopathic. Sixth nerve palsy may be associated with mastoiditis, middle ear infection, and nasopharyngeal carcinomas with skull infiltration. Cavernous sinus thrombosis is associated with sixth nerve palsy with exophthalmos and periorbital pain. Sixth nerve lesion may occur with herpes zoster ophthalmicus; third nerve palsy can also occur. Lesions in the region of the superior orbital fissure may affect the sixth, third, and fourth nerves. Sixth nerve lesion may occur with minor infections, especially in children. Gradenigo syndrome is from mastoid infection and is characterized by sixth, seventh, eighth, and occasionally fifth nerve lesions.

TRIGEMINAL NERVE

The trigeminal nerve exits the pons and travels anteriorly into Meckel cavity where the sensory neuron cell bodies form the trigeminal ganglion. After the nerve fibers exit the ganglion, they divide into the ophthalmic (CN V1), maxillary (CN V2), and mandibular (CN V3) divisions.

The ophthalmic division (CN V1) travels through the cavernous sinus and enters the orbit through the superior orbital fissure. In the cavernous sinus, CN V1 is in proximity to CN III, IV, and VI and also to CN V2 in the posterior aspect of the cavernous sinus. The ophthalmic division has no motor function; sensory function is to the forehead and scalp forward of the vertex, upper eyelid, upper aspect of the cornea, much of the nasal cavity, and lacrimal glands.

The maxillary division (CN V2) travels through the posterior aspect of the cavernous sinus, exits the skull via the foramen rotundum, and enters the orbit through the inferior orbital fissure. It then passes beneath the globe and exits onto the face via the infraorbital foramen. There is no motor function. The maxillary division provides sensation to the nose, upper lip, cheek, and lower half of cornea and conjunctiva. The maxillary sinus, upper teeth and gums, palate, and lower aspect of the nasal cavity are also supplied by this division.

The mandibular division (CN V3) is joined by the small motor fascicle of the trigeminal nerve and exits the skull via the foramen ovale. Motor supply is to the masseter, temporalis, pterygoids, tensor tympani, and mylohyoid muscles. Sensory innervation is to the lower lip, chin, floor of the mouth, lower jaw and gums, and anterior tongue.

FACIAL NERVE

The facial nerve is the predominant supply of innervation to muscles of the face, but the nerve also has other functions. Precise documentation of affected functions can accurately localize a lesion; this localization depends on accurate knowledge of facial nerve anatomy.

The facial motor nucleus is in the caudal pons. Efferent fibers arc dorsally around the abducens nucleus, then exit the ventral surface of the brainstem. The motor nerve is joined by fibers from the superior salivatory nucleus and nucleus of the solitary tract; it then joins CN VIII in the internal auditory canal (IAC). The facial nerve enters the facial canal at the terminus of the IAC. The nerve extends into the geniculate ganglion, which contains cell bodies of fibers in the nervus intermedius. The nerve leaves the geniculate ganglion and travels toward the middle ear, where it gives rise to the nerve to the stapedius muscle and the chorda tympani. The facial nerve then passes through the stylomastoid foramen to the face. The posterior auricular nerve separates from the facial nerve near the stylomastoid foramen. The main trunk of the facial nerve passes through the parotid and divides into several named branches.

The chorda tympani carries taste from the anterior two-thirds of the tongue to the nucleus of the solitary tract. Also, it carries the preganglionic parasympathetic fibers innervating the submandibular and sublingual glands.

The nervus intermedius carries the taste afferents and parasympathetic efferents that compose the chorda tympani, plus cutaneous afferents from the pinna, mastoid region, and external auditory canal (EAC). It also contains mucosal afferents from the nose, palate, and pharynx. These neurons have their cell bodies in the geniculate ganglion.

VESTIBULOCOCHLEAR NERVE

The eighth nerve serves sensory function from the vestibular apparatus and cochlea. The vestibular apparatus consists of three semicircular canals organized roughly orthogonally in the x, y, and z planes, and the semicircular canals detect head rotation in these planes. In addition, there are organs that sense head tilt and horizontal acceleration (utricle) and vertical acceleration (saccule). Deformation of cellular processes (kinocilia) produces activation of the cells in the vestibulocochlear nerve.

The cochlea transduces auditory input into action potentials in CN VIII. Vibration in the air creates vibration of the tympanic membrane; the vibration is then conducted mechanically to the ossicles and cochlea through the oval window, which in turn sets up vibration in the perilymph and basilar membrane. Hair cells have their bodies on the basilar membrane, and the hairs project into the tectorial membrane. The basilar membrane is organized through its length so that high frequencies are transduced near the oval window and low frequencies are transduced near the apex.

Output from the vestibular apparatus and cochlea is conducted in the eighth nerve through the IAC to the brainstem where fibers from the cochlea project to the cochlear nuclei. Efferents from the cochlear nuclei cross and ascend in the contralateral lateral lemniscus. Some project to the superior olivary complex, and others to the reticular formation bilaterally. Ascending fibers terminate in the inferior colliculi, which in turn projects to the medial geniculate. Efferents from the medial geniculate ascend to the primary auditory cortex, area 41 on the temporal lobe (discussed later). Throughout much of this pathway, the auditory projections are organized tonotopically, that is, they are spatially arranged according to frequency.

Vestibular outflow enters the brainstem and terminates in the vestibular nuclei, which are actually a complex of nuclei. Vestibular input is used by several systems including the cerebellum for error correction during movement, the spinal cord for control over antigravity muscles, and for eye movement control mechanisms.

GLOSSOPHARYNGEAL NERVE

Cranial nerve IX exits from the brainstem in the medulla and then exits the cranial vault through the jugular foramen. Subsequently it nears the carotid artery and jugular vein and terminates in the pharynx.

CN IX supplies the stylopharyngeus muscle and, in conjunction with CN X, the constrictors of the pharynx. Sources of sensory supply include the posterior pharynx, soft palate, tonsillar pillars, posterior nasopharynx, and posterior one-third of the tongue. The ninth nerve also carries taste from the posterior third of the tongue. The sensory fiber cell bodies are in the petrous ganglion in the distal aspect of the jugular foramen.

VAGUS

The dorsal motor nucleus of the vagus sits on the floor of the fourth ventricle in the brainstem. It gives rise to preganglionic parasympathetic fibers that have widespread projections from the pharynx to thoracic and abdominal organs. The nucleus ambiguus in the medullary reticular formation supplies all of the striated muscles of the pharynx and larynx innervated by the vagus.

Vagal afferents serving general visceral sensation from the pharynx, larynx, and thoracic and abdominal organs terminate in the nucleus solitarius and have their cell bodies in the nodose ganglion. Vagal afferents serving taste from the posterior pharynx also terminate in the nucleus solitarius with cell bodies in the nodose ganglion. Vagal afferents serving sensation from the ear terminate in the spinal tract of CN V and have their cell bodies in the jugular ganglion.

The vagus exits the brainstem in the lateral medulla, near the exit of the glossopharyngeal nerve. It exits the skull via the jugular foramen, after which it divides into functionally distinct divisions: The auricular ramus supplies skin of the external ear; the meningeal ramus supplies some of the dura intracranially; and the pharyngeal ramus innervates muscles of the pharynx and soft palate, the superior laryngeal nerve (which serves as a motor to the cricothyroid and sensory input to the larynx), and the vagal nerve.

The vagal nerve descends in the neck and has branches supplying the heart (cardiac rami) and recurrent laryngeal nerves. The recurrent laryngeal nerves innervate the vocal cords but take different paths through the chest; the left passes beneath the aortic arch, and the right moves past the subclavian artery. Together they innervate most of the muscles of the larynx. The right and left vagal nerves descend through the mediastinum and enter the abdomen through the esophageal opening in the diaphragm. The vagal divisions innervate the large and small intestine, stomach, pancreas, and liver.

ACCESSORY NERVE

The accessory nerve is composed of motor axons that originate in the accessory nucleus in the cervical spinal cord. The accessory nucleus is an elongated column of cells that extends from spinal levels C1 to C5. Neurons from C1 and C2 mainly innervate the sternocleidomastoid, whereas neurons from C3 and C4 mostly innervate the trapezius.

Small rootlets exit the medulla and brainstem at multiple levels and join to form the accessory nerve, which exits the skull via the jugular foramen. The most prominent function of the accessory nerve is innervation of the sternocleidomastoid and trapezius muscles. The axons from the nucleus ambiguus form separately from the main trunk of the accessory nerve to join the vagus in innervating muscles of the pharynx and larynx.

Supranuclear innervation of the muscles is somewhat uncertain, but it is believed that the motor neurons to the trapezius receive predominantly crossed upper motor neuron innervation while the neurons to the sternocleidomastoid receive bilateral upper motor neuron innervation.

HYPOGLOSSAL NERVE

The hypoglossal nucleus is on the floor of the fourth ventricle and contains the motor neurons that innervate the tongue. The nucleus is elongated, and multiple rootlets exit along a line between the pyramid and olive of the medulla. The rootlets converge to form the hypoglossal nerve, which exits the skull via the hypoglossal canal.

The hypoglossal nerve travels through the neck, passing near the internal carotid artery, to the base of the tongue where it divides into multiple branches. The hypoglossal nerve supplies innervation to the tongue and the genioglossus and geniohyoid muscles.

CHAPTER 2.5

Spinal Cord

Karl E. Misulis and Eli E. Zimmerman

Spinal Cord Organization

The spinal cord serves as a conduit for information relayed between the brainstem and peripheral nervous system. In addition to this purely conductive function, there is substantial neural processing at segmental levels of the spinal cord.

This discussion presumes basic knowledge of spinal cord anatomy and physiology. We review clinically important basic information where it applies to clinical localization and diagnosis.

There is a multiplicity of tracts ascending and descending the spinal cord, as shown in Fig. 2.5.1 and detailed in Table 2.5.1. Only the most important tracts are discussed here:

- Corticospinal tract
- Bulbospinal tracts (including rubrospinal, reticulospinal, tectospinal, and vestibulospinal tracts)
- Anterolateral tracts
- Dorsal columns
- Spinocerebellar tracts

The clinically most important aspects of tract anatomy are as follows:

- The corticospinal tract is mostly already crossed, so the descending axons project to ipsilateral motor neurons.
- The dorsal columns convey large-fiber sensations of vibration and proprioception and ascend uncrossed.
- The anterolateral tracts convey pain and temperature sensation and cross before ascending.

Note that there is processing of sensory and motor information at segmental levels; for sensory information, segmental relays often ascend or descend a few levels before joining the major ascending tracts.

CORTICOSPINAL AND BULBOSPINAL TRACTS

Motor control begins in the cerebral cortex and projects to two major targets. The corticospinal tracts (CST) project directly from the cortex to target spinal cord segments. Corticobulbar tracts terminate in the brainstem and predominately control cranial nerve function (described in Chapter 2.4). Bulbospinal tracts (BST) project from the brainstem to the spinal cord. Although a simplification, CST is responsible for control of muscle movement and BST controls muscle tone.

CST neurons originate from the cerebral cortex and descend through the cerebral peduncles and brainstem. Most of them decussate in the medulla and form the contralateral lateral CST. These neurons terminate in the spinal gray matter to innervate motor neurons and interneurons of the spinal cord segments. The uncrossed minority CST axons descend in the anterior CST. At various levels, axons leave the anterior CST; some cross in the ventral commissure to the contralateral side, and the remainder are uncrossed and project to the ipsilateral anterior horn.

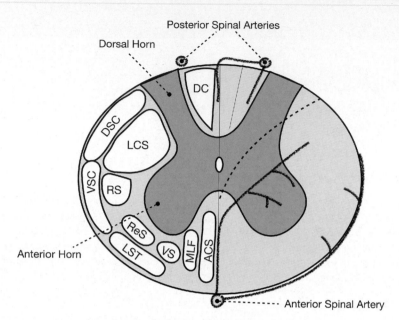

Fig. 2.5.1 Spinal cord tracts. Cross-sectional anatomy of the spinal cord shows some major tracts on the left side of the figure. The lateral corticospinal (*LCS*), anterior corticospinal (*ACS*), rubrospinal (*RS*), reticulospinal (*ReS*), medial longitudinal fasciculus (*MLF*), and vestibulospinal (*VS*) are descending tracts. The dorsal columns (*DC*), lateral spinothalamic (*LST*), dorsal spinocerebellar (*DSC*), and ventral spinocerebellar (*VSC*) are ascending tracts. The motor neurons (*MN*) are in the anterior horns. "The dashed line is the approximate biorder between anterior and posterior spinal artery distributions.

TABLE 2.5.1 ■ **Spinal Cord Tracts**

Tract	Function	Deficit
Anterolateral	Pain and temperature; poorly localized touch	Loss of pain and temperature sensation; preserved touch though different quality
Bulbospinal	Postural stability; activation of axial and appendicular muscles	Isolated lesion uncommon
Corticospinal	Initiation and maintenance of movement; especially important for fine, precise movement	Weakness; spasticity; upgoing plantar response
Dorsal columns	Vibration and proprioception; localized touch sensation	Loss of vibration and proprioceptive sensation
Spinocerebellar	Proprioception; touch; perception of body in physical space	Ataxia with fragmented appendicular movements; isolated lesion uncommon

The crossed lateral CST axons innervate principally appendicular muscles. The bilaterally projecting anterior CST axons innervate mainly axial muscles. We can envision that the lateral CST is responsible for task-directed limb movement, whereas the anterior CST is responsible for axial stabilization.

BSTs project from the brainstem bilaterally to spinal cord segments. There are three principal components of the BST; these are the reticulospinal, rubrospinal, and vestibulospinal tracts. The vestibulospinal tract is mainly involved in control of head movement with change in body position in space, so it does not project below the upper thoracic cord. The rubrospinal tract, from the red nucleus, has a role in motor function that is better understood in animals than humans. Considering the robust input to the red nucleus from the cerebellum, a role in coordination of movement is presumed. The reticulospinal tract axons project from the reticular formation to the spinal cord and are principally involved in automatic adjustments of motor power to maintain balance and posture.

ANTEROLATERAL TRACTS

Anterolateral tracts are a group of tracts that carry ascending sensory information rostrally. They include the spinothalamic tract, spinoreticular tract, and spinomesencephalic tract. They are involved predominantly in pain and temperature sensation and in poorly localized nonnociceptive information.

Spinothalamic tracts are divided into two subdivisions: the anterior and lateral divisions. The anterior division carries poorly localized touch information, and the lateral division carries mainly pain and temperature sensation. Second-order neurons cross the spinal cord at the anterior commissure and ascend in the adjacent anterior and lateral divisions of the tract.

The spinoreticular tract ascends adjacent to the adjacent lateral spinothalamic tract. Exact function of this tract is not known, but the fields of these neurons are much greater than those in the other spinothalamic tracts.

The spinomesencephalic tract is predominantly composed of the spinotectal tract, which may have a role in modulation of pain perception.

DORSAL COLUMNS

The dorsal columns form the dorsal funiculus. They are composed of central axons of primary afferent neurons with cell bodies in the dorsal root ganglia, with a small contribution of ascending neurons with cell bodies in the dorsal horn. These neurons carry tactile sensation, including the large-fiber sensations of vibration and proprioception in addition to touch. The dorsal columns are topographically organized with the legs being represented medially and the arms proximally in upper cord regions.

The dorsal columns terminate in the dorsal column nuclei. Axons from the leg terminate in the nucleus gracilis. Axons from the arm terminate in the nucleus cuneatus where they synapse on neurons whose axons cross and form the medial lemniscus, which projects to the thalamus.

Damage to the dorsal columns results in sensory deficits depending on the site of the lesion. Damage before crossing results in loss of vibration and proprioception below the lesion, ipsilateral to the pathology. Damage above the crossing results in loss contralateral to the lesion. Some causes of dorsal column damage include demyelinating disease, including multiple sclerosis and neuromyelitis optica, transverse myelitis, intraspinal tumors, and spinal trauma.

SPINOCEREBELLAR TRACTS

The spinocerebellar tracts are involved in control of movement of the body in physical space and movement of body parts in relation to each other. Spinal afferents carrying proprioceptive and touch information enter and synapse within the dorsal horn. The second-order neurons ascend in the spinocerebellar tracts, which are located in the most lateral aspect of the spinal cord. The ascending fibers from the dorsal spinocerebellar tract enter the brainstem and then enter the cerebellum via the inferior cerebellar peduncle. The axons of the ventral spinocerebellar tract ascend higher in the brainstem and then turn to descend into the cerebellum via the superior cerebellar peduncle.

Vascular Anatomy of the Spinal Cord

The arterial supply to the spinal cord is from multiple levels, beginning with branches of the vertebral arteries that descend and then fuse to form the anterior spinal artery, which runs along the anterior or ventral side of the cord. This artery receives additional vascular supply from segmental vessels. A major vessel is the artery of Adamkiewicz, which arises from the aorta and usually enters between T9 and L2 and supplies the anterior spinal artery.

The anterior spinal artery supplies the anterior two-thirds of the spinal cord, including most of the gray matter, descending tracts, both lateral and anterior spinothalamic tracts, and the spinocerebellar tracts. The posterior spinal arteries lie on the posterior or dorsal surface of the spinal cord but are not as continuous as the anterior cerebral artery. Looking at the dorsal surface of the cord, the posterior spinal arteries appear to be major components of a network of vessels with interconnections. These vessels supply the dorsal columns and part of the dorsal horns.

Spinal cord infarction often involves the anterior spinal artery or artery of Adamkiewicz. Given the structural network of the posterior spinal arteries, isolated infarction of one of these arteries is uncommon.

Anterior spinal artery infarction damages the anterior cord, sparing the dorsal columns. As with strokes anywhere, lesions are often incomplete because of some residual blood flow and because of collateral arterial supply near boundary zones of vascular supply.

Artery of Adamkiewicz infarction impacts arterial supply to the anterior spinal artery of the lower thoracic and lumbosacral cord. In most people, this artery arises from the aorta; in some people, it arises from a lumbar artery.

Damage to the artery of Adamkiewicz or directly to the anterior spinal artery produces weakness below the level of the lesion with relative preservation of sensation in most circumstances. Aortic surgery can result in this type of infarction.

Essentials of Localization

A lesion of the spinal cord is suspected in the presence of one or more of the following:
- Bilateral leg motor and/or sensory loss without arm involvement; differential diagnosis includes a parasagittal cerebral lesion
- Crossed motor and sensory finding, that is, upper motor neuron signs on one side and pain and temperature loss on the other side
- Dissociated sensory loss, that is, loss of one modality (e.g., pain) and preservation of another (e.g., vibration sense).
- Sensory level on the trunk, that is, a level on the torso below which there is sensory loss.
- Back pain and neurologic deficit below the level of the pain
- New onset of back pain in a patient with a known malignancy on opposite sides of the body

Details of diagnosis and differential diagnosis are in Chapter 3.5, but the key is to recall the findings that suggest spinal cord pathology and to have good mastery of spinal cord anatomy. With this knowledge, localization is easier.

Diagnosis of a cord lesion at a specific level is facilitated by identifying:
- Weakness in muscles innervated distal to a certain level. This weakness may be incomplete because spinal cord lesions are often incomplete. Spasticity should be present below the level of the lesion unless the lesion is very recent.
- Sensory deficit below a certain level. Note that this is an imperfect indicator because sensory level may be somewhat below the level of the pathology. Also, sensory levels are notoriously difficult to localize precisely and consistently on examination.
- Bowel and bladder control issues. These are much more likely with spinal cord lesions than brain lesions.
- Back pain at a certain level.

Peripheral Nerves, Neuromuscular Junction, and Muscle

Karl E. Misulis and Eli E. Zimmerman

Anatomy of the Peripheral Neuromuscular System

The essential features of the peripheral neuromuscular system are motor nerves, sensory nerves, autonomic nerves, the neuromuscular junction (NMJ), and muscle fibers.

Motor neurons originate in the spinal cord and brainstem and innervate skeletal muscle (Fig. 2.6.1). Each motor neuron innervates many muscle fibers, but each muscle fiber is innervated by only one motor neuron. The innervation ratio is the number of muscle fibers innervated by a single motor neuron for a particular muscle; the innervation ratio is lowest for extraocular muscles and greatest for large antigravity muscles. The inset of Fig. 2.6.1 shows a diagrammatic representation of a motor nerve innervating a muscle fiber. With denervation, there is loss of motor axons, so surviving axons sprout processes to innervate the denervated muscle fibers; this process increases the innervation ratio.

Sensory neurons have cell bodies in the dorsal root ganglia or sensory ganglia of the cranial nerves. Most sensory neurons are bipolar, with peripheral projections transducing sensory input into action potentials and central projections conducting action potentials to the spinal cord and brainstem. Fig. 2.6.1 shows sensory nerve endings and their projections through afferent nerve fibers.

Peripheral nerves are surrounded by processes of Schwann cells, which form myelin sheaths around the nerves.

The NMJ transduces action potentials of the motor nerves into muscle fiber action potentials. Acetylcholine (ACh) is released by the presynaptic terminal when it is depolarized. The ACh crosses the synaptic cleft and binds to ACh receptors (AChR); this binding causes channels to open and allows ionic flux in and out of the cell. The preponderance of ionic flux is sodium into the cell, which depolarizes the muscle fiber membrane to the point that it reaches threshold; a muscle fiber action potential is then produced.

The muscle fiber membrane conducts action potentials to the T-tubule system, which triggers release of calcium (Ca^+) from the sarcoplasmic reticulum. Calcium binds to troponin, producing a conformational change in the actin and allowing interaction with myosin, thereby producing muscle shortening.

Normally, each motor neuron action potential produces one action potential in each of its muscle fibers. Many disorders interfere with this one-to-one transmission; these include disorders of the NMJ and of peripheral nerve and muscle. Most disorders cause failure of muscle fiber potential generation, although a few (e.g., myotonia) cause repetitive discharge of muscle fibers innervated by a single axon.

The subsequent discussion in this chapter concerns organization of this peripheral system. Detailed discussion of diagnosis and disorders is presented in Chapter 3.6. In preparation for that discussion, we present the essentials of clinically relevant anatomy. As with the remainder of this book, this discussion assumes basic knowledge of neuroanatomy and neurophysiology.

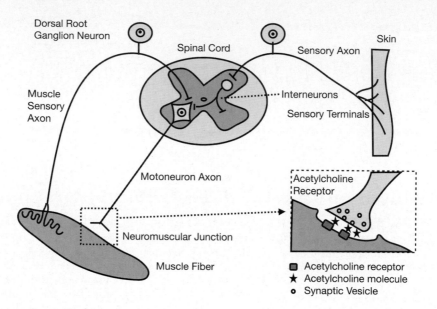

Fig. 2.6.1 Motor and sensory neurons. Diagram representing some of the principal motor and sensory connections to the spinal cord.

Brachial Plexus

The brachial plexus is formed from cervical nerve roots from C4 to T2, although the contributions from C4 and T2 are minor. The output from the brachial plexus is the major nerves radial, median, ulnar, and musculocutaneous and a host of smaller nerves, the most important of which are dorsal scapular, suprascapular, upper and lower subscapular, and lateral pectoral nerves.

We recommend committing to memory the anatomy of the brachial plexus and their formation of the major nerves.

Fig. 2.6.2 shows the anatomy of the brachial plexus. Table 2.6.1 shows the contribution of different portions of the root and plexus system to peripheral nerves. Clinical and diagnostic details of some of the important pathological entities are described in Chapter 5.5.

Some of the important anatomical details to remember include the following:
- Upper plexus lesions produce mainly deltoid and biceps weakness due to damage to C5 and C6 nerve roots.
- Lower plexus lesions produce mainly C8 and T1 distribution motor and sensory deficits with prominent weakness of intrinsic muscles of the hand.

Disorders of the brachial plexus and the lumbosacral plexus are discussed in Chapter 5.5.

lumbar and Sacral Plexus

The lumbar and sacral plexuses are often referred to as a single entity, the lumbosacral plexus, because they are considered together. The lumbar plexus is formed from nerve roots T12 to L5. The sacral plexus is formed from roots L4 to S5, although most of the portions of the examination that can be performed do not concern roots below S1.

Fig. 2.6.3 shows the lumbosacral plexus anatomy from nerve roots to formation of the proximal nerves.

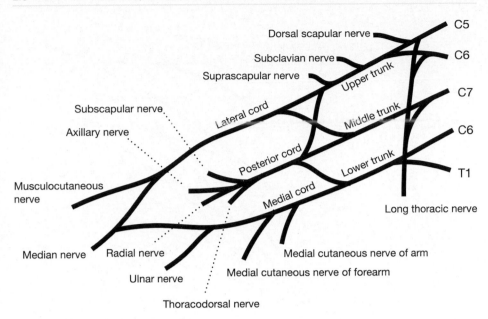

Fig. 2.6.2   Brachial plexus. Diagram of the connections of the brachial plexus. The trunks, cords, and nerves are not in precise in situ placement to illustrate connections.

TABLE 2.6.1 ■ **Brachial Plexus Innervation**

Nerve	Plexus	Motor Deficit	Sensory Deficit
Median	LC, MC; C5–T1	Finger flexors,	Lateral palmar hand
Ulnar	LT, MC; C8–T1	Intrinsic hand muscles, grip	Medial palmar hand
Radial	LT, MT, PC; C5–T1	Wrist and finger extension	Posterior-lateral forearm
Musculocutaneous	UT, LC, C5–6	Elbow flexion	Lateral forearm
Axillary	UT, PC, C5–6	Arm abduction	Lateral shoulder

UT, upper trunk; *MT*, middle trunk; *LT*, lower trunk; *LC*, lateral cord; *PC*, posterior cord; *MC*, medial cord.

Table 2.6.2 shows the contribution of different portions of the lumbosacral plexus to peripheral nerves of diagnostic value.

Some important details regarding the lumbosacral plexus include the following:

- Most patients with lumbosacral plexus lesions present with posterior pain and motor and sensory symptoms that span distribution of a single nerve.
- Plexus lesion is suspected rather than nerve root lesion when more than one nerve root distribution is seen.

Peripheral Nerves

There are innumerable peripheral nerves, but only a limited number are important in routine clinical practice.

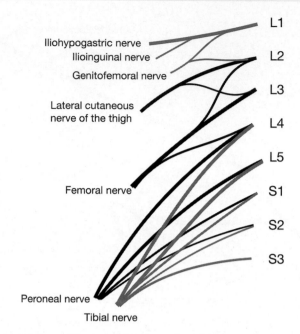

Fig. 2.6.3 **Lumbosacral plexus.** Diagram of the connections of the lumbosacral plexus. Note that the elements of the plexus are not in the precise anatomic position they would be in situ to highlight connections.

TABLE 2.6.2 ■ **Lumbosacral Plexus Innervation**

Nerve	Plexus	Motor Deficit	Sensory Deficit
Peroneal	SP; L5–S1	Foot drop	Mid and lower calf and top of foot
Tibial	SP; S1–2	Foot extension	Lateral heel if sural unaffected
Femoral	LP; L2–4	Knee extension	Anterior thigh, medial calf
Sciatic	LP, SP; L4–S3	Peroneal and tibial deficits	Peroneal and tibial deficits
Obturator	LP; L2-4	Lweg adduction	Medial thigh

LP, lumbar plexus; *SP*, sacral plexus.

Median nerve is formed from roots C5 to T1 and takes supply from the medial and lateral cords. It does not supply any muscles in the upper arm, but it supplies many of the finger and hand flexors in the forearm. The abductor pollicis brevis is a key muscle innervated in the hand. The most common median neuropathy is carpal tunnel syndrome with compression at the wrist.

Ulnar nerve is formed mainly from roots C8 and T1, which travel in the medial cord of the brachial plexus, across the medial aspect of the elbow, and into the arm. In the arm, it supplies many of the flexors of the wrist and hand and intrinsic muscles of the hand that are not supplied by the median nerve. The first dorsal interosseus (FDI) is a muscle of interest because it is easily testable clinically and on electromyography. The ulnar nerve is most sensitive to compression as it passes the medial epicondyle of the humerus.

Radial nerve is formed broadly from roots C5 to T1. The nerve continues from the posterior cord of the brachial plexus after take-off of the axillary nerve, which supplies the deltoid. The radial nerve innervates the triceps in the upper arm. In the arm, the radial nerve innervates mainly the wrist and finger extensors. The radial nerve is most likely to be damaged at the spiral groove in the distal forearm, classically described as "Saturday night palsy."

Sciatic nerve is formed from lumbosacral nerve roots L4 through S3 and exits the pelvis through the sciatic notch. It descends in the posterior thigh to the popliteal fossa at the knee where it divides into the tibial and peroneal (fibular) nerves which have different functions. In the thigh, the peroneal division innervates the short head of the biceps femoris, whereas the tibial division innervates the long head of the biceps femoris. The sciatic nerve is most likely to be damaged as it leaves the pelvis from direct injury through acute trauma, leg positioning during procedure, or needle-stick.

Tibial nerve arises from the sciatic nerve and prominently innervates the gastrocnemius and soleus muscles. Sciatic nerve injury results in dysfunction of tibial-innervated muscles, but the tibial nerve is uncommonly injured in isolation. Tarsal tunnel syndrome is damage to the tibial nerve distally as it enters the foot. In that case, only muscles of the foot are affected, although sensory symptoms are more common with this.

Peroneal (fibular) nerve is also formed from the sciatic nerve and is more commonly damaged than the tibial nerve, being the most common mononeuropathy of the leg. The peroneal nerve innervates predominantly the anterior muscles of the lower leg, including tibialis anterior among others. Damage results in foot drop.

Femoral nerve is formed from L2 through L4. After passing through the pelvis, it passes into the thigh under the inguinal ligament. This is the principal innervation of the anterior thigh which extend the leg. Damage is most common in the abdomen from hematoma formation, compression from mass lesions, pregnancy, or positioning during procedures. Most typical findings are weakness of knee extension and reduced knee reflexes.

Anatomy of the Neuromuscular Junction

STRUCTURE AND FUNCTION OF THE NEUROMUSCULAR JUNCTION

Motor neurons enter the muscle and synapse on the muscle fiber membrane at the NMJ. Depolarization of the terminal results in opening of calcium channels. Influx of calcium facilitates release of ACh. These channels are the voltage-gated calcium channels (VGCC). ACh binds to receptors on the postsynaptic muscle membrane, which produces electrical activation of muscle fibers and muscle contraction.

COMMON LESIONS OF THE NEUROMUSCULAR JUNCTION

Defects in the NMJ are multiple, and all cause weakness. In myasthenia gravis (MG), autoantibodies are made against the receptor or against a muscle-specific kinase (MuSK), which is a tyrosine kinase and is one of a number of proteins responsible for maintenance of the AChR. Because of the type of defect, strength is usually relatively preserved on first effort but sustained effort fails.

Myasthenic syndrome is due to impaired release of transmitter from the motor neuron terminal. Hence, the defect is presynaptic rather than postsynaptic as with MG. Repetitive activation results in enhanced influx of calcium and thereby enhanced release of transmitter. The clinical picture is facilitation of muscle action with repetitive effort rather than fatigue.

Many so-called nerve agents are blockers of acetylcholinesterase, thereby resulting in the absence of metabolism and enhanced action of ACh, essentially overstimulation. Neuromuscular effects include weakness and fasciculations, which when combined with excessive salivation are the usual clues to organophosphate cholinesterase inhibitor poisoning. In addition, there are central effects including seizures and coma.

Lesions affecting the NMJ are discussed in more depth in Chapter 3.7, and details of specific disorders are discussed in Chapter 5.5.

Anatomy of Muscle

STRUCTURE AND FUNCTION OF SKELETAL MUSCLE

NMJ activation of the postjunctional membrane causes depolarization of the muscle fiber membrane that is conducted through the fiber. This depolarization results in release of calcium from stores in the sarcoplasmic reticulum that then, in conjunction with adenosine triphosphate (ATP), facilitates actin and myosin binding and thereby shortening of the muscle. Eventually, the calcium is taken back up into the sarcoplasmic reticulum resulting in cessation of contraction and relaxation of the muscle.

COMMON LESIONS OF MUSCLE

Disorders of muscle include a wide range of myopathies. These involve muscle degeneration, which can be the final result of a host of different metabolic disorder. Weakness occurs because there is defective shortening of the actin-myosin complexes. Damage to the membranes results in release of muscle enzymes in most disorders; creatine kinase and aldolase are commonly measured as markers of this degeneration.

Muscular dystrophies are typically genetic and are caused by defective build and maintenance of the muscles. Age of onset varies substantially as does distribution and progression of the disorder. These details help with the differential diagnosis.

Inflammatory myopathies are usually autoimmune. They are sometimes associated with other autoimmune disorders or as a paraneoplastic condition in association with cancers.

Periodic paralyses are a family of disorders that present with episodic weakness. Details of the pathophysiology, clinical presentation, management, and course vary widely between types.

Localization by Anatomy

Cerebrum

Howard S. Kirshner and Eli E. Zimmerman

The uniqueness of the human brain derives from the higher mental functions, such as reasoning, memory, language, speech, calculations, praxis, recognition of objects (gnosis), and the asymmetrical organization of these functions in the cerebral hemispheres. Cerebral dominance, or the specialization of one cerebral hemisphere in specific functions, relates to the unique cytoarchitectural organization of the brain.

The cerebral cortex is a large, complex, convoluted structure and is the site of higher mental functions. The cortex makes up an area of about 2.5 ft^2 and contains as many as 20 billion neurons, arranged in a wrinkled assembly of gyri that allows a vast surface area of cortex to be enfolded into the small space within the human skull. The information stored in the cerebral cortex rivals that of major libraries and computer systems. As many as 70% of neurons in the human central nervous system reside in the association cortex, the site of higher functions. The cortex is composed of vertical modules, usually containing six layers. The precise anatomy varies with the function of the area. For example, the motor cortex contains large pyramidal cells, whereas sensory cortex lacks pyramidal cells but has many more granular cells. The visual cortex has a visible white matter bundle called the line of Gennari, visible to the naked eye. Areas of the cortex were numbered by Brodmann, a system still in wide use today.

The motor cortex principally involves the precentral gyrus, the supplementary motor area in the medial frontal lobe, and the prefrontal cortex. The prefrontal area is involved in the planning and initiation of movement.

Sensory cortices include the postcentral gyrus for somatosensory function, the auditory cortex (Heschl gyrus) in the superior temporal lobes, the visual cortex in the occipital lobes, and olfactory (basal frontal) and probably gustatory cortices.

Beyond this basic anatomy, the brain is divided into four primary lobes: frontal, parietal, temporal, and occipital. Each lobe has a relatively constant cortical anatomy and is divided by sulci or fissures into discrete gyri.

Functional Localization

Clinical data obtained from imaging studies such as magnetic resonance imaging (MRI), positron emission tomography (PET), and from patients undergoing surgical ablation of brain structures for epilepsy or brain tumor have helped reveal the functional anatomy of the brain in terms of the four major lobes and their cortical gyri. Within these gyri are modules dedicated to specific functions. The modules are organized not as individual centers but as parts of interconnecting networks in disparate regions of the brain. The cortical modules also connect with subcortical centers, such as the basal ganglia and other deep brain structures.

In general, the cerebral cortex is divided into primary motor areas, primary sensory areas (for vision, hearing, touch, smell, and possibly taste), and association areas. The association cortex is divided into unimodal association cortices, such as the visual and auditory association cortices, and heteromodal association cortices. The heteromodal cortical areas include the parietal cortex, a sensory association area for interaction among the senses, and the frontal cortex, which supports the executive function for the entire brain. Executive function refers to the processes that determine which of the many incoming sensory stimuli should receive attention and in what priority and what responses should be activated and in which order. These heteromodal association cortices represent the areas of largest expansion of the brain from apes to humans, and they are critically important in enabling the extraordinary cognitive and behavioral capabilities that human beings have attained.

FRONTAL LOBE

The posterior portion of the frontal lobe, on the lateral convexity of the brain, is the precentral gyrus, which contains motor cells of the primary motor cortex (Brodmann area 4). This cortical strip carries a map of the contralateral side of the body (homunculus), with cells programmed to produce contractions of specific muscles or specific movements. The motor homunculus has its face and lips in the most inferior part of the gyrus, just above the sylvian fissure; the hand and arm lie above that, and the foot and leg extend over the superior part of the gyrus and continue downward on the medial aspect of the hemisphere. Stimulation of cells in the motor cortex produces specific muscle contractions in contralateral parts of the body. The relatively large size of the cortical representation of the thumb, fingers, and hand, compared to the arm, indicates the importance of fine finger movements. Similarly, the large space reserved for the mouth and lips reflects the importance of speech.

Anterior to the primary motor cortex is the premotor cortex, which is involved in the initiation and planning of skilled motor acts. Anterior to the face area of the motor strip is the cortical Broca area (area 44), thought to program patterned movements of the vocal apparatus to produce phonemes and words. Damage to this area results in Broca aphasia, a syndrome of nonfluent speech and partially preserved comprehension (see Chapter 5.2). Area 8, in the superior frontal lobe, controls the movement of the head and eyes to the contralateral side. Damage to this region produces a "gaze preference" in which the eyes tend to look to the ipsilateral side. On the other hand, seizure activity emanating from this cortical region produces rhythmic turning of the head and eyes to the contralateral side. The supplementary motor cortex, on the medial side of the hemisphere anterior to the motor leg area, produces complex postures or patterned movements. Lesions in this area also disrupt the initiation of speech. Another function of the dorsolateral frontal lobe, the frontal heteromodal association cortex of the brain, is related to executive functions. The dorsolateral frontal lobe is also important for working memory, also termed immediate memory or attention span.

Functions of the prefrontal cortex anterior to the premotor area and the orbitofrontal cortex are complex and incompletely understood. Lesions of the frontal cortex may produce disinhibition of speech and other behaviors, known as the frontal lobe syndrome. Patients with lesions of the orbitofrontal cortex may have normal intelligence and memory, but families may state that the individuals have totally changed personality; examples of such personality changes are short temper, irritability, poor impulse control, antisocial personality, and a general tendency to act out.

The lateral frontal convexities also are involved in the initiation of behavior. Bilateral lesions of this area result in a reduction or cessation of behavior, often referred to as akinetic mutism or abulia. Patients may sit and stare passively, not speaking, or may respond only in a whisper or after a delay. This type of frontal lobe syndrome is referred to as "Pseudodepression". In general, frontal lobe syndromes resemble psychiatric disorders because they involve profound alterations of behavior and personality, but basic cognitive functions such as memory, language, and visuospatial functioning, as well as elementary motor and sensory functions, remain intact.

On the medial surface of the frontal lobe lies the cingulum or cingulate gyrus. This gyrus is a part of the limbic system, or Papez circuit, of projections from the hippocampus via the septum and fornix to the mamillary bodies and then to the anterior thalamic nuclei. Projections then emanate from the thalamus to the cingulate gyrus and then back to the hippocampus. This circuit is important for memory and for elementary limbic functions, such as motivation and drive. The cingulate gyrus is also important for the experience of pain.

PARIETAL LOBE

The parietal lobe consists of a superior and inferior parietal lobule. The anterior part of the parietal lobe contains areas 3, 1, and 2 devoted to sensory function. In the inferior parietal lobule are areas 39 and 40, the angular and supramarginal gyri. The inferior parietal lobule in the left hemisphere is tied to language function, especially reading and naming; to calculations and arithmetic; and to distinguishing left from right. This region is the second part of the heteromodal association cortex, along with the dorsolateral frontal lobe. The parietal association cortex may be thought of as a center for the association of information from different sensory modalities, such as vision, hearing, and touch.

Gerstmann associated four deficits with lesions of the left inferior parietal lobule: agraphia, acalculia, right–left confusion, and finger agnosia (loss of the ability to know which finger is which). The inferior parietal lobule in the right hemisphere is involved with the body schema. Right inferior parietal lobe lesions produce neglect of the left side of the body. The superior parts of the parietal cortex are devoted to visuospatial and constructional functions and higher level cortical sensory functions, such as stereognosis (recognition of palpated shapes) and graphesthesia (ability to recognize letters or numbers drawn on the skin).

Lesions of the right parietal lobe produce important neurobehavioral deficits, including neglect of the left side of the body, denial of deficit (anosognosia), and dressing apraxia (inability to don garments correctly in relation to the body). Other spatial and topographical dysfunctions associated with right parietal lobe lesions are difficulty finding one's way around and an inability to draw or read a map. The retrosplenial part of the occipital lobe, behind the splenium of the corpus callosum, is also related to topographical reasoning. Constructional tasks, such as copying figures, drawing a clock or house, and bisecting a line, may reveal difficulty with spatial relationships or neglect of the left side of space.

Although speech and language are relatively well-preserved in patients with right parietal lesions, the emotional intonation of speech may be lacking, as may the ability to comprehend emotional tone in the speech of others. Patients with strokes or other pathology in the right parietal region may fail to grasp sarcasm or humor. They also may fail to respect the proper turn-taking of a normal conversation, or they may respond to questions asked of the patient in the next bed.

The right hemisphere, although it is less involved with language, does affect the pragmatics of communication as opposed to semantics (meanings) or syntax (grammar). Such deficits may result in the patient understanding what is said, but not how it is said; in other words, the patient understands the literal meaning of the words but not the emotional, humorous, ironic, or sarcastic context. Such "paralinguistic" deficits are disabling to patients in the social world and affect communication, even when speech and language functions are preserved.

Emotional indifference often characterizes the mood of these patients; they may be undisturbed by left-sided paralysis or by the impending loss of ability to work. These right hemisphere deficits, expressed over time, change the personality of affected individuals. Families often have more difficulty accepting a change in personality after a stroke or brain injury than they do in accepting handicaps such as the inability to speak or understand language that are seen after left hemisphere injuries.

TEMPORAL LOBE

The superior temporal gyrus of each hemisphere contains the primary auditory cortex (areas 41 and 42), which lies buried within the sylvian fissure. Lesions of the primary auditory cortex on both sides cause cortical deafness. Such patients are rarely totally deaf and often hear some pure tones. In some patients, bilateral superior temporal damage results in pure word deafness (inability to understand spoken words, with preserved pure tone hearing and recognition of nonverbal sounds). Another bitemporal syndrome is auditory agnosia or the inability to recognize nonverbal sounds. Finally, phonagnosia refers to the inability to recognize familiar voices.

The left superior temporal gyrus contains the Wernicke area, which is critical to the comprehension of spoken language. There may be a language comprehension area in the inferior temporal gyrus and adjacent fusiform gyrus, as identified by electrical stimulation (the basal temporal language area [BTLA]). It is interesting that surgical ablation of this area usually does not cause lasting aphasia. Therefore, the BTLA may be part of a network involved in understanding language but may not be a necessary component to the functioning of the language comprehension system. Recent information from primary progressive aphasia or other neurodegenerative disorders affecting language (see Chapter 5.2), suggests that the anterior temporal lobe is also involved in comprehension.

The right temporal lobe is a silent or "noneloquent" area of the brain because surgical resection of this area produces only subtle deficits. Acute lesions of the right temporal lobe, however, can produce acute confusion and delusional thinking, or delirium.

Appreciation of rhythm and musical qualities may be affected by right temporal lesions, along with deficits in nonverbal memory. In general, the medial temporal areas, such as the hippocampus, together with their connections to the thalamus, septal area, and cingulate gyri of the medial frontal lobes are most clearly related to memory.

Bilateral lesions produce lasting loss of new learning and recent memory. Unilateral left medial temporal lesions produce disorders of verbal memory, whereas unilateral right temporal lesions produce nonverbal memory loss.

OCCIPITAL LOBE

The most posterior, medial poles of the occipital lobes are the primary visual cortices (area 17). Damage to this cortex on one side produces a contralateral hemianopic visual field defect in both eyes. Damage to both sides may produce cortical blindness. Some patients with cortical blindness are unaware of their blindness and confabulate descriptions of objects and scenes they claim to see (Anton syndrome).

In recent years, emphasis has been placed on dorsal versus ventral visual pathways. The dorsal pathway, through the parietal lobe, is involved with spatial aspects of visual perception, such as seeing where something is. The ventral visual pathway, through the temporal lobe, is involved in identifying what one sees. Areas adjacent to the primary visual area (areas 18 and 19) are called the visual association cortex and are thought to contribute to complex visual analysis. Lesions of these areas on both sides produce a complex visual syndrome called visual agnosia, to be discussed later in this chapter.

Cerebral Dominance and Functional Specialization

Since Broca's publication in 1861, we have known that in most humans the left hemisphere is dominant for language. Virtually 99% of right-handed people and most left-handed people have left hemisphere dominance for language. Handedness is correlated with cerebral dominance, so left-handed individuals are more likely than right-handed people to have right hemisphere language dominance. However, most left-handers still become aphasic if the left hemisphere is damaged, and only a few become aphasic if the right hemisphere is damaged, a phenomenon called "crossed aphasia." Some left-handed individuals appear to have mixed

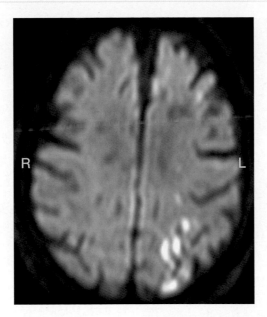

Fig. 3.1.1 **Magnetic resonance imaging (MRI) showing multifocal watershed infarction.** MRI with diffusion weighted imaging, showing multiple small areas of acute infarction in the "watershed" area of the left parietal lobe. Clinical details in the text.

dominance, such as having speech expression in the left hemisphere and comprehension in the right hemisphere.

The right hemisphere serves many nonlanguage functions. As discussed with reference to the parietal lobes, right hemisphere functions include visuospatial and constructional tasks, knowledge of maps and topography, dressing, emotional feeling and processing, production of emotional intonation of speech, and music appreciation. Reading and writing music, on the other hand, appear to be left hemisphere functions.

Cerebral dominance may have structural correlates including a longer planum temporale in the left hemisphere than in the right. Similar asymmetries have been described in newborn infants, suggesting that these anatomic asymmetries are genetically programmed, not acquired through use. Cerebral asymmetries also have been reaffirmed using computed tomography (CT) and MRI studies. The relationship of such asymmetries to language dominance holds true in groups, but it is not sufficiently definite to be predictive of dominance in individual patients.

Speech and language functions are discussed in Chapter 5.2 and will not be considered further here. Apraxia, agnosia, and dementing illnesses will be discussed in Chapter 5.1.

Fig. 3.1.1 shows a brain MRI with diffusion weighted imaging, with multiple small areas of acute infarction in the "watershed" area of the left parietal lobe. The patient presented with acute confusion, difficulty with naming, calculations, and reading, which are elements of the Gerstmann syndrome. This was secondary to severe stenosis of the left internal carotid artery, and the syndrome improved after carotid endarterectomy.

Fig. 3.1.2 shows a brain MRI with diffusion weighted imaging; left, showing acute infarction R temporal-parietal lobe and FLAIR MRI; right and below, showing old infarctions in the right medial frontal lobe and L frontal lobe. This 82-year-old man had a stroke in the right anterior

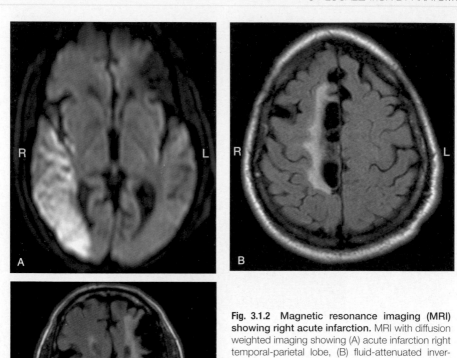

Fig. 3.1.2 Magnetic resonance imaging (MRI) showing right acute infarction. MRI with diffusion weighted imaging showing (A) acute infarction right temporal-parietal lobe, (B) fluid-attenuated inversion recovery (FLAIR) MRI showing prior stroke, and (C) MRI FLAIR image showing old infarctions in the right medial frontal lobe and left frontal lobe. Clinical details in the text.

cerebral artery (ACA) territory in 1999, secondary to atrial fibrillation, leaving him with a residual left leg weakness. In 2010, he presented with confusion and impaired memory. An MRI disclosed the old right anterior cerebral artery (ACA) territory infarction but also an "old" left frontal infarction and an acute infarction in the right temporal-parietal region. This is a classic case of vascular cognitive impairment, of the type sometimes referred to as "multiinfarct dementia."

Basal Ganglia and Thalamus

Karl E. Misulis, Eli E. Zimmerman, and Martin A. Samuels

Basal Ganglia

Lesions of the basal ganglia typically produce movement disorders, with the predominant results being abnormalities of tone and involuntary movement. For clinical purposes, the important classification is into the following two categories:

- Akinetic rigid syndromes (too little movement)
- Involuntary spontaneous movements (too much movement)

AKINETIC RIGID SYNDROMES

"Akinetic" refers to the lack of movement, and "rigid" refers to muscle stiffness. Important entities in this category are Parkinson disease (PD), which is responsible for about 80% of this category, drug-induced parkinsonism, progressive supranuclear palsy, and multiple system atrophy–parkinsonian type (MSA-P), along with some lesser-known entities (Table 3.2.1). The differential diagnosis includes paratonia, which is increased muscle tone due to cerebral cortical damage, particularly in the frontal region.

Akinetic-rigid syndromes have a pattern of movement where spontaneous movements are slow, and passive movements are impaired by increased tone. Corticospinal tract signs are not present, such as hyperreflexia and extensor plantar responses.

INVOLUNTARY SPONTANEOUS MOVEMENTS

Involuntary spontaneous movements include essential tremor, Parkinson tremor, dystonia, dyskinesias, chorea, athetosis, and ballism. Important involuntary movements are presented in Table 3.2.2.

The pattern of movements varies widely, but by far the most common is tremor. Of the tremors, action and postural tremor are typical of essential tremor, whereas rest tremor is typical of PD. Despite these generalizations, sometimes additional study is needed to differentiate between them.

It is impossible to classify each disease purely into one category. For example, PD is mainly an akinetic-rigid syndrome, but tremor is an important feature. Huntington disease presents with chorea in adults, but it may present with rigidity with juvenile onset. These disorders are discussed in more detail in Chapter 5.7.

Dystonia is an abnormality of tone not due to spasticity, which typically produces abnormal positions and postures. Possible causes of dystonia are many, but the most important can be broken down into the following classes:

- Structural
- Degenerative
- Metabolic
- Drug-induced
- Idiopathic

TABLE 3.2.1 ■ **Akinetic-Rigid Syndromes**

Disorder	Features
Parkinson disease (PD)	Bradykinesia; rigidity; resting tremor; postural instability
Vascular parkinsonism	Increased tone; less tremor; often corticospinal tract signs
Drug-induced parkinsonism	Increased tone often with orofacial dyskinesias
Dementia with Lewy bodies (DLB)	Parkinsonism and dementia developing within a year of each other; often prominent hallucinations
Multiple system atrophy (MSA)	Multiple System Atrophy–Parkinsonian type: Parkinsonism and autonomic dysfunction; lean to one side (Pisa syndrome); bulbar deficits Multiple System Atrophy–Cerebellar type: Parkinsonism with cerebellar dysfunction especially gait; autonomic dysfunction
Progressive supranuclear palsy (PSP)	Stooped posture with propensity to falls; ophthalmoparesis with reduced upgaze, resulting in head extension

TABLE 3.2.2 ■ **Involuntary Spontaneous Movements**

Movement	Clinical Features	Etiologies
Essential tremor	Arm tremor evoked by action and posture	Idiopathic; genetic
Chorea	Rapid and irregular movements of especially arms and trunk	Hereditary (Huntington); neurodegenerative; basal ganglia stroke; pregnancy induced
Athetosis	Slow, writing movements	Stroke; dopaminergic medications; cerebral palsy
Ballism	High-amplitude rapid movements of the extremities, usually unilateral	Infarction of the subthalamic nucleus or other region of the basal ganglia

Structural causes include infarction, hemorrhage, tumor, abscess, vascular malformation, postsurgical complications, and trauma. Degenerative causes include Huntington disease, PD, progressive supranuclear palsy (PSP), multiple system atrophy (MSA), and olivopontocerebellar atrophy (OPCA). Dopa-responsive dystonia probably falls into this category.

Metabolic causes include Wilson disease, some amino acid defects, metachromatic leukodystrophy, neurodegeneration with iron accumulation, Leigh disease, ataxia telangiectasia, Niemann-Pick disease, and Lesch-Nyhan syndrome. Drug-induced dystonia is most often caused by neuroleptics, but it can also be caused by dopamine agonists used for treatment of parkinsonism.

Idiopathic dystonia includes several syndromes that may ultimately be found to belong in the degenerative or metabolic categories:
- Focal dystonias, including writer's cramp, cranial dystonia, and torticollis
- Dystonia musculorum deformans (generalized dystonia)
- Dopa-responsive dystonia
- Paroxysmal dystonia

Dyskinesia is spontaneous movements unintended by the patient. They can have various manifestations, and all of the disorders discussed in the following paragraphs are forms of dyskinesia. Medications are the most common cause followed by genetics and stroke.

Athetosis, chorea, ballism, and tremor are abnormal spontaneous movements that, strictly speaking, fit under the heading of "dyskinesia." Athetosis has been considered a slow version of chorea. All of these hyperkinetic disorders have been reported to occur from stroke.

Athetosis is a slow writhing movement that is most prominent distally. It is most commonly seen in Huntington disease but can also be seen in hypoxic damage and in a host of less common disorders including autoimmune.

Chorea is a rapid jerky movement, mainly of distal muscles that patients frequently blend into volitional activity. Huntington disease is the prototypic cause.

Ballism is violent flinging movements. The unilateral version is hemiballismus. The most common cause of hemiballismus is infarction of the subthalamic nucleus. Bilateral ballism is extremely rare and usually due to bilateral basal ganglia damage, without focus on the subthalamic nucleus.

Thalamus

All sensory information ascending to the cortex passes through the various nuclei of the thalamus, so it follows that lesions of the thalamus can cause sensory deficits as well. Patients with thalamic lesions may experience thalamic pain syndrome; in the chronic phase of injury, patients have severe pain contralaterally. This pain is often quite intractable.

There are multiple types of lesions, and some of the clinical findings are discussed previously and in other chapters. A brief synopsis is presented here.

Thalamic infarction occurs because of damages mainly to the branches of the posterior cerebral artery (PCA) with mainly sensory findings. In some individuals, the vessels to both sides arise from one PCA via an anatomical variant artery of Percheron; in this circumstance, unilateral vascular lesion can result in bilateral thalamic infarction. Because the thalamus is supplied by the posterior circulation, associated findings often include midbrain damage from infarction in a basilar distribution and/or hemianopia due to PCA occlusion. Infarction in the anterior circulation (i.e., the branches of the internal carotid, including the middle cerebral artery) do not produce thalamic damage. The sensory deficit from thalamic infarction can affect the entire contralateral body, including face, arm, leg, and trunk. Other findings include neglect, which may resemble that seen with parietal lobe damage of the right hemisphere damage.

Thalamic pain syndrome is characterized by severe pain contralateral to a lesion in the thalamus. The pain is present at rest but is exacerbated by sensory stimulation. Sensory detection thresholds are elevated. Infarction is the most common cause of thalamic pain. Involvement of the posterior ventrobasal region is thought to be necessary for generation of thalamic pain.

MENTAL STATUS CHANGES

In some patients with dementia and decreased levels of consciousness, the main finding on studies is bilateral degeneration of the thalamus. There are often associated eye findings, including pupillary abnormalities. Patients with top-of-the-basilar syndrome present with deficits in short-term memory associated with cortical blindness.

Language disturbance can develop after dominant hemisphere thalamic infarction. Patients develop a transcortical aphasia with impaired naming, word searching, and word substitution but preserved repetition. The transcortical feature of this language disturbance is helpful in differentiating thalamic from cortical lesions. The aphasia is usually transient.

Motor Disorders

Patients with thalamic lesions are not paralyzed, but they often have difficulty moving; this difficulty probably reflects connection of the thalamus with the basal ganglia. This finding is most common with lesions that involve the ventrothalamic and subthalamic regions. Formal testing reveals essentially normal strength of muscles when they are tested individually, but there is decreased tone and a tendency to not use the muscles voluntarily (a form of neglect). This condition is likely due to a deficit in the sensory feedback responsible for maintaining normal movement.

Cerebellum

Eli E. Zimmerman and Karl E. Misulis

Diagnosis of Cerebellar Lesions

The first important distinction in clinical practice is among lesions that primarily affect the vermis, that primarily affect the cerebellar hemispheres, or that diffusely affect the cerebellum. The second important distinction is between lesions that affect only the cerebellum and lesions that affect the brainstem and/or other neural structures.

Diagnosis of cerebellar dysfunction depends on history and examination, as with any neurological structure. Acute onset of cerebellar ataxia suggests a vascular insult, whether infarction or hemorrhage. Slowly progressive ataxia has a wide differential diagnosis, although the most important causes are alcoholic cerebellar degeneration, tumors, and hereditary cerebellar degeneration.

Lesion of the vermis produces gait ataxia characterized by a broad-based stance and impaired placing of the limbs when walking. Compensatory movements can produce a truncal tremor with stance and gait. Movements of the individual limbs show good coordination. Nystagmus is sometimes seen.

Lesion of the cerebellar hemisphere produces limb ataxia ipsilateral to the lesion. Movements are jerky and often fragmented. Gait is broad-based, and the patient tends to fall to the side of the lesion. Repetitive movements are irregular, lacking the rhythm and consistency of normal movements. Tremor of the ipsilateral limbs that is prominent with movement can develop, as seen on finger-nose-finger testing.

Localization of Deficits

Just as the cerebral cortex has a homunculus for its primary motor and primary somatosensory cortices, so does the cerebellar cortex. More specifically, the spinocerebellum has the representation of the body for its control over coordination of ongoing movement. There are dual representations in the cerebellum—one in the anterior lobe and one in the posterior lobe.

Dysfunction of the median zone (or vermis) causes difficulty with midline functions. Postural instability and truncal ataxia are common, as are difficulties with speech and eye movements.

Dysfunction of the intermediate zone causes difficulty with control of the extremities, causing ataxia of the upper or lower limbs or difficulty with rapid alternating movements, called dysdiadochokinesia.

Dysfunction of the lateral zone differs because much of the lateral zone of the cerebellum (i.e., the neocerebellum) has no part of the homunculus. These portions of the cerebellum serve higher order purposes, such as learned movements and the planning and sequencing of complicated tasks. It is becoming more recognized that patients with dysfunction of the lateral zones of the cerebellum can have cognitive difficulties as well (like the "ataxia" of thought). This is termed the cerebellar cognitive affective syndrome (CCAS), which can produce a multimodal disorder of cognitive function and sometimes even psychotic features.

Cerebellar Stroke

Cerebellar stroke presents with acute onset of cerebellar ataxia, often associated with vertigo, nystagmus, and other signs referable to brainstem dysfunction. Infarction can directly involve the brainstem in addition to the cerebellum; hemorrhage can result in brainstem compression and is a neurosurgical emergency. Clinical differentiation of hemorrhage from infarction of the cerebellum is imperfect. Presumption of infarction may delay the surgery necessary for cerebellar hemorrhage, so early imaging is necessary in patients with cerebellar stroke.

INFARCTION PRODUCING CEREBELLAR ATAXIA

The cerebellum receives its blood supply via the superior cerebellar artery (SCA), anterior inferior cerebellar artery (AICA), and posterior inferior cerebellar artery (PICA). These three vessels anastomose extensively on the surface of the cerebellum.

AICA infarction produces ipsilateral ataxia from damage to the cerebellar hemisphere and peduncle, along with brainstem findings such as vertigo, nystagmus, and ipsilateral Horner syndrome. Patients may have ipsilateral facial weakness from cranial nerve VII involvement, and deafness due to ischemia of inner ear structures, and facial sensory loss due to trigeminal nucleus and tract involvement, with loss of the corneal reflex. Superior cerebellar artery infarction produces ipsilateral ataxia plus nystagmus, vertigo, Horner syndrome, and intention tremor and may produce contralateral hearing loss due to involvement of the crossed lateral lemniscus.

Cerebellar ataxia develops as a result of many brainstem stroke syndromes; in some patients, the cerebellum is directly infarcted, whereas in others the ataxia is due to damage to cerebellar inflow or outflow tracts. For example, midbrain infarction with damage to the red nucleus can produce contralateral cerebellar ataxia, and lateral medullary infarction with damage to the inferior cerebellar peduncle causes ipsilateral cerebellar ataxia. In patients with acute onset cerebellar ataxia thought to be secondary to stroke, associated brainstem signs must be sought; these signs will aid in localizing the area of damage.

CEREBELLAR HEMORRHAGE

Cerebellar hemorrhage may present with cerebellar ataxia but many patients have signs referable to mass effect, which produces brainstem compression. Common symptoms include occipital headache, vertigo, gait and/or limb ataxia, nausea with or without vomiting, and diplopia. Signs include nystagmus, gaze palsies, skew deviation, ataxia, hyperreflexia with upward plantar responses, facial weakness, and decreased level of consciousness. Early on, cerebellar hemorrhages near the midline may not present with any neurological abnormality if the patient is examined lying on a stretcher. Getting the patient up to walk may be diagnostic and is an essential part of the examination, even in the emergency department.

Cerebellar Degenerations

Cerebellar degeneration is not common, and it is frequently not recognized. Many patients are misdiagnosed as having Parkinson disease or stroke. The degeneration may be hereditary, paraneoplastic, or of unknown etiology.

Patients present with gradually progressive ataxia that affects gait and limb movements indicating diffuse cerebellar involvement. Cerebellar degeneration is suggested by prominent cerebellar ataxia, with other neurologic deficits being less impressive. Important cerebellar degenerations are discussed in the next section; in these degenerations, the cerebellar signs are only a portion of the neurologic findings.

ALCOHOLIC CEREBELLAR DEGENERATION

Patients who abuse alcohol may develop gait ataxia due to degeneration of the rostral vermis. This degeneration has a characteristic appearance at autopsy, which may be seen even on magnetic resonance imaging (MRI) sagittal images of the vermis; atrophy of the rostral segments is far out of proportion to atrophy of the remainder of the vermis.

Patients present with gait ataxia with little or no arm ataxia. Leg coordination is impaired on heel-knee-shin testing.

INHERITED ATAXIAS

Ataxias are classified by genetics, age of onset, and pathophysiology. This section presents a few key disorders and guides to suspicion and diagnosis. There are dozens of genetically distinct disorders in this category.

Friedreich ataxia is an autosomal recessive disorder characterized by cerebellar degeneration and other neurologic findings, including peripheral neuropathy, corticospinal tract signs, and cardiomyopathy. Patients have an increased incidence of optic atrophy, diabetes mellitus, and sensorineural deafness. Onset is usually between 8 and 15 years of age. Patients present with cerebellar symptoms and signs; on examination, associated findings are detected. Family history must be taken in these patients, as in all patients with progressive cerebellar ataxia. Diagnosis is by clinical findings. Patients with Charcot-Marie-Tooth disease or hereditary motor-sensory neuropathy may be misdiagnosed as having Friedreich ataxia, since they may appear ataxic because of their severe neuropathy.

Ataxia-telangiectasia is a progressive cerebellar ataxia combined with eye and skin telangiectasias and immunodeficiency. Inheritance is autosomal recessive. Presentation is usually in childhood with ataxia and later eye movement disruption, especially with saccades and pursuit movement. The immunodeficiency predisposes to hematologic malignancies and infections.

Progressive myoclonic ataxia usually has autosomal recessive inheritance. Patients present with cerebellar ataxia plus myoclonus and seizures. Note that this is sometimes called Ramsay-Hunt syndrome, although this eponym is more commonly used for herpes zoster affecting the facial nerve, which is yet another problem with use of eponyms.

Autosomal dominant ataxias comprise a host of spinocerebellar ataxias. They exhibit progressive cerebellar ataxia and have various contributions of other manifestations including corticospinal, extrapyramidal, or cognitive dysfunction.

MULTIPLE SYSTEM ATROPHY–CEREBELLAR TYPE

Multiple system atrophy–cerebellar type (MSA-C) is associated with multiple motor system involvement, with cerebellar dysfunction and a prominent component. This can be gait and/or appendicular ataxia and dysarthria. A clue to this diagnosis is also cerebellar dysfunction affecting eye movements such as saccadic pursuit and prominent gaze-evoked nystagmus.

PARANEOPLASTIC CEREBELLAR DEGENERATION

Cerebellar ataxia occurs in children with neuroblastoma as a remote effect of tumor. Patients show gait and limb ataxia plus opsoclonus.

Cerebellar ataxia occurs in adults with cancers of the lung, breast, and/or gastrointestinal tract and with lymphoma. Patients develop a rapidly progressive gait and limb ataxia with nystagmus. Degeneration of Purkinje cells of the cerebellum is found at autopsy.

Diagnosis is made clinically after imaging studies fail to show tumor in the posterior fossa. Circulating antibodies may make the diagnosis in life. This is an example of a paraneoplastic syndrome, in which specific antibodies can sometimes be found.

PERI-INFECTIOUS CEREBELLAR DYSFUNCTION

Acute cerebellar ataxia can develop after viral infection, especially varicella. Patients appear with cerebellar ataxia affecting appendicular and gait function, nystagmus, and occasionally opsoclonus and head tremor. Except for the cerebellar signs, the neurologic examination is usually normal. It is unclear whether this ataxia is mediated directly by the virus or by an immune-mediated attack. This syndrome is more common in children than in adults.

Tumors

Tumors may affect the midline or hemispheres of the cerebellum. Tumors of the midline will primarily affect gait, whereas tumors of the hemispheres will produce limb ataxia. The mass effect of all cerebellar tumors can result in global cerebellar dysfunction and ultimately distortion of the brainstem with resultant brainstem signs. Obstructive hydrocephalus can develop with deformation and eventual obliteration of the fourth ventricle.

Cerebellar tumors in children are usually primary and include pilocytic astrocytomas in the hemispheres, ependymoma, primitive neuroectodermal tumors invading the midline of the cerebellum, and medulloblastoma. Cerebellar tumors in adults are more frequently metastatic and may be midline or lateral. Meningiomas can produce cerebellar appendicular or gait ataxia, depending on location. A large proportion of meningiomas are incidental findings on imaging studies in patients being imaged for other reasons. Oligodendrogliomas are rare in the posterior fossa.

Brainstem and Cranial Nerves

Eli E. Zimmerman and Karl E. Misulis

Brainstem Dysfunction

MIDBRAIN

Isolated cranial nerve (CN) III or CN IV palsy is rarely due to a midbrain lesion, despite the location of the nuclei. Midbrain lesions can produce partial or complete palsies of these cranial nerves plus hemiparesis from involvement of the cerebral peduncle or ataxia from damage to the red nucleus. In addition to these direct effects of midbrain lesions, many such lesions can obstruct the aqueduct, producing hydrocephalus affecting the lateral and third ventricles but sparing the fourth ventricle.

Important lesions of the midbrain include infarctions, intrinsic tumors, and extrinsic compression by tumors in the pineal region. Some of these are discussed in the following sections. Basilar thrombosis and top-of-the-basilar syndrome affect the midbrain, but they affect other structures as well, so they are discussed at the end of this chapter.

Parinaud Syndrome

Parinaud syndrome is due to dysfunction of the rostral aspect of the dorsal midbrain. The most common cause is a tumor in the pineal region, but infarction or hemorrhage can also cause the syndrome. Hydrocephalus can produce downward displacement of tissue in the midbrain region, also producing Parinaud syndrome. The lesion affects the pretectal region of the midbrain, the posterior commissure, and the interstitial nucleus.

Patients present with supranuclear difficulty with vertical gaze; there is defective voluntary gaze but preserved vertical vestibuloocular reflexes. Pupillary response is impaired to light but relatively preserved to accommodation (light-near dissociation). Other classic findings are convergence-retraction nystagmus, lid retraction, and lid lag. Convergence-retraction nystagmus consists of rhythmic convergence and divergence movements induced by upward gaze.

Partial lesions are often seen, making identification of the entire clinical syndrome uncommon. In practice, defective vertical gaze with light-near dissociation, often with unequal pupils, suggests the lesion. Because many patients with this syndrome have tumors, extension into the hypothalamic region can produce diabetes insipidus. Lesion of the caudal midbrain at the level of the inferior colliculus can produce defective downward gaze with preservation of pupillary responses.

Weber Syndrome

Weber syndrome is contralateral hemiparesis with ipsilateral oculomotor palsy that does not spare the pupil. It is due to damage to the cerebral peduncle and oculomotor nerve. The most common cause is posterior circulation ischemia, although tumors can produce the symptoms.

Syndrome of Benedikt

The syndrome of Benedikt consists of contralateral hemiparesis, ipsilateral oculomotor palsy, and contralateral cerebellar ataxia. The ataxia is a combination of corticospinal dysfunction and damage to the red nucleus. Case reports of this have been reported with strokes, tumors, or infection (tuberculoma) affecting the midbrain.

PONS

Pontine lesions can produce varied lesions depending on the rostrocaudal and dorsal-ventral extent of the damage. Important symptoms suggesting a pontine lesion include lateral gaze palsy from paramedian pontine reticular formation (PPRF) dysfunction, facial or abducens nerve palsy, and signs of parenchymal damage, such as corticospinal tract dysfunction. Lesions of the pons that produce predominantly ocular motor abnormalities were discussed earlier in the section on cranial nerves.

Millard-Gubler Syndrome

The Millard-Gubler syndrome is due to a lesion in the pons affecting the sixth nerve nucleus, corticospinal tract, and intra-axial portion of the seventh nerve. Clinical findings include ipsilateral lateral rectus palsy, contralateral hemiplegia, and ipsilateral facial weakness. The seventh nerve palsy is typical of lower motor neuron seventh nerve palsies.

Foville Syndrome

A lesion in the pons can affect the PPRF, corticospinal tract, and intraaxial portion of the facial nerve. Patients present with an ipsilateral facial palsy, contralateral hemiparesis, and gaze palsy to the side of the lesion.

Locked-In Syndrome

Locked-in syndrome is most commonly due to basilar artery thrombosis, although it can also be due to pontine hemorrhage or infarction or to central pontine myelinolysis. It is also called osmotic demyelination syndrome, related to rapid correction of hyponatremia.

Patients present with quadriplegia and facial weakness. Often, the only voluntary motor power is of vertical eye movements and eye closure. Patients are often misdiagnosed as being in a coma because of the absence of response to verbal command; but if the examiner is careful to test by eye blink or eye movement, the patient is found to be awake and able to take in sensory information. Patients quickly learn to communicate by a code with these minimal movements if given the opportunity.

The differential diagnosis of locked-in syndrome includes other causes of quadriparesis including Guillain-Barré syndrome and other neuropathies, botulism, myasthenia gravis, and profound metabolic derangement. The differential diagnosis also includes true coma, persistent vegetative state, and akinetic mutism.

Pure Motor Hemiparesis

Lacunar infarction of the ventral aspect of the pons, the basis pontis, can especially damage the corticospinal tract fibers, leaving more dorsally located cranial nuclei and nerves spared. This condition results in contralateral hemiparesis with few or no associated signs.

The pons derives arterial supply from the basilar artery, which in turn sends circumferential arteries around the pons. These arteries send penetrating branches into the pons. Occlusion of one of these penetrating vessels is thought to be responsible for brainstem lacunar syndromes. The differential diagnosis of pure motor hemiparesis includes infarction in the ventral pons or the internal capsule.

Clumsy Hand-Dysarthria Syndrome

Lacunar infarction of the basis pontis may involve not only the corticospinal tract, as with pure motor hemiparesis, but also the facial nerve. Patients present with dysarthria, dysphagia, clumsiness, and corticospinal tract signs. Differential diagnosis includes lesions of the internal capsule.

MEDULLA

Lateral Medullary Syndrome

Lateral medullary (Wallenberg) syndrome is usually due to occlusion of the posterior inferior cerebellar artery (PICA), which is a branch of the vertebral artery or the vertebral artery itself. Findings include ipsilateral ataxia due to damage to the inferior cerebellar peduncle and cerebellum, ipsilateral Horner syndrome from involvement of the intrinsic sympathetic axons that descend into the cervical cord, and vertigo with nausea with or without vomiting from damage to the vestibular nuclei. Ipsilateral pharyngeal and laryngeal dysfunction due to damage to the nucleus ambiguus produces dysarthria and dysphagia. Ipsilateral trigeminal involvement produces sensory loss on the face. Damage to the ascending spinothalamic tract produces decreased pain and temperature sensation contralateral to the lesion.

Medial Medullary Syndrome

The medial medullary syndrome is less common than the lateral medullary syndrome. Infarction of the medial medulla is due to occlusion of branches of the vertebral artery, which project to form the anterior spinal artery. These penetrating branches can be occluded, infarcting the pyramids, medial lemniscus, and hypoglossal nerve. Patients present with contralateral hemiparesis, contralateral loss of position and vibratory sensation, and ipsilateral paresis of the tongue.

CRANIAL NERVE DYSFUNCTION

Cranial nerves are discussed individually except for the oculomotor, trochlear, and abducens, which together control ocular movement. Lesions affecting one cranial nerve solely or predominantly are discussed under the respective nerve. Brainstem lesions producing cranial nerve dysfunction in addition to other neurologic dysfunctions are discussed at the end of the chapter.

OLFACTORY NERVE

Anosmia (lack of smell) is produced by peripheral or central processes. Head injury is a common cause of anosmia due to disruption of the small olfactory nerves that penetrate the cribriform plate. Tumors of the olfactory grove compress the inferior frontal region, producing few neurologic signs. Patients may present with mood alteration. Although patients rarely complain of olfactory abnormalities, examination can reveal anosmia. Other important causes of anosmia include increased intracranial pressure and some neurodegenerative diseases, including Parkinson disease and Alzheimer disease.

Sinusitis can impair flow of air to the sensory regions and is a more common etiology than any of the others discussed here.

OPTIC NERVE

Optic nerve lesions usually produce monocular visual loss, and subacute deficits may not be initially noticed by the patient. Formal testing may reveal reduced visual acuity that cannot be improved by correcting for refractive error. Color vision is often impaired. If a focal portion of the optic nerve is compressed or otherwise damaged, there may be a monocular abnormality in visual fields. Fig. 1.3.1 (in Chapter 1.3) shows changes in visual fields with lesions of the optic nerves, chiasm, and tracts.

Important causes of optic neuropathy include the following:

- Optic neuritis
- Multiple sclerosis (MS)

- Neuromyelitis optica (NMO) spectrum disorder
- Anti-myelin oligodendrocyte glycoprotein Anti-MOG disease
- Ischemic optic neuropathy (arteritic and nonarteritic)
- Tumors
- Malnutrition (alcohol tobacco amblyopia)
- Trauma

Optic neuritis is characterized by inflammation and demyelination of the optic nerve. This finding is usually idiopathic, although approximately 50% of patients with optic neuritis subsequently develop MS. Clinical features cannot clearly differentiate isolated optic neuritis from MS-associated optic neuritis.

For the diagnosis of MS, history or examination has to indicate evidence of other neurologic lesions that could be due to central demyelination. Magnetic resonance imaging (MRI) is helpful to rule out optic nerve compression and also to look for signs of white matter changes in the brain. See Chapter 5.9 for a discussion of the clinical criteria for MS.

Tumors can affect the optic nerves, and the three most important are gliomas, meningiomas, and pituitary tumors. Optic nerve gliomas can occur as isolated entities or in association with neurofibromatosis. Patients present with progressive visual loss. The tumor location can be identified based on details of the visual fields. Proptosis (forward protrusion of the eye) suggests involvement of the nerve in the orbit, and pituitary tumors produce deformation of the optic chiasm, resulting in junctional scotomata.

Trauma commonly damages the eye or optic nerves, and detailed evaluation must be performed as soon as possible after the injury. Periorbital edema may make ocular examination impossible by 24 to 48 hours after the injury.

OCULAR MOTOR SYSTEM

Detailed eye movement examination is warranted in every patient with subjective diplopia or who has signs of an ocular motor defect on neurologic examination.

The following should be done as part of the ocular motor examination:
- Movements of each eye are tested in all of the primary directions of gaze.
- Diplopia is assessed with different directions of gaze.
- Pupillary responses to light and accommodation are assessed.
- The swinging-flashlight test is done to test for an afferent pupil.

The eyes are tested together, although the examiner should concentrate on the specific responses of each eye. Nystagmus of one eye should prompt examination of the eyes individually. The examiner must use knowledge of neuroanatomy during the examination to determine whether the defects are best explained by a defect in cranial nerves, brainstem, brain, or extraocular muscles.

The precision of eye movement may limit the ability of the examiner to detect subtle divergence of gaze; therefore, the patient should be asked about diplopia evoked by directions of gaze.

Pupillary response is elicited by shining a bright light into each eye of the patient, one eye at a time. The diameter of each pupil before and during light exposure is noted. When the light is shone in one eye, both eyes should constrict equally.

The swinging-flashlight test examines pupillary responses from both eyes. The room must be dark enough that the eyes are not constricted, yet light enough that the diameter of the pupils can be determined. A bright light is shone first into one eye then quickly into the other. The normal response is constriction of both pupils when the light is initially shone into one eye. Quickly moving the light between the eyes should result in no alteration in diameter. If both pupils constrict more when light is shone into one eye than the other, the eye eliciting the lesser constriction is described as having an afferent defect, which points to an optic nerve or orbital lesion.

Optokinetic nystagmus (OKN) is elicited by the movement of a patterned background. The typical real-life stimulus is passing scenery as a car drives through the countryside. The eyes fix on an object of interest, and the image moves toward the rear of the vehicle. When fixation can no longer be maintained, gaze is redirected toward the front of the vehicle, and a new target is selected. The fast phase of the nystagmus is toward the front of the vehicle. In clinical practice, OKN is tested by passing a striped tape in front of the eyes at a constant velocity. The nystagmus is analogous to the eye movements elicited by the vehicle movement OKN is normally symmetric with movement of the tape in either direction. Lesion of one hemisphere in the parietooccipital region produces an abnormal or absent OKN when the tape is moved toward the side of the lesion. An even more compelling stimulus is movement of a mirror held close in front of the patient. Compensatory movements are virtually impossible to suppress.

One of the most important uses of OKN is for diagnosis of psychogenic blindness. Patients who are blind will not develop OKN, whereas patients with psychogenic blindness often will.

Differential Diagnosis of Ocular Motor Abnormalities

Examination of the eyes is complex if more than one cranial nerve is affected; although multiple cranial neuropathies must be considered, central lesions and neuromuscular lesions should be considered as well. The deficits associated with single lesions are listed in Table 3.4.1. Ocular motor defects and associated anatomic localizations are presented in Table 3.4.2.

Cerebral Lesions

The anatomy of cerebral control over eye movement was discussed earlier. Massive lesions of one hemisphere are associated with a contralateral hemiparesis plus gaze preference to the side of the lesion, that is, the side opposite to the hemiparesis. With oculovestibular reflexes, the eyes can

TABLE 3.4.1 ■ Focal Lesions of the Ocular Motor System

Lesion	Findings
Left frontal lobe destructive lesion	Left gaze preference, often with right hemiparesis
Left frontal lobe irritative lesion (e.g., seizure)	Right gaze preference, sometimes with nystagmoid movements of eyes
Left parietooccipital region lesion	Defective smooth pursuit in both horizontal directions of gaze in the contralateral hemifield
CN III palsy	Ptosis and impaired upward gaze and adduction; extrinsic compression lesions affecting pupil early; nerve ischemia often spares pupil
CN IV palsy	Impaired depression of the ipsilateral eye while in adduction; head tilt to the side opposite the lesion due to external rotation of eye
CN VI palsy	Impaired abduction of eye
Medial longitudinal fasciculus	Internuclear ophthalmoplegia; impaired adduction of ipsilateral eye with gaze to side opposite lesion; nystagmus of the contralateral (abducting) eye
Pontine lesion (Millard-Gubler syndrome)	Ipsilateral CN VI palsy, facial palsy, and contralateral hemiparesis
Midbrain lesion (Parinaud syndrome)	Impaired upgaze with dilated and nonreactive pupils

TABLE 3.4.2 ■ Localization of Ocular Motor Defects

Defect	Features	Localization and Type of Lesion
Downbeat nystagmus	Vertical nystagmus with fast phase downward; accentuated by downgaze and suppressed by upgaze	Craniocervical junction, e.g., tumor, malformation, cerebellar lesion
Horner syndrome	Miosis, ptosis, often with ipsilateral hypohydrosis	Ipsilateral brainstem, spinal cord, lower brachial plexus, or cervical sympathetic chain
Left gaze preference	Eye looks left but may be driven across midline by vestibuloocular reflex	Left frontal lobe if preference can be overcome with doll's head maneuver; right pons if not
Millard-Gubler syndrome	Ipsilateral CN VI and VII palsy and contralateral hemiparesis	Ipsilateral pons affecting CN VI nucleus, intraaxial portion of CN VII, and corticospinal tract
Ocular bobbing	Jerking of eyes with a fast phase downward and slow return	Pons—though some diffuse brainstem lesions may also do this
Parinaud syndrome	Impaired upgaze with dilated and nonreactive pupils	Midbrain, usually compressive lesion, e.g., pineal region tumor
Skew deviation	Vertical diplopia with one eye persistently elevated	Brainstem or cerebellum; lower eye is on the side of the lesion
Internuclear ophthalmoplegia	Impaired adduction of the contralateral eye with gaze to one side	Medial longitudinal fasciculus on side of the eye that fails to adduct
Horizontal nystagmus	Fast deviation of eyes to one side with slower return to the opposite side	Brainstem of vestibular system, e.g., many brainstem tumors or stroke

usually be brought across the midline. More restricted lesions of the hemisphere will result in smaller deficits, usually due to frontal lobe damage.

Frontal Lobe Lesions

Frontal lobe lesions result in gaze preference to the side of the lesion. Because the hemisphere is important for pursuit to the side of the lesion, pursuit is impaired as well. Surviving neurons may compensate for the gaze preference within hours, if there are incomplete lesions; more typically, the gaze preference lasts days and then corrects.

Some patients are seen with eye deviation toward the side of the paralysis. These patients often have deep lesions involving the thalamus.

Frontal lobe irritative lesions affecting the frontal eye fields may cause paroxysms of gaze toward the side contralateral to the lesion. Seizures would be a typical example. Following the seizure, the gaze would likely be to the side ipsilateral to the lesion as a postictal phenomenon.

Parietal and Occipital Lobe Lesions

The parietooccipital cortex is involved in smooth pursuit (i.e., in directing attention to an object of interest) in addition to its role in visual perception. Optic radiations through the parietal and occipital lobes project to the striate cortex of the occipital lobe; the prestriate region of the cortex is involved in analysis of this input. Lesions in this parietooccipital region result in impaired pursuit movements in both directions of horizontal gaze in the contralateral visual field.

Brainstem Lesions

Brainstem lesions that predominantly affect eye movements are discussed here, whereas those that produce other deficits are discussed in the brainstem section. Some important entities affecting eye movements discussed elsewhere include Parinaud syndrome, Millard-Gubler syndrome, and Foville syndrome.

Horner Syndrome

Horner syndrome consists of miosis (pupil constriction) plus ptosis and is a manifestation of damage to sympathetic fibers. Associated findings may include ipsilateral anhidrosis (impaired sweating), enophthalmos, and, in congenital cases, hypopigmentation of the iris. Although the pupil is small, it reacts normally to light and accommodation. Causes of Horner syndrome include lesions at the following levels:

- Brainstem
- Spinal cord
- Brachial plexus
- Sympathetic chain

Brainstem lesions affect the sympathetic fibers as they descend into the spinal cord. The sympathetic pathway is adjacent to the spinothalamic tract, so Horner syndrome due to a brainstem lesion is often associated with contralateral loss of pain and temperature sensation. Symptoms associated with specific brainstem syndromes are discussed in the following paragraph; many of them are associated with Horner syndrome.

The sympathetic fibers descend in the lateral aspect of the cervical cord, and lesions in this region can produce Horner syndrome.

Central cord lesions may produce bilateral Horner syndrome, which is clinically difficult to recognize. Ptosis and miosis with no other ocular motor abnormality suggest this syndrome.

The sympathetic efferents exit the spinal column at T1; they briefly join the brachial plexus and then ascend in the cervical sympathetic chain. Lesions affecting the T1 root may include intervertebral disc lesions, avulsion injuries, cervical rib lesions, and tumors.

The cervical sympathetic chain ascends with the carotid artery into the skull, then through the cavernous sinus, and then into the orbit. Lesions of these axons can occur with neck and skull-base tumors and carotid surgery. Lesions can also be found in the cavernous sinus and posterior aspect of the orbit.

Horner syndrome may occur with cluster headache and occasionally migraine. Diagnosis is by typical history and exclusion of other causes.

Internuclear Ophthalmoplegia

Internuclear ophthalmoplegia (INO) is characterized by a defect in adduction of one eye with lateral gaze. The abducting eye has nystagmus. The lesion is in the medial longitudinal fasciculus (MLF) in the brainstem, which connects the PPRF to the third nerve nuclear complex. The MLF crosses shortly after leaving the PPRE, so the lesion is ipsilateral to the eye that exhibits the difficulty with adduction.

Convergence is usually preserved in INO. Associated findings may include upward or torsional nystagmus and skew deviation.

Common causes of INO are MS and infarction. Because of the proximity of the MLF to the midline, INO is often bilateral.

One-and-a-Half Syndrome

The one-and-a-half syndrome is a gaze palsy with an INO. It is due to a lesion in the pons affecting the PPRF, sixth nerve nucleus, and ipsilateral MLF. The only intact horizontal eye movement

TABLE 3.4.3 ■ Diagnosis of Central Versus Peripheral Vertigo

Clinical Feature	Peripheral Etiology	Central Etiology
Latency	0-40 s	None
Duration	Brief; mean 7.8 s	Long; may be persistent
Intensity	Severe	Mild to moderate
Nystagmus	Limited duration; consistent direction	Persistent; changing direction
Nausea ± vomiting	Severe	Mild

is abduction of the contralateral eye. The most common causes of this syndrome are MS and infarction.

Skew Deviation

Skew deviation is characterized by vertical diplopia that cannot be explained by a cranial nerve palsy or extraocular muscle lesion. The lesion is in the brainstem or cerebellum. The most common cause is infarction. The lower eye is on the side of the lesion.

Horizontal Nystagmus

Horizontal nystagmus can be of central or peripheral origin. The differential diagnosis is aided by examination of the characteristics of the nystagmus. Vestibular dysfunction produces nystagmus with a slow component toward the side of the lesion. Gaze toward the side opposite the lesion accentuates the slow phase of the nystagmus.

Lesions of the brainstem commonly produce nystagmus. Nystagmus of central origin is differentiated from nystagmus of peripheral origin by several features:

- Central nystagmus is not suppressed by fixation, whereas peripheral nystagmus is suppressed.
- Central nystagmus rarely has a torsional component, whereas peripheral nystagmus commonly does.
- Latency to evoked nystagmus with the Barany maneuvers is shorter with central lesions than with peripheral lesions (Table 3.4.3).
- Duration of evoked nystagmus with the Barany maneuvers is longer with central lesions than with peripheral lesions (see Table 3.4.3).

Nystagmus is common with many lesions of the brainstem, especially strokes and tumors; these are discussed in the brainstem section. A few beats of nystagmus at extremes of gaze are considered normal and should not be confused with clearly abnormal movements.

Downbeat Nystagmus

Downbeat nystagmus is evident in the primary position and is accentuated by downward gaze. Upward gaze suppresses the nystagmus. Lesion is classically at the cervicomedullary junction, although other brainstem lesions can produce this finding. The differential diagnosis is extensive and includes tumors, craniocervical subluxation, Chiari malformation, basilar invagination, and hydrocephalus. Cerebellar degeneration can be associated with downbeat nystagmus in the absence of direct cervicomedullary pathology.

Ocular Bobbing

Ocular bobbing is characterized by a rapid conjugate downgaze followed by a slower return to the primary position; this movement is similar to that of a fishing bob on the surface of the water. The defect is usually bilateral. Lesion is of the pons and can be due to tumor, infarction, or hemorrhage within the substance; less frequently, extrinsic compressive lesions are found. Uncommon causes are encephalitis and central pontine myelinolysis. Inverse ocular bobbing, with the fast phase upward, is less likely to be due to a focal structural lesion and is more likely to be due to anoxia or prolonged status epilepticus.

Oculogyric Crisis

Oculogyric crisis is an uncommonly recognized disorder characterized by spasmodic conjugate ocular deviations, usually upward and sometimes lateral. It is most commonly caused by neuroleptics, but it can also be seen with carbamazepine, lithium, and head injury. The patient can often voluntarily suppress the deviation, but only briefly.

Individual Cranial Nerve Lesions

CN III Palsy

Lesions of the third nerve are most common in the following locations:

- Intracranial segment near the posterior cerebral artery
- Intracranial segment near the tentorium cerebellum
- Intracranial segment, independent of a structural lesion
- Cavernous sinus
- Orbit

Proximity of the nerve to the posterior cerebral and posterior communicating arteries makes it susceptible to compression by aneurysms. This is the prime concern of clinicians when they observe a large, poorly reactive pupil.

The third nerve can be compressed by transtentorial herniation of the uncus with increased intracranial pressure. Fibers serving pupillary response may be affected before ocular movements because of their peripheral location on the nerve.

The third nerve is commonly damaged by ischemia as it passes through the subarachnoid space. Ischemia is seen most commonly with diabetes and hypertension. Pupillary fibers may be spared because their peripheral location protects them from infarction by vessels penetrating the nerve. Therefore, pupil response is an important differentiating feature: Early pupillary dilation favors a compressive lesion, whereas a pupil-sparing third nerve palsy is more commonly ischemic. However, this is not an absolute differentiating feature, and pupil-sparing third nerve palsies with compressive lesions are not infrequent.

In the cavernous sinus, the third nerve is near the carotid artery and trochlear, abducens, and trigeminal nerves. There is a rostrocaudal anatomical organization as well, which influences the effect of lesions depending on whether they are nearer the orbit or the brain. Lesions that can affect the oculomotor nerve in the cavernous sinus include aneurysms, thrombophlebitis, and extension of nasopharyngeal tumors.

Lesion in the orbit can affect the superior and/or inferior divisions of the oculomotor nerve; in addition, it can interfere with movement of the globe because of mechanical effects. Pain and proptosis are common in this setting.

CN IV Palsy

Trochlear nerve palsy produces vertical diplopia plus head tilt to the side opposite the lesion. The head tilt compensates for diplopia due to extortion of the eye produced by the superior oblique palsy. The most common cause of fourth nerve palsy is trauma, which accounts for 34% of all cases; 20% of these are bilateral. Infarction of the nerve can occur in diabetes mellitus and atherosclerotic disease. Most other causes result in signs referable to midbrain or other cranial nerve(s). Other cranial neuropathies suggest a meningeal process. Involvement of CN III and/or VI suggests a lesion in the cavernous sinus or superior orbital fissure. Corticospinal tract signs or ataxia suggests a midbrain lesion.

CN VI Palsy

Abducens palsy can be due to lesion at almost any point from the nucleus to the distal nerve as it enters the lateral rectus in the orbit. Nuclear sixth lesions are more common than third or fourth nerve palsies. Because of the proximity to the PPRF and the intraaxial portion of the facial nerve, conjugate gaze palsy and facial weakness often accompany the lateral rectus weakness. Lesion of the subarachnoid portion of the abducens nerve may develop from increased intracranial pressure, head injury, nerve infarction from diabetes or atherosclerotic disease, and meningitis.

Extraocular Muscle Lesions

Extraocular muscles may be affected directly by lesions, which must be differentiated from ocular motor nerve lesions. Careful examination reveals a pattern of weakness that cannot be explained by lesions of a single cranial nerve or combination of nerves. Common causes of extraocular muscle disease include the following:

- Trauma
- Thyroid ophthalmopathy
- Myasthenia gravis

Trauma can affect the ocular motor muscles by entrapment, which is common with orbital fractures. The defect may initially be missed because of periorbital edema, which impedes examination.

Thyroid ophthalmopathy is due to inflammation and fibrosis of ocular muscles. Exophthalmos is associated with this and usually precedes the ocular motor disorder. The most severely affected muscles include the inferior rectus, with the medial rectus, superior rectus, and obliques affected to a lesser extent.

Myasthenia gravis is associated with weakness of the ocular muscles that cannot be explained by single neural lesions. The medial rectus is commonly affected, but any muscle may be involved. The pattern of abnormality may be variable or worse with fatigue, and ptosis of the eyelids is often involved.

Ptosis is common and is usually asymmetric. The defects are exacerbated by sustained gaze using affected muscles. Diagnosis is supported by improvement with edrophonium injection, although neurogenic lesions may show some improvement with this treatment as well.

Pupillary Abnormalities

The control of pupil diameter has been discussed, and pupillary abnormalities in relation to many lesions have also been presented. This section concerns problems that are confined to the pupil, with no other ocular motor abnormalities.

In physiologic anisocoria, there is a difference in pupil diameter at rest. There is a visible difference in pupil size in about 20% of patients, although it is usually a discrepancy of less than 1 mm. Both pupils react to direct and consensual stimulation, and both react to accommodation. There should be no lid or other ocular motor abnormalities.

Afferent pupillary defect is a defect in response with stimulation of one eye due to damage to one optic nerve or eye itself. The pupils should be equal; in a darkened room when light is shone in the unaffected eye, both pupils should constrict, but when light is shone in the affected eye, neither eye should constrict. In fact, when illumination of the good eye is removed, both eyes should dilate. This is also termed Marcus-Gunn pupil.

CN III palsy affecting pupil as well as other ocular motor function shows the pupil on the affected side larger than the other. There should be ptosis, reduced elevation, adduction, and depression of the eye. Light in either eye produces constriction of the pupil on the unaffected side.

Horner syndrome is dysfunction of the sympathetic supply to the affected side, and is discussed elsewhere. A pitfall with diagnosis of Horner syndrome is the assumption that the larger pupil is the abnormal one; the examiner is anchoring the diagnosis on a potential CN III palsy.

Tonic (Adie) pupil is where a pupil is slow to react to light but reacts better to accommodation. Tonic pupil is dilated at rest and does not react to flashes of light. With sustained bright light, the pupil slowly constricts. It does not immediately dilate on discontinuation of the light. Accommodation results in better constriction than light does, because accommodation is a stronger physiological stimulus for constriction. The lesion with tonic pupil is usually of the ciliary ganglion or nerves from the ganglion to the eye. The disorder can be idiopathic (Adie syndrome) or due to trauma or local orbital lesions (tumor, infection). It can also be a manifestation of peripheral neuropathy with autonomic symptoms.

Afferent pupil (Gunn pupil) is caused by a lesion of the optic nerve. The motor outflow to the pupils is normal, and the pupils are of equal size and react when the patient enters bright light. The defect is only evident when the eyes are tested individually. The swinging-flashlight test, discussed earlier, is particularly helpful in this diagnosis. With an afferent defect, the direct response is less prominent than the consensual response: As the light is alternated between eyes, illumination of the eye with the optic nerve lesions results in dilation of both pupils. In contrast, with partial third nerve lesions, the pupil responds incompletely to direct or consensual stimulation, but the contralateral side responds normally. The differential diagnosis of optic nerve lesions includes tumor, optic neuritis, and trauma. Retinal lesions can also produce an afferent defect, although the lesion is usually more severe and retinal abnormalities are often apparent on funduscopic examination.

Argyll Robertson pupil is small, irregular, and unresponsive to light, although it responds to accommodation. The Argyll Robertson pupil is seen in meningovascular syphilis, but it can also be seen with tumors compressing the dorsal midbrain (such as pinealomas), diabetes, brainstem encephalitis, sarcoidosis, Adie syndrome, amyloidosis, and glaucoma. The disparity between the responses to light and accommodation is probably due to a difference in the pathways involved in the reflexes.

Oculomotor Apraxia

Oculomotor apraxia is the inability to make voluntary saccades when the basic mechanisms for eye movements are intact. Reflexive eye movements are intact. Oculomotor apraxia can be congenital or acquired.

Congenital oculomotor apraxia presents in childhood with thrusting head movements during which the eyes close; this movement compensates for the saccadic deficit. Other neurologic deficits are frequently seen, including strabismus and developmental delay.

Acquired oculomotor apraxia can develop in patients with bilateral parietal damage and may be a manifestation of diffuse cerebral disease, such as hypoxic-ischemic encephalopathy. Patients may manifest some of the same head thrusting as seen in children with congenital oculomotor apraxia, but it is less marked.

VESTIBULOCOCHLEAR SYSTEM

Lesions of CN VIII can affect one or both sensory modalities, that is, vestibular and/or auditory. Vestibular dysfunction causes vertigo, nausea and vomiting, and imbalanced walking; nystagmus is found on examination with no objective signs of brainstem dysfunction. Auditory dysfunction presents with hearing loss and often tinnitus, which is frequently the earliest sign of CN VIII dysfunction.

Differentiation between a brainstem lesion and a vestibulocochlear nerve lesion can be difficult. Both can present with the nonspecific complaint of dizziness, which may mean vertigo, presyncope, ataxia, orthostasis, panic-attack response, and/or other vague disorders. Vertigo, a perception of movement of the patient or environment, is the relevant finding.

Vestibulocochlear nerve lesion is suggested by the following findings:
- Latency of several seconds between head movement and symptoms
- Symptoms lasting less than one minute
- Fatigue with repetitive provocation
- Severe vertigo, often with nausea and vomiting, which may be incapacitating
- No associated signs of brainstem dysfunction

Brainstem lesion is suggested by the following findings:
- Immediate onset of symptoms after head movement
- Long-lasting and/or persistent symptoms after head movement
- Frequent lack of fatigue with repetitive provocation
- Mild to moderate sensation of vertigo
- Often other associated signs of brainstem dysfunction

Ataxia of gait is common with central and peripheral disorders, but patients with peripheral disorders usually have good coordination of individual limbs.

Vestibular Schwannoma

This condition, also known as acoustic neuroma, is a schwannoma of the vestibular portion of the eighth nerve. Common presenting symptoms include tinnitus and hearing loss. Pressure on surrounding structures can produce ataxia, facial pain (from trigeminal involvement), facial weakness (from facial nerve involvement), and other brainstem signs (from direct compression). Despite the vestibular branch origin, vertigo is uncommon. Confirmation of diagnosis requires MRI with special attention to the internal auditory canal (IAC) and cerebellopontine angle.

Benign Paroxysmal Positional Vertigo

Benign positional vertigo is characterized by paroxysms of vertigo triggered by a certain position or certain direction of head movement. Table 3.4.3 presents guidelines for differentiating between central and peripheral vertigo.

Peripheral Vestibulopathy

Peripheral vestibulopathy encompasses the diagnoses of vestibular neuronitis and labyrinthitis; although some experts make a distinction between the two, this differentiation is blurred in practice. Patients present with episodes of vertigo interspersed with periods without neurologic symptoms. Peripheral vestibulopathy is differentiated from benign paroxysmal positional vertigo by the absence of a precise positional component. Many patients seek medical attention with their first episode, which may lead to concern over other possibilities, including brainstem infarction, tumor, and demyelinating disease.

Ménière Disease

Ménière disease is characterized by attacks of vertigo associated with a roaring sound. The attacks abate within a day or so but are followed by hearing loss. The auditory symptoms are key to the diagnosis.

Multiple Sclerosis

Dizziness is a common early symptom in MS. The dizziness may be a vague disequilibrium or true vertigo. The key to diagnosis is evidence of other neurologic lesions on history and examination. In practice, the diagnosis is rarely made at the first encounter.

Diagnosis depends on documentation of multiple lesions in space and time. MRI shows areas of increased signal intensity in the white matter on T2-weighted images. Cerebrospinal fluid studies can be supportive.

MOVEMENT AND SENSATION OF FACE, THROAT, AND HEAD

Facial Nerve

The most important differentiation for facial nerve dysfunction is between a central and a peripheral lesion. Because of the long and circuitous route of the facial nerve within the pons, brainstem lesions may produce what appears to be peripheral facial palsy.

Peripheral facial weakness is differentiated from central weakness by distribution and associated findings. The entire face is affected with peripheral lesions, whereas the lower face is predominantly affected with central lesions. This difference occurs because supranuclear input to the facial nuclei is bilateral for neurons controlling the upper face and mainly unilateral for neurons controlling the lower face.

A lesion of the facial nerve within the brainstem is usually associated with other neurologic findings, such as an abducens nerve palsy or contralateral weakness; these findings in conjunction with a peripheral CN VII palsy suggest a lesion in the caudal pons. Cerebral lesions producing lower facial weakness usually do not cause other brainstem signs and commonly produce arm weakness or incoordination ipsilateral to the facial palsy. Weakness contralateral to the facial palsy suggests a pontine lesion on the side of the facial weakness.

Bell Palsy

Bell palsy is idiopathic facial palsy with no other cranial neuropathies. The cause is not completely known, although some individuals believe that it can be due to zoster or other herpes viruses. Isolated facial palsy can be the first sign of Guillain-Barré syndrome.

The onset of idiopathic facial palsy is usually heralded by pain around and posterior to the ear, followed by weakness of the upper and lower face that may progress over several days. Associated symptoms may include hyperacusis and loss of taste over the ipsilateral anterior two-thirds of the tongue, depending on the location of the lesion. Hyperacusis is an apparent increase in sound volume perceived by the ipsilateral ear. It is due to damage to the nerve to the stapedius, which arises from the facial nerve in the facial canal.

Peripheral facial nerve palsy is differentiated from a central lesion by involvement of the upper and the lower face; central lesions mostly affect the lower face. Brainstem lesions usually produce dysfunction of other cranial nerves or brainstem structures. Lacrimation is affected if the facial nerve lesion is proximal to the greater petrosal nerve.

Ramsay-Hunt Syndrome

Ramsay-Hunt syndrome in this context refers to zoster of the geniculate ganglion. Patients present with severe ear pain and usually have a vesicular eruption in the external auditory canal (EAC). The facial palsy usually follows the onset of pain by 1 to 3 days. Diagnosis can be missed if the vesicles are not observed or are attributed to otitis externa. A typical history of ear pain with "otitis externa" followed by facial weakness suggests Ramsay-Hunt syndrome. Occasionally, other cranial nerves may be affected, including the trigeminal and glossopharyngeal nerves. Sensory loss on the face and palate are symptoms associated with these lesions, respectively.

Hemifacial Spasm

Hemifacial spasm involves episodic clonic activity of one side of the face. It often begins in the region of the orbicularis oculi and then spreads to surrounding muscles innervated by the facial nerve. The location of the lesion is thought to be the facial nerve because hemifacial spasm can occur after Bell palsy, with tumors affecting the facial nerve, or after local facial trauma. Some patients develop hemifacial spasm due to pulsation of a small artery against the facial nerve.

Trigeminal Nerve

The trigeminal nerve can be damaged in the posterior fossa intraaxially by tumors, vascular disease, vascular malformations, or demyelinating disease. Tumors or vascular structures can cause extra-axial involvement. Isolated lesions of the trigeminal nerve are unusual; the most common disorder is trigeminal neuralgia. Trigeminal nerve fibers can be affected by disorders affecting other structures, which are discussed elsewhere; some of the most important are the lateral medullary syndrome and lateral pontine syndrome.

Trigeminal Neuralgia

Trigeminal neuralgia is characterized by unilateral paroxysms of pain on the face. The pain is usually lancinating and follows one of the trigeminal divisions. Occasionally, the pain follows more than one division.

The localization of the lesion with trigeminal neuralgia is usually not determined; the patient's history strongly suggests the diagnosis. Examination is normal, although some patients report subjective sensory loss in the affected distribution. Trigeminal neuralgia is, therefore, usually considered idiopathic, although it may be seen in patients with vascular compression of the trigeminal ganglion, demyelinating disease, and tumors with compression.

Zoster of the Trigeminal Ganglion

Zoster of the trigeminal ganglion, which is uncommon, can result in severe pain and paresthesia in the distribution of the trigeminal nerve. In contrast to trigeminal neuralgia, real sensory loss can occur with zoster.

Raeder Paratrigeminal Neuralgia

This rare condition is characterized by pain in a trigeminal distribution with ipsilateral ptosis and miosis. Associated findings may include fourth or sixth nerve palsies. This condition is usually due to lesions in the vicinity of the trigeminal ganglion, including tumors, infections, and vascular malformations.

Glossopharyngeal Nerve

Lesions of the ninth nerve are unusual and difficult to identify. The stylopharyngeus muscle cannot be tested by routine examination. The gag and palatal reflexes use CN IX afferents but the efferents are via CN X.

Glossopharyngeal Neuralgia

Glossopharyngeal neuralgia is a rare condition characterized by severe lancinating pain in the posterior pharynx, usually in the region of the tonsils. It is occasionally associated with syncope, which is attributed to activation of carotid sinus afferents. Glossopharyngeal neuralgia is usually idiopathic, but structural lesions must be considered, including tumors and vascular malformations at the cerebellopontine angle.

Nasopharyngeal Lesions

Nasopharyngeal lesions may produce glossopharyngeal deficits in conjunction with lesions of any or all of CN X, XI, and XII. The most common pathology is probably neoplastic, but infections, trauma, and postoperative deficits account for many of these cases.

Glomus Jugulare Tumors

Glomus jugulare tumors arise from the chemoreceptors of the jugular bulb. They can present with CN IX deficits, including impaired gag reflex. Typical symptoms include pulsatile tinnitus and hearing loss from CN VIII involvement. The patient may have headaches due to increased intracranial pressure, which is associated with obstruction of jugular vein outflow. Erosion of surrounding bone and vascularization may produce a pulsatile vascular structure in the external auditory canal (EAC). Accessory nerve involvement may produce sternocleidomastoid and trapezius weakness. CN X involvement may produce dysphonia and signs of vocal cord paralysis.

Vagus

Isolated lesion of the whole vagus nerve is uncommon. Several brainstem syndromes may result in vagal dysfunction.

Recurrent Laryngeal Nerve Palsy

This is the most commonly diagnosed vagal dysfunction in clinical practice and should be a red flag for chest pathology. Patients present with hoarseness, which may be initially attributed to bronchitis or sinusitis. However, the persistence of the hoarseness leads to further medical evaluation. Laryngoscopy reveals unilateral vocal cord paralysis. Chest radiograph or computed tomography confirms the diagnosis. Common causes of recurrent laryngeal nerve palsy include tumors affecting the mediastinum and aneurysms of the subclavian artery or aortic arch. No cause is identified in some patients.

Vincristine has been implicated in some cases of unilateral recurrent laryngeal nerve palsy, although infiltration by the cancer for which the patient was given the drug must be ruled out. Peripheral neuropathy uncommonly affects vagal nerves; when it does, it produces bilateral deficits.

Pseudobulbar Palsy

Pseudobulbar palsy is impairment of bulbar function due to bilateral supranuclear lesions. Bilateral lesions are required for this palsy to be seen because of the bilateral descending innervation of the motor nuclei. Bifrontal infarctions or contusions are common causes of pseudobulbar palsy, although the differential diagnosis is wide. Patients present with dysphagia and dysarthria. Associated features unrelated to brainstem function include emotional volatility with uncontrollable and often inappropriate laughing and crying.

Accessory Nerve

Pure lesions of the accessory nerve are unusual in clinical practice; when present, they are usually due to local tumor infiltration or surgery. Catheterization of the internal jugular has been reported as a cause. Accessory nerve damage results in weakness of the ipsilateral sternocleidomastoid and trapezius. The ipsilateral sternocleidomastoid weakness causes impaired turning toward the side opposite the lesion. Many causes of accessory palsy also cause dysfunction of other cranial nerves; they are discussed at the end of this chapter.

Hypoglossal Nerve

Isolated lesion of the hypoglossal nerve is uncommon; usually, multiple lower cranial nerves are affected. These syndromes are discussed in the following sections. Lesion of the hypoglossal nerve results in impaired movement of the tongue, with resultant dysarthria and dysphagia. The tongue deviates to the side of the lesion because of impaired protrusion. Neck injuries, tumors, and infections can result in unilateral hypoglossal lesions with only partial paralysis of the tongue.

Supranuclear lesions have little effect on many pharyngeal muscles unless the lesions are bilateral. However, unilateral corticobulbar lesion can result in deviation of the tongue, which protrudes toward the side of the hemiparesis. Supranuclear lesions are differentiated from nuclear and nerve lesions by the absence of atrophy on examination and the absence of denervation on electromyography (EMG).

Clinical Syndromes

CHIARI MALFORMATIONS

The Chiari malformations are disorders of early development of the craniocervical junction in which the cerebellar tonsils extend through the foramen magnum. In many patients, this malformation is an incidental finding on MRI, but it can become symptomatic through compression of the cervico-medullary junction or via hydrocephalus. Chiari malformations are divided into the following types:

Type I: Herniation of the cerebellar tonsils with no other neurologic involvement

Type II: Herniation of the cerebellar tonsils along with caudal displacement of the medulla (Arnold-Chiari malformation)

Type III: Cervical spina bifida with a cerebellar encephalocele

Type IV: Agenesis of the cerebellum (Dandy-Walker syndrome)

Type III is usually obvious at birth. Diagnosis of types I and II is less obvious and should be considered in patients with symptoms of hydrocephalus and/or cervicomedullary junction lesion, including headache with nausea with or without vomiting, truncal ataxia, head tilt, pain in the neck and shoulders, and dysfunction of the lower cranial nerves. Corticospinal tract signs may be present. Nystagmus is common with medullary compression. Type IV may be an incidental finding.

DANDY-WALKER SYNDROME

Dandy-Walker syndrome is agenesis of the cerebellar vermis with a cystic region in the dorsal aspect of the posterior fossa that communicates with the fourth ventricle. Hydrocephalus develops in childhood or in adult life.

Patients present in childhood with macrocephaly. Associated neurologic findings include ataxia, corticospinal tract signs, nystagmus, and cranial nerve palsies. If the hydrocephalus develops in adult life, patients present with typical signs of hydrocephalus. The majority of patients have other neurologic developmental disorders, including agenesis of the corpus callosum, heterotopias, aqueductal stenosis, and pachygyria of the cerebral cortex.

FOSTER KENNEDY SYNDROME

The Foster Kennedy syndrome is usually due to a tumor affecting the inferior frontal region, including meningiomas of the olfactory groove or sphenoid ridge. The clinical triad consists of the following:

- Ipsilateral anosmia
- Ipsilateral optic atrophy
- Contralateral papilledema

Anosmia is due to involvement of the olfactory bulb or tract. Optic atrophy is from chronic compression of the ipsilateral optic nerve. Contralateral papilledema is from pressure on the other optic nerve, which is less affected than the ipsilateral nerve because of distance from the origin of the lesion.

CAVERNOUS SINUS SYNDROME

The cavernous sinus contains the internal carotid artery, the venous sinus itself, and CN III, IV, V, and VI. All of these can be affected by a lesion in the cavernous sinus. Of the divisions of the trigeminal nerve, CN V1 (ophthalmic division) is most likely to be involved, whereas V3 (mandibular division) is least likely to be involved because of its short course in the sinus before exiting.

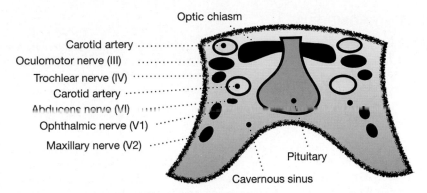

Fig. 3.4.1 **Cavernous sinus.** Anatomy of the cavernous sinus showing proximity of key structures.

Cavernous sinus lesions may cause painful or painless ophthalmoplegia. Occasionally, the pain may precede the ophthalmoparesis

TOLOSA-HUNT SYNDROME

Tolosa-Hunt syndrome is due to a lesion in the region of the cavernous sinus. Patients present with retroorbital pain and have a combination of palsies of the trochlear nerve, the abducens nerve, and the ophthalmic and maxillary divisions of the trigeminal nerve. The differential diagnosis includes other cavernous sinus lesions, pituitary tumors, and pituitary apoplexy (Fig. 3.4.1).

SUPERIOR ORBITAL FISSURE SYNDROME

Superior orbital fissure syndrome resembles cavernous sinus in that all three ocular motor nerves may be affected. However, proptosis is common, and the maxillary division of the trigeminal nerve is spared.

CEREBELLOPONTINE ANGLE SYNDROME

Lesions at the cerebellopontine angle may include acoustic schwannomas, meningiomas; vascular malformations; nerve sheath tumors of the trigeminal, facial, or glossopharyngeal nerves; intrinsic tumors of the brainstem such as gliomas; and chronic meningeal involvement of tumor or an infectious agent.

Symptoms depend on the structures involved, but common symptoms include ipsilateral facial numbness from trigeminal involvement, ipsilateral hemiataxia from involvement of the cerebellum or cerebellar peduncle, tinnitus, and hearing loss. Tinnitus is a common presenting complaint, but hearing loss is often only found on examination. Facial nerve involvement can occur but is uncommon, especially early in the course. Compression or infiltration of the brainstem can produce contralateral weakness with corticospinal tract signs.

GRADENIGO SYNDROME

Gradenigo syndrome is dysfunction of the ophthalmic nerve (V1) and the abducens nerve (VI), usually due to involvement where the two nerves are near one another in the temporal bone. Patients have pain in a V1 distribution associated with lateral rectus palsy.

BASILAR THROMBOSIS

Thrombosis of the basilar artery results in extensive infarction of the pons and midbrain and is often fatal. Patients present with coma, quadriplegia, and horizontal gaze palsies. Some patients with less extensive damage may develop the locked-in syndrome. Basilar thrombosis is suspected by the bilateral brainstem signs, with localization at and above the level of the pons.

MULTIPLE SYSTEM ATROPHY

Multiple system atrophy (MSA) is the term for a group of diseases that have autonomic defect as a commonality. This is in combination with either parkinsonism (MSA-P) or cerebellar dysfunction (MSA-C). MSA includes the disorders previously diagnosed as olivopontocerebellar degeneration (OPCA), Shy-Drager syndrome, and striatonigral degeneration. These latter terms have been retired.

MSA-P is more common than MSA-C.

MSA-P is characterized by parkinsonism with rigidity, bradykinesia, and autonomic insufficiency with orthostatic hypotension. MSA-P is differentiated from Parkinson disease by an action and postural tremor not typically seen in Parkinson disease; only a minority of patients exhibit resting tremor. MSA-P patients can have other abnormal movements including myoclonus or dystonias or dyskinesias.

MSA-C is characterized by predominant cerebellar signs on presentation with limb and gait ataxia as well as dysarthria, dysphagia, and ocular motor abnormalities including diplopia and difficulty with visual tracking, especially smooth pursuit.

TOP-OF-THE-BASILAR SYNDROME

Top-of-the-basilar syndrome is due to occlusion of the distal basilar artery as it bifurcates into the left and right posterior cerebral arteries. The occlusion is usually due to an embolus ascending in the vertebral arteries to the basilar arteries. Symptoms and signs are mainly due to infarction of the occipital lobes and midbrain, thalamus, and medial aspect of the temporal lobe. Findings include cortical blindness from bilateral occipital lobe damage, pupil and eye movement defects from midbrain damage, and memory dysfunction from temporal lobe damage. Damage to descending corticospinal tracts can produce corticospinal tract signs. Sensory findings can be due to damage to ascending tracts and thalamic damage.

Eye movement abnormalities include paralysis of vertical gaze, convergence, and skew deviation. Pupillary abnormalities include irregular or asymmetric pupils, often with decreased responsiveness. If the occipital lobe involvement is incomplete, patients may have hemianopia or other incomplete visual field defects.

Spinal Cord

Karl E. Misulis and Eli E. Zimmerman

Spinal Cord Anatomy and Localization

Localizing a lesion to a specific location within the cord is key to diagnosis. The differential diagnosis is narrowed by deciding exactly how the cord is affected through the following signs:

- Corticospinal tract deficits
- Segmental cord deficits
- Nerve root deficits

Corticospinal tract signs indicate damage to these tracts and include hyperreflexia and abnormal reflexes such as extensor plantar response, increased amplitude of the tendon reflexes, often spread of the reflexes to adjacent muscle groups, and clonus elicited by tendon reflex or passive movement. Corticospinal tract signs are commonly seen in demyelinating diseases, such as transverse myelitis and multiple sclerosis (MS) and can be an early sign of any cause of extrinsic cord compression.

Spinal cord damage affects the level(s) of cord involvement directly and affects the ascending and descending tracts passing through the area. Gray matter damage results in weakness of muscles innervated by segmental nerves due to damage to the anterior horn cells. Atrophy of muscles innervated by one segmental level is usually due to nerve root involvement; but if the denervation spans two or three levels and is bilateral, then a midline gray matter lesion is suspected. Gray matter lesions include syrinx and intraparenchymal tumors.

Segmental damage to the posterior horns produces loss of most sensation at the levels of the injury but also affects the sensation below the level of the injury, with exact involvement depending on which of the sensory tracts is affected, the uncrossed dorsal columns and/or the crossed spinothalamic tracts.

Nerve root damage results in pain and sensory disturbance in the distribution of the root and weakness of innervated muscles.

Spinal cord level helps to determine etiology. Generally, dysfunction is most evident below the level of the lesion, although there may be signs at the level. Motor deficits below the lesion are upper motor neuron. Motor deficits at the level of the lesion are lower motor neuron.

A guide to rostrocaudal localization of spinal lesions is as follows:

- Cervical spine damage results in spastic weakness of the legs with weakness in the arms at and below the lesion.
- Thoracic spine damage results in spastic weakness of the legs with preservation of all arm and neck function unless there is another lesion.
- Lumbar spine damage results in leg weakness with a distribution appropriate to the level of the weakness. Sphincter dysfunction is common.
- Sacral cord lesion results in dysfunction of hip muscles with some leg muscle involvement, although patients are usually able to walk. Sphincter dysfunction is expected with little or no control.

The motor and sensory levels of the deficit are usually fairly accurate in localizing the rostrocaudal extent of the lesion; however, a lesion may be significantly above the level of the deficit.

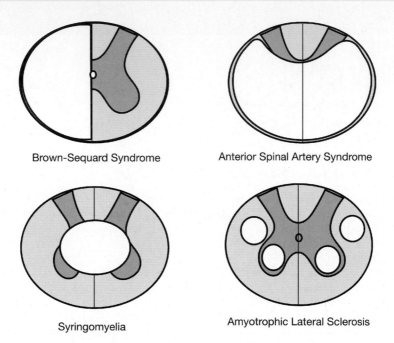

Brown-Sequard Syndrome   Anterior Spinal Artery Syndrome

Syringomyelia   Amyotrophic Lateral Sclerosis

Fig. 3.5.1   Spinal cord disorders. Diagram of stylized lesions of the spinal cord with specific pathologies.

For example, leg weakness with a sensory level in the midthoracic region may be due to a lesion low in the cervical cord; imaging only the thoracic region will miss the lesion. Fig. 3.5.1 shows the regions of the spinal cord affected by some important disorders. The level of sensory involvement does not exactly correlate with neuroanatomic maps because sensory afferents project up and down a few segments. Also, the maps of the dermatomes are not exact, with fuzzy sensory boundaries and variability between patients. Table 3.5.1 shows clinical findings associated with some important lesions of the spinal cord.

Bowel and bladder control issues can develop with damage at any level of the spinal cord, but they are especially likely when there is damage to the lumbosacral cord. The pattern of damage differs depending on the level of the injury.

Localization of Spinal Lesions

Any level of the spinal cord can be affected by disease, but the common causes differ at various levels of the neuraxis. For example, cervical myelopathy is commonly due to disc disease and spondylosis, whereas these are uncommon causes of myelopathy in the thoracic regions. In the thoracic regions, the clinician should more readily suspect other pathology, such as tumors. Disorders of the individual nerve roots, including cervical and lumbar radiculopathy, are discussed in Chapter 5.5.

CRANIOCERVICAL JUNCTION LESIONS

Craniocervical junction lesions present with varied symptoms and signs depending on the severity of the lesions. Mild disease presents with gait difficulty and sensory loss that is most prominent across the shoulders and extends to the upper arms; dysesthesias extending to the hand can occur.

TABLE 3.5.1 ■ Spinal Lesions

Lesion	Findings
Anterior spinal artery syndrome	Paralysis and loss of pain and temperature sensation below the lesion; preservation of vibration and proprioception; level usually between T9 and L1
Brown-Séquard (spinal hemisection) syndrome	Ipsilateral: Segmental lower motor neuron dysfunction; loss of vibration and proprioception below lesion; corticospinal tract signs below level of the lesion Contralateral: Loss of pain and temperature sensation
Cauda equina syndrome	Asymmetric pain and sensory loss affecting caudal nerve roots, especially L4–S2; bowel and bladder changes with severe disease
Central cord syndrome (usually cervical spine)	Weakness of arms with relative preservation of legs; corticospinal tract signs in legs but not arms; frequently painful in arms
Neoplastic cord compression	Pain in spine region; ultimately, weakness and sensory loss below level of lesion
Neoplastic meningitis	Multifocal motor and sensory loss in distribution of individual dermatomes; pain common with nerve root infiltration
Spinal stenosis	Back pain, often exacerbated by walking; patchy weakness and reflex changes in the legs, usually in a dermatomal distribution
Syrinx	Loss of pain and temperature sensation at level of the lesion, followed by lower motor neuron signs and then long track signs and more definite myelopathy

More severe disease produces quadriparesis with spasticity and sphincter dysfunction, palsies of cranial nerve (CN) IX to CN XII, and downbeat nystagmus. Dysfunction of higher cervical roots produces weakness of paraspinal muscles that, in conjunction with accessory palsy, can produce impairment of head posture.

Common causes of craniocervical junction lesions include tumors at the craniocervical junction and subluxation or fracture of C1. Differential diagnosis includes cervical cord and brainstem lesions. Cord lesions do not produce palsies of the lower CNs. Lower cervical cord lesions spare proximal upper extremity motor function and do not affect phrenic nerve function. Brainstem lesions typically produce alterations in consciousness, except for the locked-in syndrome. In craniocervical lesions, the deficits in CN VII and CN VI nerve function are evident.

CERVICAL CORD

Central Cord Syndrome

Central cord syndrome is usually due to trauma, although it can be due to intrinsic lesions of the cord, including tumors and syringomyelia. When due to trauma, it is usually from hyperextension of the neck. The patient presents with weakness of the arms with relative preservation of the legs, which is called man-in-a-barrel syndrome. Some degree of quadriparesis is almost always present, including hyperreflexia and upward plantar responses in the legs. The reflexes may be depressed in the arms, especially early in the course. Pain in the hands and arms is common and may be severe.

The clinical findings of central cord syndrome are probably due to damage to the central gray matter. Quadriparesis suggests damage to the lateral corticospinal tracts. There may be dissociated sensory loss in the arms; that is, there may be a deficit in pain and temperature sensation with preservation of touch, vibration, and proprioception. This combination occurs because of involvement of the crossing axons of the anterolateral tracts.

Cervical Spondylosis

Spondylosis is growth of osteophytes resulting in ankylosis, or loss of mobility, of the spine. Encroachment on the spinal canal produces damage to segmental nerve roots and compression to the spinal cord. Neurologic symptoms can be from radiculopathy due to damage to individual nerve roots at affected levels or from myelopathy due to damage to descending tracts.

Cervical spondylosis is most common at the C5 to 6 level, with less common involvement at the C6 to 7 and C4 to 5 levels. C5 to 6 spondylosis results in weakness and atrophy of muscles innervated by these roots, especially the biceps and deltoid. Biceps reflex is usually depressed. If there is myelopathy, reflexes below this level will be brisk with upward plantar responses. Corticospinal tract dysfunction often produces incoordination of the hands.

Differential diagnosis of cervical spondylosis includes other causes of myelopathy including tumors. Amyotrophic lateral sclerosis (ALS) is commonly mistaken for cervical spondylosis with myelopathy because ALS frequently presents with weakness of the hands and corticospinal tracts in the legs. Many patients with ALS undergo imaging studies of the cervical spine to rule out spondylosis. A differentiating feature is the prominent wasting of intrinsic muscles of the hand seen in most ALS patients; this finding is distinctly absent in cervical spondylosis, which rarely affects C8 and T1 nerve roots. However, if there is any doubt as to the correct diagnosis, imaging should be done because cervical spondylosis is potentially treatable.

THORACIC CORD

Causes of lesions in the thoracic region include vascular occlusion, tumors, disc disease, trauma, transverse myelitis, MS, and abscess. Pain as an early symptom suggests an extrinsic lesion producing cord compression, whereas absence of pain suggests an intrinsic lesion, whether neoplastic or inflammatory. The anterior spinal artery syndrome is the most common vascular lesion in the thoracic cord.

Lesions of the upper thoracic cord may have few findings other than those that would help define a sensory level, along with corticospinal tract signs when white matter tracts are affected. Lesions of the lower thoracic cord, especially below T9, may preserve function of the upper abdominal muscles; this condition can result in rostral movement of the umbilicus with a sit-up maneuver (Beevor sign). Testing of the abdominal reflexes can be helpful in these cases.

LUMBAR CORD

The most common lesions affecting the lumbar cord region are lumbar radiculopathy and spinal stenosis. Tumors and other compressive lesions can affect the cauda equina and conus medullaris.

Lumbar Spondylosis and Spinal Stenosis

Spondylosis develops in the lumbar area, just as it does in the cervical spinal cord. Degenerative changes include osteophyte formation, hypertrophy of the posterior ligaments, disc protrusion, and facet hypertrophy. Spondylolisthesis is forward slippage of a vertebral body on the bone beneath. The defect can be degenerative or congenital.

Spinal stenosis is characterized by reduced caliber of the spinal canal, usually due to severe degenerative changes. Spondylosis, ligamentum flavum hypertrophy, and disc protrusion encroach on the subarachnoid space. Patients complain of back pain, often exacerbated by walking, and leg pain with standing and walking (neurogenic claudication). The spinal claudication is probably due to direct nerve compression rather than ischemia of the lower cord and/or nerve roots. A vascular component is possible since ambulation causes venous engorgement, resulting in reduced effective caliber of the canal and resultant increased compression of the vascular and neural elements.

Diagnosis of spinal stenosis is confirmed by magnetic resonance imaging (MRI), computed tomography (CT), or myelography of the lumbar spine. Postmyelographic CT scanning can clearly demonstrate the absence of subarachnoid space at affected levels.

An important differential diagnosis is vascular claudication of the legs because both spinal stenosis and vascular claudication can produce pain with walking. No clinical features are diagnostic, but there are some general guidelines.

Spinal stenosis is suggested by the following:
- Pain most prominent in the thigh
- Neurologic symptoms with exertion, including weakness and dysesthesias
- Improvement over at least several minutes during sitting but not during standing after cessation of exertion
- Positional nature of exertional pain, for instance, greater difficulty walking downhill than uphill but little difficulty bicycling
- Stooped posture
- Peripheral pulses usually present

Vascular claudication is suggested by the following:
- Pain most prominent in the calf
- No or only vague neurologic symptoms with exertion
- Improvement within seconds to a few minutes after cessation of exertion; sitting usually not required
- No positional nature of exertional pain
- Peripheral pulses usually absent

Cauda Equina and Conus Medullaris Lesions

The cauda equina (literally, horse's tail) consists of the lower lumbar and sacral nerve roots. Lesions of the cauda equina produce asymmetric pain and sensory loss in the caudal roots; most symptoms are due to dysfunction of L4 to S2. The ankle tendon reflex is commonly absent. Bowel and bladder symptoms develop with severe disease. Important lesions affecting the cauda equina are lumbar disc disease and spondylosis, ependymoma, metastatic tumors, and trauma with subluxation.

The conus medullaris is the terminal portion of the spinal cord; it is the origination of the most caudal nerve roots. Patients present with bowel and bladder dysfunction early in the disease, whereas these symptoms develop later in cauda equina lesions. Sensory loss in the perineal region may develop. Involvement of the conus medullaris may produce corticospinal tract signs, including upward plantar response and hyperreflexia of the Achilles tendon reflex. At the same time, weakness of distal muscles and loss of knee reflexes suggest a lower motor neuron lesion. Important lesions affecting the conus medullaris are the same as those affecting the cauda equina.

SACRAL CORD

S1 is the sacral root most commonly damaged by degenerative disease of the lumbar spine. Patients present with weakness of the gastrocnemius and intrinsic muscles of the feet. Sensory loss affects the sole of the foot.

S2 lesion produces weakness, which is most prominent in the intrinsic muscles of the feet, but it may be subtle. Sensory loss affects the saddle area.

Lower sacral lesions are rare; they may be caused by trauma or tumors involving the sacrum. Bowel and bladder symptoms and impotence predominate; there are no leg symptoms or signs.

Clinical Correlations

MECHANICAL MYELOPATHIES

Compressive myelopathies are often due to protrusion of intervertebral discs; intraspinal tumors; or invasion into the cord by tumors involving spinal bony structures, intraspinal infection, or hematomas.

These are usually suspected by a development of motor and sensory deficits that conform roughly to a level. The speed of development is a clue to the diagnosis. Epidural hematoma would be rapid in onset and would often occur after lumbar puncture or other instrumentation, whereas meningioma produces slowly progressive deficits as it grows. Lesions associated with more severe spine pain are likely to be inflammatory (e.g., abscess), more rapidly developing, or associated with bony destruction, although this general guide is not definitive.

Spinal Cord Trauma

Trauma is a common cause of spinal cord injury. In a young patient, motor vehicle accidents are the most common cause. In older patients, falls are most common. Other etiologies can include sports, assault, and others.

Spinal cord injury following a sports injury can be suggested by:
- Leg weakness more than arm weakness.
- Sensory disturbance below the lesion.
- Early hyporeflexia followed by hyperreflexia and corticospinal tract signs such as extensor plantar responses.
- Local spinal region pain.

Diagnosis of spinal cord trauma is focused first on stabilizing the patient and then on determining whether emergent surgical intervention is needed. CT and MRI are commonly used for this purpose, although myelography is still occasionally done especially when other imaging modalities cannot be performed or are inconclusive.

Tumors Affecting the Spinal Cord

Tumors affecting the spinal cord can be classified into the following categories:
- Extradural
- Intradural but extramedullary
- Intramedullary

Extradural tumors are the most common, and they are usually due to metastases from systemic neoplasms. Lung, breast, renal, and gastrointestinal tumors first metastasize to the bone and subsequently expand into the spinal canal, producing extrinsic cord compression. Involvement of a local nerve root may result in radicular pain, weakness, and sensory loss. The vast majority of tumors affecting the spine have associated back pain, so absence of back pain would be strong, though not absolute, evidence against a spinal tumor. Lymphomas extend from the paravertebral region through a nerve root foramen into the spinal canal, also producing cord compression. Radicular symptoms are expected.

Intradural but extramedullary tumors are usually neurofibromas or meningiomas. They produce all of the signs and symptoms of extrinsic cord compression, although there may be signs of nerve root compression as well.

Intramedullary tumors are usually gliomas. They frequently produce initial symptoms by involvement of the gray matter. With progression, there is involvement of the white matter with subsequent development of corticospinal tract signs. Back pain may be present, but it is less common than with extradural tumors. Radicular pain is unusual with intramedullary tumors.

Diagnosis of spinal tumors is usually by MRI. If the expected lesion is not found, complete myelography may be indicated.

Syringomyelia

Syringomyelia is a cyst in the spinal gray matter that extends longitudinally over several segments. It is different from hydromyelia, which is abnormal enlargement of the central canal. Syrinx is commonly due to a Chiari malformation, which is thought to produce the cyst by causing blockage of cerebrospinal fluid flow, pressure waves within the central canal, subsequent rupture of the central canal into the surrounding parenchyma, and ultimate formation of the cyst. The mass effect of the syrinx will initially damage the crossing fibers destined for the anterior spinothalamic tract, which convey pain and temperature sensation. Subsequently, damage to the gray matter at the levels of the syrinx will produce motor neuron degeneration. With more severe enlargement, compression of white matter tracts will produce signs below the level of the lesion, including spasticity and sensory loss.

Patients present with loss of pain and temperature sensation at the levels of the lesion; with cervical syrinx, this loss occurs across the shoulders and arms, sometimes described as a cape or shawl distribution. Weakness from lower motor neuron degeneration at the level of the lesion develops. With white matter compression, spasticity below the lesion and sensory loss below the lesion develops; at this stage, it is difficult to differentiate a syrinx on clinical grounds from other causes of myelopathy.

Differential diagnosis includes other causes of myelopathy including tumors. Intraparenchymal tumors, usually gliomas, may present in a fashion indistinguishable from syrinx. Diagnosis is by MRI.

Brown-Séquard Syndrome

Spinal cord hemisection is known as Brown-Séquard syndrome. The classic description is based on complete surgical section of one lateral half of the cord, and it is a lesion rarely seen in clinical practice. However, elements of the Brown-Séquard syndrome are seen in some patients with traumatic injuries, tumors, demyelinating diseases, asymmetric spondylosis, and, rarely, infections of the spine.

Ipsilateral findings at the level of the lesion include weakness of muscles innervated by this dermatome. Below the level of the lesion, deficits of vibration and proprioception, muscle weakness, and corticospinal tract signs are seen. There are no contralateral findings at the level of the lesion; however, below the level of the lesion, there are deficits in pain and temperature sensation.

The most important clinical findings for diagnosis of the syndrome are those below the level of the lesion. Deficit and pain help localize the dermatomal level of the lesion.

VASCULAR DISEASE

Vascular disease of the spinal cord is uncommon; when present, it can be difficult to diagnose clinically. History is as important as physical examination. The abrupt onset of a deficit localized to the spinal cord in the absence of trauma suggests a vascular event. The most important spinal vascular syndromes are infarction due to occlusion of the anterior spinal artery and hemorrhage from vascular malformations and trauma.

Anterior Spinal Artery Syndrome

Probably the most common spinal vascular syndrome is infarction due to direct compression of the vessels by mass lesions, which is the reason mass lesions may produce acute onset or worsening of symptoms. Occlusion of the anterior spinal artery produces infarction of most of the spinal cord, excluding the dorsal aspect of the dorsal horn and dorsal columns. The occlusion is commonly due to damage to the artery of Adamkiewicz; the artery can be occluded as it arises from the aorta. Cross-clamping of the aorta is a common cause of infarction.

Patients present with paralysis below the level of the lesion. Sensory findings are important and include deficit in pain and temperature sensation below the level of the lesion with relative preservation of vibration and proprioception due to lack of involvement of the dorsal columns. Light touch is preserved, although patients often report that touch feels different. When the artery of Adamkiewicz is occluded, the rostral level of the lesion is between T9 and L1. When the anterior spinal artery is directly occluded, a lesion in the upper thoracic or upper lumbar region is more common.

Anterior spinal artery syndrome is differentiated from other causes of myelopathy by the preservation of vibration and proprioception. Few other causes of myelopathy present with as abrupt an onset.

Posterior Spinal Artery Occlusion

Infarction due to occlusion of the posterior spinal arteries is much less common than infarction due to occlusion of the anterior spinal artery. Posterior spinal artery occlusion presents with loss of vibration and proprioception below the level of the lesion.

Hemorrhage

Arteriovenous malformations and venous angiomas can occur in the spinal column in the subarachnoid space or in the parenchyma of the spinal cord. Symptoms develop because of hemorrhage with subsequent mass effect and infarction; the malformation of Foix-Alajouanine often produces symptoms by thrombosis. Patients present with back pain, weakness of the legs, and sensory symptoms that may be intermittent. Symptoms may develop after trauma or childbirth and may be incorrectly attributed solely to spinal injury. Diagnosis is usually made by MRI.

Aneurysms can occur in the spinal column but are responsible for less than 1% of subarachnoid hemorrhages. Patients present with acute onset of back pain, and the pain quickly extends to involve other spinal regions and the head. When the patient presents obtunded, there may be no clue that the origin was spinal; however, a spinal source should be considered if arteriography is unrevealing.

Spinal epidural and subdural hematomas may occur due to seemingly trivial trauma. Children are more likely to develop hemorrhage in the cervical region, whereas adults develop hemorrhage in the thoracic and lumbar regions. Patients present with severe spinal pain in the affected region followed by development of motor and sensory symptoms appropriate to the level of the lesion.

Intraparenchymal hemorrhage not due to vascular malformation can develop after spinal injury, and it can present with a central cord syndrome or myelopathy. The location of the lesion is a determinant of the symptoms.

TOXIC, METABOLIC, AND NUTRITIONAL DISORDERS

The spectrum of toxic, metabolic, and nutritional myelopathies is not as broad as for encephalopathy, but there are some important causes.

Vitamin B12 Deficiency

Vitamin B12 deficiency can present neurologically with various combinations of neuropathy, cognitive disorder, and myelopathy. The damage to the spinal cord is predominately of the dorsal and lateral columns producing motor deficits of myelopathy along with sensory deficits. Many, but not all, patients will have macrocytic anemia.

Presenting symptoms are often diffuse limb weakness and sensory loss and are often associated with cerebellar ataxia. Corticospinal tract signs may be present. B12 deficiency is considered when patients present with both peripheral neuropathic and corticospinal tract signs.

Copper Deficiency

Copper deficiency can produce myelopathy. Causes include defects in absorption and excessive zinc intake. This is another cause of combined peripheral neuropathic and myelopathic deficits. Findings of the myelopathy are both motor with corticospinal tract signs and sensory with deficits, especially in vibration and proprioception sensation. Findings of the peripheral neuropathic involvement include distal sensory loss and suppressed distal reflexes. With B12 deficiency, this is a cause of extensor plantar responses and absent ankle reflexes.

Copper deficiency is suspected when patients exhibit the peripheral and central findings. However, both do not have to be present, so copper deficiency can be missed when the deficit is predominately myelopathic. Copper levels are low in most patients, although borderline deficiency probably can produce symptoms. When copper deficiency is suspected, B12 should be checked and vice versa.

Vitamin E Deficiency

Vitamin E deficiency is uncommon and is more often due to malabsorption than deficient nutritional intake. Vitamin E deficiency can produce myelopathy, and associated findings can suggest a spinocerebellar syndrome.

Nitrous Oxide Toxicity

Nitrous oxide is often used as an anesthetic but more often is toxic when used recreationally. Clinical manifestations are almost identical to those of B12 deficiency because nitrous oxide interferes with the intracellular function of B12. Myelopathy is often associated with peripheral neuropathy and cognitive dysfunction, as can be seen with B12 deficiency.

INFECTIOUS AND INFLAMMATORY DISORDERS

Poliomyelitis

Polio is infection of the spinal cord and brainstem by an enterovirus. Polio is occasionally seen in nonimmunized patients. In immunized patients, polio is due to either incomplete inactivation of the virus contained in the vaccine or a type of virus not included in the vaccine.

The virus infects motor neurons of the spinal cord and/or brainstem, producing weakness and atrophy of affected muscles. The weakness is commonly asymmetric, with preferential involvement of distal muscles. Reflexes are depressed and are usually absent, differentiating this finding from the results of a central lesion.

Bulbar involvement occurs in about 15% of patients with polio. CNs prominently affected are the facial, glossopharyngeal, and vagus. Involvement of the reticular formation produces impaired respiration. Patients may develop encephalitis with impaired level of consciousness, but this is a rare occurrence.

Transverse Myelitis

Transverse myelitis is a clinical syndrome that may include several disorders. Patients present with an onset of myelopathy that progresses over hours to days. Back pain and vague sensory symptoms may precede objective signs of myelopathy. A minority of patients will report a preceding febrile illness, but this is not a useful clinical feature.

Transverse myelitis is an isolated entity in most patients. Only some 7% subsequently develop MS.

Multiple Sclerosis

MS is characterized by zones of demyelination with preservation of axons. The spinal cord is often though not invariably involved, producing myelopathy that resembles transverse myelitis. The diagnosis is suspected by medical history or examination of other demyelinating lesions either in the past or subsequent to the myelopathy. Common associated symptoms include visual loss, hemiparesis or hemisensory loss, and ataxia.

Diagnosis of MS is established by clinical criteria and MRI. When a patient presents with myelopathy, MRI of the brain is often ordered. Areas of spinal demyelination that are longer that three spinal segments are known as longitudinally extensive lesions, the presence of which raises the suspicion of a disorder other than MS. These disorders include neuromyelitis optica (NMO) (Devic disease) due to the anti-aquaporin-4 (water channel) antibody or subacute combined degeneration caused by vitamin B12 deficiency or copper deficiency.

Neuromyelitis Optica Spectrum Disorder

Neuromyelitis optica spectrum disorder (NMOSD) is an inflammatory disorder characterized mainly by demyelination but also by axonal loss. The name is derived from the predilection to affect the spinal cord and optic nerves. For many years, the disorder was known as NMO or Devic disease. As experience identified involvement other than spinal cord and optic nerves, "spectrum disorder" was added to the name. The brainstem is the most commonly affected region outside of spinal cord and optic nerves, but there can be other involvement. NMOSD is not MS, which is pathophysiologically distinct.

NMOSD is considered when a patient presents with transverse myelitis or optic neuritis. As such, patients present with visual loss in one or both eyes and/or myelopathy. Diagnosis is established by clinical presentation supported by MRI evidence of demyelination and laboratory tests including antibody to aquaporin-4 (AQP4) or myelin oligodendrocyte glycoprotein (MOG).

Tabes Dorsalis and Syphilitic Myelitis

Tabes dorsalis is due to involvement of the dorsal roots by late neurosyphilis. This is rarely seen. There is meningeal inflammation and inflammatory changes in the dorsal roots. Damage to these axons results in atrophy of the dorsal root ganglia and dorsal columns. Patients present with sensory ataxia; their balance and gait difficulties are due to lack of correct sensory information regarding limb position. Classically there is a slapping gait. Reflexes are depressed, as is common with sensory deficits.

Involvement of the ventral roots may produce weakness and atrophy, but these findings are much less prominent than the sensory findings. Associated neurologic findings are clues to the diagnosis. The Argyll Robertson pupil is discussed in Chapter 3.4, and other pupillary abnormalities can be seen as well. Charcot joints are joints that have been destroyed due to absence of detection of pain. Other cranial neuropathies may be present, producing ptosis, facial weakness, and/ or hearing loss. Bowel and bladder reflexes are impaired because of damage to afferents. However, there are no findings to suggest corticospinal damage.

A rarer cause of spinal cord dysfunction is syphilitic myelitis, which presents as progressive weakness and spasticity below the level of involvement. This condition tends to occur earlier in the course of syphilis than tabes dorsalis.

DEGENERATIVE DISORDERS

Motor neuron diseases are prominent degenerative disorders affecting spinal cord neurons. These include spinal muscular atrophy (SMA), ALS, progressive muscular atrophy (PMA), and primary lateral sclerosis (PLS).

Spinal Muscular Atrophy

SMA usually presents in young life, from the neonatal period to young adulthood; age of onset probably reflects rate of progression of the motor neuron degeneration rather than different pathophysiological entities Nevertheless, SMA is considered to be three entities: infantile-onset SMA (Werdnig-Hoffman disease), juvenile onset SMA (Kugelberg-Welander disease), and adult-onset SMA. All three are characterized by progressive degeneration of motor neurons.

Adults and older children present with progressive proximal weakness and muscle atrophy, especially in the legs. Infants present with hypotonia and weakness of facial and pharyngeal muscles. Tendon reflexes are reduced because of the decreased number of functioning motor units. Sensory function is normal.

SMA is most commonly inherited through autosomal recessive inheritance, although some patients with adult onset and rare patients with juvenile onset have autosomal dominant inheritance.

Differential diagnosis of SMA includes many myopathies and neuropathies. The purely motor character of the findings eliminates most neuropathies. Proximal predominance is common in SMA, so this cannot be used to differentiate it from myopathies. Electromyography (EMG) shows different patterns in myopathy and motor neuron degeneration and therefore can confirm clinical differentiation between motor neuron diseases, such as SMA, and myopathy.

Differentiation of SMA from ALS is by absence of corticospinal tract signs. Differentiation of adult-onset SMA from PMA is difficult, but the latter usually presents with very asymmetric weakness, which often involves only one limb for years. Bulbar involvement with PMA is unusual.

Primary lateral sclerosis

PLS is an upper motor neuron degeneration that usually presents initially with weakness and spasticity in the legs. Unlike ALS, there is no lower motor neuron involvement, at least initially. With time, there is often bulbar motor involvement. Also, there may be development of lower motor neuron findings later in the disease.

Diagnosis is suspected when a patient presents with mainly leg weakness and spasticity with no signs of fasciculations on examination or denervation on EMG.

Progressive Muscular Atrophy

PMA is thought to be a variant of ALS, and it accounts for approximately 10% of patients with ALS. Patients present with atrophy and weakness of limb muscles. Later in the course, generalized muscular atrophy and fasciculations develop.

PMA is suspected with lower motor neuron deficits without sensory findings and with no upper motor neuron deficits. Later in the disease course, many patients do develop upper motor neuron findings.

Amyotrophic Lateral Sclerosis

ALS is characterized by degeneration of spinal and bulbar motor neurons and degeneration of upper motor neurons. As a result, patients have weakness, atrophy, and fasciculations characteristic of lower motor neuron disease plus upper motor neuron signs, including hyperreflexia and extensor plantar responses. Differential diagnosis includes SMA; ALS is differentiated from SMA by the presence of corticospinal tract signs in ALS. Differentiation from cervical spondylosis is discussed in the section on cervical spondylosis earlier in this chapter.

Peripheral Nervous System

Karl E. Misulis and Eli E. Zimmerman

Approach to Diagnosis

Neuromuscular disorders have specific clinical findings, as discussed here, but part of the task of neuromuscular localization is ruling out a lesion of the spinal cord or brain. Central disorders producing peripheral manifestations usually affect systems other than the peripheral nervous system or have an anatomic distribution that would be unusual with a peripheral lesion. For example, weakness in a left median distribution would suggest a peripheral lesion. Weakness in a median and ulnar distribution would suggest a single lesion at the level of the brachial plexus or higher. If the ipsilateral leg is also weak, a single lesion would have to be in the central nervous system (CNS). Once the disorder has been identified as being neuromuscular, differential diagnosis depends on detailed anatomical localization, which requires distinguishing among lesions in the following locations:

- Muscle
- Nerve
- Neuromuscular junction

Disorders of muscle and neuromuscular junction produce pure motor symptoms. Only a few nerve disorders produce pure motor symptoms, and those include motor neuron diseases and multifocal motor neuropathy. Reflexes are commonly preserved in disorders of muscle and the neuromuscular junction, unless the weakness is severe. Severe hyporeflexia or areflexia suggests neuropathy and is most common in sensory neuropathy.

NERVE CONDUCTION STUDIES AND ELECTROMYOGRAPHY

Nerve conduction velocity (NCV) and electromyography (EMG) aid with the differential diagnosis by localizing and classifying the defect by differentiating muscle from nerve from neuromuscular junction dysfunction (Table 3.6.1). For patients with neuropathy, the studies can differentiate axonal from demyelinating syndromes and determine which nerves are affected.

Neuropathy typically produces slowing of peripheral NCV and/or reduced amplitude of the compound motor action potential (CMAP) and sensory nerve action potential (SNAP). With chronic denervation, EMG shows fibrillation potentials and positive sharp waves due to spontaneous action potentials in denervated muscle fibers and shows large-amplitude polyphasic motor unit potentials indicative of reinnervation of muscle fibers by surviving motor axons. Acutely, EMG may only show reduced numbers of functioning units. Neuropathy may be characterized by degeneration mostly of axons, neuron cell bodies, or myelin sheath.

Myopathy produces normal nerve conductions, except that the CMAP may be reduced because of the reduced number of muscle fibers activated by the action potentials. Motor unit potentials are small for the same reason, and they are often polyphasic because of dispersed action potential activation and propagation in the muscle fiber membrane. This combination is often called the brief, small-amplitude polyphasic potential.

119

TABLE 3.6.1 ■ **Neurodiagnostic Findings With Lesion Locations**

Lesion	CMAP	SNAP	Motor NCV	Sensory NCV	EMG
Motor neuropathy	Reduced	Normal	Normal or near normal	Normal	Denervation
Sensory neuropathy	Normal	Low amplitude	Normal	Mild slowing or absent	Normal
Axonopathy	Reduced	Reduced or absent	Normal or near normal	Normal or near normal	Denervation
Demyelinating neuropathy	Dispersed	Dispersed or absent	Slow; conduction block	Slow or absent	Normal or denervation
Myopathy	Normal or low amplitude	Normal	Normal	Normal	Myopathic pattern
Neuromuscular transmission defect	Normal or low amplitude	Normal	Normal	Normal	Normal or myopathic

CMAP, Compound motor action potential; *EMG,* electromyography; *NCV,* nerve conduction velocity; *SNAP,* sensory nerve action potential.

Neuromuscular transmission defects have normal NCVs except for reduction of CMAP amplitude, especially in myasthenic syndrome. Repetitive stimulation produces a changing CMAP; the effect of repetitive stimulation differs with individual disorders and stimulation frequency (discussed later).

MUSCLE AND NERVE BIOPSY

Muscle biopsy is indicated for patients in whom the following diagnoses are suspected:
- Muscular dystrophy
- Inflammatory myopathy
  - Polymyositis
  - Dermatomyositis
  - Infectious or parasitic myopathy
- Mitochondrial myopathy
- Glycogen and lipid storage disorders
- Vasculitis

Muscle biopsy shows infiltration in most patients with inflammatory myopathies. Dermatomyositis classically features atrophy of the fibers at the periphery of the fascicles, individual fibers undergoing degeneration and regeneration, and perivascular inflammation; however, dermatomyositis may sometimes not show such classic features. Muscular dystrophies are characterized by degenerating and regenerating muscle fibers and replacement of muscle tissue by connective tissue. Sural nerve biopsy is indicated for patients in whom the following diagnoses are suspected:
- Vasculitis
- Some demyelinating neuropathies
- Amyloidosis
- Some familial and suspected metabolic neuropathies

For individuals with storage disorders, assays for specific enzymes may be revealing. Focal regions of vascular inflammation suggest vasculitis. Leprosy shows infiltration of white blood cells into nerve segments, and the bacteria may be demonstrated on special stains.

LABORATORY TESTS

Creatine kinase (CK) is elevated in most patients with inflammatory myopathy, and it is modestly elevated in some patients with denervating diseases. CK is normal in most neuropathies and in all predominantly sensory neuropathies. CK is often normal in metabolic myopathies. Duchenne muscular dystrophy is associated with a marked elevation in CK, but the increase may be less marked or absent in other dystrophies. Aldolase is also increased in many myopathies; it is less increased in other neuromuscular conditions.

Laboratory tests depend on the type of neuropathy, although many clinicians perform a general battery of tests without regard to the type of neuropathy. The following list of tests may be adapted to the specific type of neuropathy:

- Complete metabolic profile (CMP)
- Complete blood count
- Vitamin B12 and folate levels
- Thyroid function (free T4 and thyroid-stimulating hormone)
- Rapid plasma reagin (RPR)
- 24-hour urine for heavy metals
- Serum protein electrophoresis, serum immunoelectrophoresis, and urine immunoelectrophoresis

Depending on clinical findings, additional tests may be indicated, including human immunodeficiency virus (HIV), red cell cholinesterase, blood lead, lactate, antinuclear antibody (ANA), erythrocyte sedimentation rate, C-reactive protein, and heavy metals. Clinicians should ideally first classify the neuropathy and then judiciously select tests to look for disorders that produce that type of neuropathy.

Neuropathies

Localization and diagnosis of some important neuropathies are presented in this section.

DIFFERENTIAL DIAGNOSIS

Anatomic localization of the lesion in patients with neuropathy is critical to the differential diagnosis. With characterization of the neuropathy, the list of possible diagnoses is narrowed. For example, a subacute demyelinating sensorimotor polyneuropathy would be most suggestive of Guillain-Barré syndrome. A chronic pure motor neuronopathy would be most suggestive of amyotrophic lateral sclerosis (ALS) or spinal muscular atrophy (SMA). Neuropathy should be classified according to the following criteria:

- Modality: Motor, sensory, autonomic, or a combination
- Chronicity: Acute, subacute, or chronic
- Pathology: Neuronal, axonal, or demyelinating
- Distribution: Focal, multifocal, or generalized
- Age at onset

Table 3.6.2 lists some important neuromuscular disorders and their classification according to this scheme.

Modality

Modalities include motor, sensory, and autonomic function. This discussion focuses on motor and sensory function. The most common neuropathies are sensorimotor, indicating damage to peripheral nerves without preference to modality. Pure motor or pure sensory neuropathies are usually due to direct neuronal damage at the soma, that is, at the motor neurons (anterior horn cells) or dorsal root ganglion neurons, respectively.

TABLE 3.6.2 ■ Important Neuropathies and Neuronopathies

Disorder	Chronicity	Distribution	Modality	Pathology
Amyotrophic lateral sclerosis	C	G	M	A
Carpal tunnel syndrome	C	F	SM	A, D
CIDP	C	MF	SM	D
Conduction block neuropathy	C	MF	M, SM	D
Diabetic neuropathy	C	G, MF, F	S, SM	A
Guillain-Barré syndrome	A or S	G	SM	D
Spinal muscular atrophy	C	G	M	A

CIDP, Chronic inflammatory demyelinating polyneuropathy. Chronicity: A, Acute; C, chronic; S, subacute.
  Distribution: F, Focal; G, generalized; MF, multifocal. Modality: M, Motor; S, sensory; SM, sensorimotor.
  Pathology: A, Axonal; D, demyelinating.

Motor neuropathies are characterized clinically by weakness often with fasciculations and muscle cramps. NCV testing shows low-amplitude CMAPs and occasionally reduced motor NCVs, depending on pathology. EMG shows denervation in affected muscles.

Sensory neuropathies are characterized clinically by loss of sensation and presence of abnormal sensations. Terminology usage can be conflicting, but terms commonly use are paresthesia and dysesthesia. In this chapter, paresthesias are abnormal perception of sensation, such as a tingling sensation. Dysesthesias are abnormal spontaneous sensations with a painful character. These are usually both spontaneous and evoked or modulated by sensory stimulation. If large-diameter axons are involved in the neuropathy, the abnormal sensation is commonly tingling, whereas if small fibers are predominantly involved, the sensation is often burning. NCV testing in pure sensory neuropathies shows reduced SNAP amplitude and often slow sensory NCV depending on pathology. EMG shows no denervation in muscle.

Sensorimotor neuropathies are characterized by the combined symptoms of motor and sensory neuropathies; however, fasciculations are unusual. NCV testing shows low-amplitude CMAPs and SNAPs with moderate to severe axonal neuropathies. Demyelinating neuropathies produce slow motor and sensory NCVs and have focal areas of conduction block early in the course.

Autonomic neuropathies are characterized clinically by vasomotor and gastrointestinal motility dysfunction; the most common effects are orthostatic hypotension and gastroparesis. Conventional NCV testing and EMG show no abnormalities unless sensory neuropathy and motor neuropathy coexist. Special studies of sympathetic function can reveal the dysfunction.

Chronicity

Most neuropathies are chronic. Neurotoxins tend to produce CNS symptoms acutely, with neuropathy as a delayed effect that often appears only after prolonged exposure. The classification of chronicity for neuropathy is a bit different from that of other deficits, such as corticospinal tract dysfunction. One useful definition is acute = 4 weeks or less, subacute = 4 to 8 weeks, and chronic = longer than 8 weeks.

By this classification, acute neuropathies are predominantly mononeuropathies, such as pressure palsies and nerve infarctions. Guillain-Barré syndrome (with the most common version being acute inflammatory demyelinating polyneuropathy; AIDP), porphyria, diphtheria, and critical illness neuropathy. Subacute neuropathies include some presentations of B12 deficiency, diabetic amyotrophy, vasculitis, and subacute inflammatory demyelinating polyneuropathy (SIDP).

Chronic neuropathies include most others, including chronic inflammatory demyelinating polyneuropathy (CIDP).

Pathology

Pathology reveals the type of neuropathy. There are three basic types: axonal, neuronal, and demyelinating. In addition, there is a classification based on the type of damage: neurapraxia, axonotmesis, and neurotmesis.

- Neurapraxia is traumatic disruption of nerve fiber function without transection of axons.
- Axonotmesis is traumatic breakage of axons with an intact connective tissue sheath.
- Neurotmesis is complete transection of the nerve.

Axonal neuropathies are caused by degeneration of the axons and form the largest group of neuropathies. Longer axons are affected more severely, so the symptoms and signs are more prominent distally. No symptoms are particularly distinctive for axonal neuropathy; differentiation from demyelination is made predominantly on the basis of NCV testing and EMG. Examination reveals preserved tendon reflexes in patients with axonal neuropathies in contrast to the depressed reflexes seen with demyelinating neuropathies. Muscle weakness is accompanied by muscle atrophy, which is more prominent with increasing chronicity.

Neuronopathies are caused by degeneration of the nerve cell body and imply a metabolic or genetic defect. Because the motor neurons and dorsal root ganglion neurons are usually not directly affected by the same pathological process, the symptoms will be motor or sensory, depending on the neurons involved. Neuronopathies are difficult to distinguish clinically from axonopathies. Features that would suggest a neuronopathy include involvement of a single modality, fasciculations, reduced CMAP or SNAP with normal NCV, and denervation of distal and very proximal muscles, such as the paraspinals.

Demyelinating neuropathies are characterized clinically by motor and sensory symptoms, especially weakness, paresthesias, dysesthesias, and sensory loss. Symptoms may be both proximal and distal, although distal musculature is predominantly affected. Demyelinating neuropathies often lack the distal symmetric ascending character of axonal neuropathies. Examination shows depressed tendon reflexes; for example, the diagnosis of is less likely if tendon reflexes are preserved, even early in the course. Depressed tendon reflexes are the main differentiating feature from axonal and neuronal degenerations. If the tendon reflexes are depressed out of proportion to the weakness, a demyelinating neuropathy is suspected. Motor and sensory NCVs are slow. CMAPs and SNAPs are low in amplitude with a dispersed waveform, in contrast to the low-amplitude preserved wave-shape seen in axonal neuropathies. Demyelinating neuropathies frequently produce prominent weakness with unimpressive atrophy compared with that seen in axonal neuropathies.

Distribution

Neuropathies are focal, multifocal, or generalized. Patients with generalized neuropathies are predisposed to develop pressure palsies, which present as focal neuropathies.

Focal neuropathies are commonly compressive, although there can be vascular causes. Common damaged areas are the median nerve at the carpal tunnel, the ulnar nerve at the ulnar groove, and the peroneal nerve at the fibular neck.

Multifocal neuropathies are usually due to a systemic disorder. Important causes include diabetes, leprosy, polyarteritis nodosa, and other vasculitides. Familial predisposition to pressure palsies may also present with the symptoms of mononeuropathy multiplex.

Generalized neuropathies usually have a distal predominance, although examination, NCV testing, and EMG reveal both proximal and distal damage. Because of the distal symptoms, upper extremity dysfunction may be revealed only on NCV testing and EMG.

Age of Onset

Many neuropathies that occur in adults do not occur in children. For example, a chronic pure motor neuronopathy in an adult would most likely be ALS; in children, it would more likely be SMA. SMA can occur later in life but does so only rarely. The presence of signs of upper motor neuron involvement would add more security to the diagnosis of ALS. Important neuropathies and neuronopathies in children include the following:

- SMA
- Metabolic disorders (e.g., storage disease)
- Juvenile diabetes with neuropathy
- Vincristine neuropathy in children with certain cancers
- Guillain-Barré syndrome
- Hereditary neuropathies
- Polyneuropathies

The most important differentiating feature in polyneuropathies is between axonal and demyelinating. Most metabolic neuropathies are axonal, including diabetes, renal neuropathy, and most drug-induced neuropathies. Demyelinating neuropathies are rarer and include the immune-mediated neuropathies.

DIABETIC NEUROPATHY

Diabetic neuropathy can be of several types, with predominance of sensory neuropathy, sensorimotor neuropathy, mononeuropathies, and mononeuropathy multiples. More uncommon is a diabetic lumbosacral polyradiculopathy.

Diagnosis depends on documentation of the elements that are affected. Is almost every nerve affected or only individual nerves? Is the affected element proximal or distal? EMG aids with documentation of the type. These are further discussed in Chapter 3.6.

IMMUNE-MEDIATED NEUROPATHIES

There are many immune-mediated neuropathies, but this discussion will focus on the most common and most important for routine neurology practice. Some of the others are discussed in more detail in Chapter 5.5.

AIDP is a rapidly progressive neuropathy with sensory and motor deficits; this is the most common subset of the group called Guillain-Barré syndrome. They are suspected with this clinical presentation, and the diagnosis is supported by finding elevated protein in cerebrospinal fluid (CSF) without another cause. Nerve conduction studies (NCS) can show the demyelination, but early studies may be normal and treatment usually does not have to wait for NCS confirmation.

CIDP is a demyelinating neuropathy that can present as AIDP but has slightly different clinical presentation, with proximal and distal involvement. More details are presented in Chapter 5.5.

SIDP is similar to CIDP but develops over 4 to 8 weeks.

When a patient presents with AIDP, they should be warned that there is the possibility that this might be a first presentation of CIDP, although the chance is relatively low. If they get worse, they should return promptly for reevaluation and additional treatment. Data are sparse, but a general impression is that 15% of patients diagnosed with AIDP are subsequently diagnosed with CIDP. Factors that correlate more with first initial presentation of CIDP included absence of provoking incident (e.g., infection) and progression beyond 4 weeks.

There are rare subtypes of Guillain-Barré syndrome that are discussed in Chapter 5.5.

HEREDITARY NEUROPATHIES

Hereditary neuropathies are a diverse group of disorders with widely varying pathophysiology and inheritance. Autosomal dominant and recessive disorders are included in this group. Penetrance can be variable. Neurophysiological studies can show axonal or demyelinating changes. Details are presented in Chapter 5.5.

Hereditary neuropathy is suspected especially if there is a family history but also if there is onset in childhood. Syndromic identification is key to the suspicion of some neuropathies.

MONONEUROPATHIES

Descriptions of mononeuropathies can be voluminous; almost every nerve in the body has at least one described syndrome. The most common and most important mononeuropathies are discussed in detail in Chapter 5.5. Cranial neuropathies are discussed in Chapter 4.2.

MONONEUROPATHY MULTIPLEX

Mononeuropathy multiplex is dysfunction of multiple single peripheral nerves. Coincidental mononeuropathies can occur; when two or more neuropathies are present, a systemic disorder is usually present. Important causes are diabetes, vasculitides (e.g., polyarteritis nodosa), and leprosy. NCV shows multifocal slowing of nerve conduction in affected nerves.

Classification of mononeuropathy multiplex in the setting of a polyneuropathy is controversial. If the severity of damage to individual nerves far exceeds the NCV and EMG abnormalities due to the polyneuropathy, then the diagnosis of mononeuropathy multiplex is probably reasonable. Some clinicians maintain that, in the presence of a polyneuropathy, multiple mononeuropathies do not have the same pathophysiological and clinical significance.

Motor Neuron Disease

Motor neurons have cell bodies in the spinal cord and brain, so they are technically part of the CNS. However, they are the motor side of the peripheral nervous system, so some motor neuron diseases are briefly discussed here. A more comprehensive discussion is in Chapter 5.5.

Motor neuron diseases spare sensory nerves and must be distinguished from myopathies, which also only produce motor symptoms. The three most important motor neuron diseases are:

- ALS in which upper and lower motor neuron degeneration presents as weakness and corticospinal tract signs;
- SMA with degeneration of lower motor neurons only;
- Poliomyelitis with viral-induced degeneration of motor neurons;
- Multifocal motor neuropathy with demyelination of motor nerves, can be confused with ALS but is not axonal.

Neuromuscular Junction and Muscle

Karl E. Misulis and Eli E. Zimmerman

Neuromuscular Transmission Defects

Neuromuscular transmission defects present with weakness and fatigability. The tendency to fatigue early and the absence of sensory symptoms are clues to these disorders.

These defects are due to impaired synaptic transmission, either from impaired acetylcholine (ACh) release from the presynaptic terminal or reduced available ACh receptors (AChRs) on the postsynaptic terminal. The essential features of the major neuromuscular transmission defects are shown in Chapter 5.5.

Myasthenia gravis is an autoimmune disorder that presents with weakness that often involves ocular motor function but then extends to involve other muscle groups, including bulbar and respiratory muscles.

Botulism is due to poisoning with the botulinum toxin and is suspected when a patient presents with rapidly progressive weakness and is found to have had recent abdominal complaints, even if there is no known etiology for the toxin entry.

Myasthenic (Eaton-Lambert) syndrome is an autoimmune disorder and is often paraneoplastic. It is suspected when a patient presents with weakness and autonomic symptoms including dry mouth.

Myopathies

Myopathies present with muscle weakness without sensory dysfunction. Myopathies are differentiated from amyotrophic lateral sclerosis (ALS) by the absence of upper motor neuron signs. Nerve conduction velocities (NCVs) are normal in myopathies, although the compound motor action potential (CMAP) may be reduced in muscles with atrophy. Electromyography (EMG) in myopathies shows abnormal motor unit potentials that are different from the potentials seen in neuropathies. See Table 3.6.1 (see Chapter 3.6) for differentiation of myopathy from neuropathy. Details on many of the disorders discussed here are presented in Chapter 5.5.

DYSTROPHIES

Muscular dystrophies are suspected when a patient presents with insidious progression of weakness and often an alteration of gait. The absence of sensory findings suggests that this is not peripheral neuropathy. There are syndrome appearances to some of these disorders.

INFLAMMATORY MYOPATHIES

Inflammatory myopathies include polymyositis, dermatomyositis, and viral myositis. These are suspected when a patient presents with weakness without sensory involvement. Classic skin changes suggest dermatomyositis. Inflammatory myopathies can be paraneoplastic, so the presence of certain known cancers raises this concern. Details of these disorders are presented in Chapter 5.5.

METABOLIC MYOPATHIES

Metabolic myopathies are considered especially when children present with multisystem disorders for which myopathy is a cone component. Chapter 5.5 details some of these disorders. These disorders present with hepatic, cardiac, and cognitive deficits.

PERIODIC PARALYSIS

Periodic paralysis includes a group of disorders characterized by episodic weakness. The exact symptoms and chemistry differ between individual disorders. Onset is in childhood or adolescence. Weakness can be profound, but ocular and respiratory muscles are unaffected.

Hypokalemic periodic paralysis presents with attacks of weakness with low potassium. Symptoms are often on awakening. They are typically provoked by preceding carbohydrate load. This is suspected especially when a young patient presents with a history of episodes of morning weakness.

Hyperkalemic periodic paralysis presents with episodes of marked weakness often precipitated by exercise or fasting. Between episodes, myotonia can be demonstrated.

Localization by Dysfunction

Mental Status

Howard S. Kirshner and Martin A. Samuels

As in every aspect of the neurologic examination, the mental status examination can help to localize a lesion in the nervous system. It can also provide crucial information about the extent and severity of the patient's deficits.

The most important aspect of the mental status examination is the importance of performing it. Some patients maintain a "cocktail party" demeanor of social conversation that can mask major deficits in orientation and memory. Focal lesions may affect only visuospatial function, only language, or even only reading or writing; the correct diagnosis cannot be made without documentation of these specific cognitive deficits. For a more detailed treatment of mental status examination, the reader is referred to a new book by Mendez (2022). Recommended mental status examination by the American Academy of Neurology for the core neurology clerkship curriculum is shown here:

- Level of alertness
- Language function
  - Fluency
  - Comprehension
  - Repetition
  - Naming
  - Reading
  - Writing
- Memory
  - Immediate
  - Short term
  - Long term
- Calculations
- Visuospatial processing
- Abstract reasoning

Level of alertness is a description of the patient's level of consciousness. Coma is designated by the lack of any meaningful response to stimulation. Stupor and obtundation are stages of alertness in which there are meaningful responses only with greater than normal stimuli. Other levels of alertness include milder states of drowsiness, normal alertness, or even hypervigilance or agitation.

Language function should be tested in detail, especially when a lesion of the left hemisphere is suspected. Testing is generally divided into six parts:

- Description of spontaneous speech, with emphasis on fluency, word or sound errors, or word-finding difficulty
- Naming
- Repetition
- Auditory comprehension
- Reading both aloud and for comprehension
- Writing

If a patient does not speak in response to invitation, the examiner can try to induce speech by requesting an automatic sequence such as naming the days of the week or counting from 1 to 10, and then transitioning to spontaneous speech, if possible. As discussed in Chapter 5.2, language abnormalities on the bedside mental status examination are useful in localizing lesions and sometimes even in pointing to a specific diagnosis.

Memory encompasses many separate cognitive operations. Immediate or "working" memory is a measure of attention. It is tested at the bedside by having the patient repeat digits forward (the normal digit span is 7) or spelling "WORLD" forward and backward. Digit span, forward or backward, also measures attention. Reverse digit span, or spelling "WORLD" backward, however, may require some short-term memory. Short-term memory is usually tested antegrade by asking the patient to immediately repeat back three words and then recall them after a delay of 5 minutes. Some mental status examinations include more short-term memory items; for example, the Montreal Cognitive Assessment (MoCA) contains five items. Short-term memory can be tested nonverbally for locations of hidden objects in the room or reproduction of visual designs (drawings). Short-term memory can also be tested informally in the interview by asking about tests the patient has just had or details of meals, doctor visits, or relative visits. Long-term memory can be tested for biographical details, provided that a family member can verify the answers, or by asking items of general knowledge such as past presidents.

Calculations are tested because arithmetical reasoning is localized in the left parietal lobe; written calculations also involve visuospatial functions that may involve the right hemisphere. Serial 7 subtractions from 100 can be used as a test of both attention (immediate memory) and calculation ability. Asking a patient to make change from a $5 bill may also be used to test calculation ability.

Visuospatial functions can be tested in several ways. The patient can be asked to bisect a line or draw a figure such as a clock (with placement of the numbers and hands to reflect a specific time). Alternative drawings can include a house, a daisy, or a three-dimensional box. The intersecting pentagons from the Mini-Mental State Examination (MMSE) is another option. Visuospatial function can also be tested by asking the patient to draw a map of the United States and locate specific cities or states.

Abstract reasoning tests the patient's ability to plan ahead and to understand the significance of facts or events. Comprehension of irony and humor also provides insight into the patient's ability to understand concepts not obvious from the literal meaning of the words. Finally, the patient's insight into the nature of the illness, and their reaction to it, provides a measure of the patient's understanding of the situation.

Several other functions are not specifically included in the standard mental status examination. The patient's emotional state is important to gauge; this includes the patient's mood (subjective emotional state) and affect (the patient's emotional state as judged by the examiner). In other words, the examiner can judge the patient's emotional state by the effect the patient has on the examiner; depressed patients make the examiner feel "down", whereas manic patients may make the examiner laugh or feel elated.

Praxis is the ability of the patient to perform learned motor acts or to pantomime them in response to command. For example, asking the patient to demonstrate how to hammer a nail or to brush their teeth with each hand can assess apraxia.

Gnosis is the patient's ability to recognize objects in specific sensory modalities; loss of this recognition is called "agnosia". Agnosias are generally specific to one sensory modality; for example, visual agnosia refers to the inability of a patient to recognize a visual object (in the presence of the ability to recognize it by touch or sound). Auditory and tactile agnosias have been recognized. Recognition of subsets of stimuli within a sensory modality, such as visual faces (prosopagnosia) or familiar voices (phonagnosia), can be impaired in isolation.

Mini-Mental State Examination

There are several standard mental status examinations. The most widely used is the MMSE of Folstein and colleagues. This examination is reproduced below. The MMSE has the advantage of a standard format and a quantitative score, but it has several limitations. First, it should not be a straitjacket that keeps the examiner from performing more detailed examinations of language and other functions, when appropriate. Second, it is heavily weighted toward orientation and verbal processes, with only one point for a visuospatial task. Third, it is heavily dependent on education. Many educated patients demonstrate a ceiling effect on this test. It is therefore not sensitive in detecting early dementia in educated patients. The items on the MMSE are given points as follows:

- Orientation to time
  - Year   1
  - Month   1
  - Date   1
  - Day   1
- Orientation to place
  - State   1
  - County   1
  - Town   1
  - Hospital   1
  - Floor   1
- Attention (serial 7s or spell "WORLD" backward)   5
- Memory
  - Register three items   3
  - Recall three items at 5 minutes   3
- Naming (pencil, watch)   2
- Repetition (no ifs, ands, or buts)   1
- Following three-step command   3
- Following printed command (e.g., close your eyes)   1
- Write a sentence   1
- Copy intersecting pentagons   1

Montreal Cognitive Assessment

The MoCA is more difficult than the MMSE. It is scored on the basis of 30 points, as is the MMSE, but scores for the same patient average about 5 points lower than on the MMSE. The test includes naming three uncommon animals, recalling five words, doing a simple Trail Making Test Part B, and copying a cube and other items.

Localization of Dysfunction

On the basis of the examination, the patient may be identified as falling into one of a few categories.

NORMAL

The spectrum of what is normal is wide. Evaluation depends on the background of the patient. In general, an unimpaired senior citizen should be able to accomplish the tasks of the testing described previously.

Cognitive changes with aging are a commonly recognized disorder but are difficult to define. There are normal changes with aging. Spheres that are particularly affected in the absence of dementia include reduction in perceptual reasoning and processing speed. Perceptual reasoning involves using visual information and solving problems. The block-design task for the Wechsler Adult Intelligence Scale (WAIS) is such a task. Processing speed decline is important to consider because this change can impair performance on other tasks that might seem to have more cognitive implications.

MILD COGNITIVE IMPAIRMENT

Mild cognitive impairment (MCI) is a condition in which there are detectable deficits, but it is not clear that there is a marked difference in functioning. Also, patients with MCI often have reversible causes. Common etiologies of this presentation are certain medications and depression. With aging, the incidence of depression approaches 14%. In the same aging population with a recent loss of a partner, the incidence of depression was approximately 50%. MCI can be a precursor to Alzheimer disease, in which case time orientation and memory are affected (amnestic MCI). Other cases of MCI have language, executive function, or other deficits not suggestive of Alzheimer disease. These are often referred to as multidomain MCI.

DEMENTIA

Dementia is decline in cognition from baseline that interferes with functioning. Dementia is distinguished from encephalopathy by the absence of a reversible cause and a different clinical presentation.

With dementia, the patient has normal alertness and responsiveness, but their performance on some of the tests are impaired. Dementia is diagnosed by careful examination and study to document the deficits and ensure no reversible cause is identified.

ENCEPHALOPATHY

Encephalopathy, including delirium, is distinguished from dementia in impairment due to a cause which is potentially reversible potentially reversible. Patients with encephalopathy are often lethargic with psychomotor slowing, although agitated encephalopathy can occur. The onset of encephalopathy is more acute than delirium, and the degree of encephalopathy can fluctuate.

Potential causes for encephalopathy include some medications, toxic substances, metabolic dysfunction (e.g., renal or hepatic), endocrine dysfunction (e.g., hypothyroid), or infection.

Stroke can present as encephalopathy without definite focal signs in patients with multiple small infarctions or as part of the cognitive deficit often seen with posterior cerebral artery infarctions, which produce visual field defects but typically not hemiplegia.

UNABLE TO ASSESS

Patients may be unable or unwilling to cooperate with formal mental status testing, in which case it is impossible to accurately assess mental status. It is useless to try to evaluate a patient for dementia when they are sick in the hospital and have delirium.

Brainstem and Cranial Nerve Dysfunction

Eli E. Zimmerman and Howard S. Kirshner

Cranial nerves are discussed elsewhere in this text. This chapter identifies some other commonly seen syndromes involving the brainstem and cranial nerves. Lesions affecting one cranial nerve solely or predominantly are discussed under the respective nerve; brainstem lesions producing cranial nerve dysfunction in addition to other neurologic dysfunctions are discussed individually. Table 4.2.1 summarizes cranial nerve function.

Brainstem Localization

Knowledge of the long tracts that ascend and descend through the brainstem and the locations of cranial nerve and other brainstem nuclei are critical for the localization of brainstem lesions. These can be considered along three important axes: rostral-caudal, dorsal-ventral, and medial-lateral. In general (with exceptions), the rostrocaudal direction reflects the different cranial nerve nuclei, the dorsal-ventral axis separates cranial nerve nuclei (dorsal) from long tracts passing through the brainstem (ventral), and the medial-lateral direction within each side of the brainstem separates motor (medial) from sensory (lateral) structures.

Localization of lesions affecting the brainstem is easier if a systematic approach is used. When faced with a difficult diagnostic problem, it is important to think systematically rather than relying on the many complicated brainstem syndromes. Important questions to ask include the following:

- Is the lesion intra-axial or extra-axial?
- What is the rostrocaudal location of the lesion?
- Is the intraaxial lesion unilateral or bilateral?
- What clinical conditions can produce damage in this localization?

Isolated single cranial nerve palsies are usually extra-axial, that is, not in the substance of the brainstem. Multiple cranial nerve palsies can still be caused by extraaxial disease. An intraaxial lesion is suggested by the combination of cranial nerve palsies and signs of damage to ascending and descending tracts. For example, an isolated CN VI palsy, which causes impaired abduction of the ipsilateral eye, is relatively common and can result from microvascular disease, trauma, and increased intracranial pressure, although it is often idiopathic. In contrast, a CN VI palsy combined with damage to the medial longitudinal fasciculus, which causes internuclear ophthalmoplegia, is caused by a lesion in the pons.

Rostrocaudal localization is most easily identified by carefully determining which cranial nerves are affected. For example, an oculomotor lesion with signs of intraaxial damage suggests a midbrain lesion, whereas glossopharyngeal and vagus damage suggests a medullary lesion.

Determination of whether the lesion is unilateral or bilateral requires understanding of which tracts are crossed and at which level. The descending corticospinal tracts cross in the medulla. The dorsal columns, which carry information about fine touch, vibration, and proprioception,

TABLE 4.2.1 ■ Cranial Nerve Function.

Number	Name	Motor Function	Sensory Function
I	Olfactory		Smell
II	Optic		Vision
III	Oculomotor	Superior, inferior, and medial recti; inferior oblique; pupil; ciliary muscles	
IV	Trochlear	Superior oblique	
V	Trigeminal	Muscles of mastication	Face; forehead; external ear; mucosa; cornea; sinuses
VI	Abducens	Lateral rectus	
VII	Facial	Muscles of face and scalp; stapedius	Soft palate; taste of anterior tongue
VIII	Vestibulocochlear		Hearing; position in space; acceleration
IX	Glossopharyngeal	Pharyngeal muscles; stylopharyngeus	Pharynx; taste of posterior tongue
X	Vagus	Pharynx, larynx, thoracic and abdominal viscera	Pharynx; larynx; external auditory canal; thoracic and abdominal viscera
XI	Accessory	Sternocleidomastoid; trapezius; some pharynx; upper larynx	
XII	Hypoglossal	Tongue; strap muscles of neck	

ascend the spinal cord uncrossed, synapse in the nucleus gracilis and nucleus cuneatus in the medulla, and then cross as they ascend through the medulla, forming the medial lemniscus. The spinothalamic tract axons, which convey pain and temperature sensation, cross within the spinal cord segment and then ascend crossed in the cord. The spinothalamic tract stays lateral in the brainstem and ascends to the midbrain where it joins with the medial lemniscus to enter the thalamus.

Once the lesion has been determined to be intraaxial and the rostrocaudal and unilateral or bilateral localization has been made, individual syndromes can be considered. Specific etiologies are suggested by associated symptoms; for example, acute onset of a deficit suggests ischemic stroke, sudden onset of headache and vomiting suggests a hemorrhage, and a slowly progressive deficit suggests an expanding mass lesion.

Disorders of Olfaction

Anosmia is usually not caused by a neurologic problem, but it can be. Chapter 3.4 discusses a number of disorders affecting the olfactory nerve. In addition, sinusitis and a host of infectious and postinfectious disorders can produce reduced or abolished sense of smell. Similarly, a wide variety of toxins can produce temporary or permanent anosmia. Neurodegenerative diseases, especially Parkinson disease, are associated with loss of smell.

Diagnosis is facilitated by determining whether there was an inciting event. If not, then other etiologies are considered, such as tumor affecting the inferior frontal region.

Visual Disorders

Visual loss is a common chief complaint in the emergency department. It is sometimes neurologic and often not. Context and history are important. Unless the diagnosis is clearly neurologic, emergent ophthalmology consultation is strongly considered because treatable ocular pathology can become irreversible if there is a delay in treatment. For example, one of our patients with multiple sclerosis (MS) presented to the emergency department with monocular visual loss. Triage assumed it was MS, but it turned out to be acute glaucoma. Other causes of acute onset of monocular visual loss include ischemic optic neuropathy, retinal detachment, and intraocular hemorrhage.

Subacute onset of monocular visual loss is less likely to be vascular and raises the differential diagnosis of optic neuritis, optic nerve compression, or primary eye pathology. Workup of suspected optic neuritis usually involves magnetic resonance imaging (MRI) of the orbits and often the brain along with an ophthalmology consultation.

Binocular visual loss has a broad differential diagnosis that is narrowed if there is a visual field defect. Hemianopia or consistent quadrant defect affecting both eyes indicates a lesion behind the chiasm; the most common location is occipital.

Dizziness and Hearing Loss

Dizziness is a vague term and has multiple meanings to patients and providers. Some mean vertigo, a spinning or moving sensation. Other symptoms that can be labeled as dizziness include presyncopal sensation, double vision, gait ataxia, and mental fogginess. Key to diagnosis is the determination of what the patient means by dizziness.

Vertigo without other deficits is usually peripheral vestibulopathy.

Vertigo with cranial nerve deficit or ataxia suggests a brainstem lesion, but additional information is needed to determine etiology. An acute onset suggests stroke. An episodic or progressive lesion can be demyelinating disease, tumor, or other structural etiology.

Patients with hearing loss are seldom referred to neurology first; usually an ear, nose, and throat clinician sees those patients. However, in the absence of a peripheral process, neurology is often asked to evaluate. Hearing loss with acute onset is often idiopathic, but it can be due to stroke, if the labyrinthine artery is affected by damage to the anterior inferior cerebellar artery. This is a form of stroke. Tempo and characteristics of the symptoms are key to diagnosis because imaging typically does not show the vascular damage.

Facial Weakness

Unilateral facial weakness is usually due to Bell palsy, an inflammatory condition of the facial nerve thought to be due to herpes simplex virus in most cases. Upper and lower facial muscles are typically affected. Differential diagnosis includes herpes zoster and is evidenced by vesicles seen in the external auditory canal ipsilateral to the facial weakness (Ramsay-Hunt syndrome). Stroke is an uncommon cause of unilateral facial weakness. When it is present, it predominantly affects the lower face, making its distinction from Bell palsy easier. Sarcoidosis is in the differential diagnosis, but this is uncommon.

Bilateral facial weakness raises concern over Lyme disease and Guillain-Barré syndrome, but it can occur in otherwise typical idiopathic facial palsy.

Dysarthria and Dysphagia

Dysarthria has a broad differential diagnosis. In the emergent evaluation of patients with dysarthria, stroke is often considered, but dysarthria in the absence of other signs would be unexpected.

Among some of the causes of dysarthria that can appear to be initially isolated are medication effect, myasthenia gravis, and structural lesion of the oropharynx, with infection being a relatively common etiology.

Dysphagia has a similar differential diagnosis and frequently coexists with dysarthria. Expert speech and swallowing evaluation can help to determine the type of defect if it is not clear on presentation. This can narrow the differential diagnosis.

Motor

Eli E. Zimmerman and Karl E. Misulis

Motor System Localization

Identification and description of motor deficits is critical for the understanding of neurologic localization. The assessment of the presence of weakness and other motor deficits provides an excellent basis for approaching the localization of brain lesions.

Elements required for localization of lesions affecting the motor system include:

- Nature of the deficit
  - Weakness
  - Incoordination
  - Stiffness
  - Tremor
  - Spasms or jerking
- Location of the motor deficit
  - Generalized
  - Focal
  - Multifocal
  - Shifting location
- Associated symptoms
  - Sensory loss
  - Visual deficit
  - Speech deficit
- Examination findings
  - Objective weakness
  - Subjective weakness without objective deficit identified
  - Spasms or clonic movements
  - Tremor
  - Rigidity
- Associated nonmotor clinical findings
  - Tendon reflex
  - Pathologic reflexes

On the basis of these findings, the deficits can be localized to one of almost innumerable locations. For example, rigidity with hyperreflexia and extensor plantar response indicates a corticospinal tract lesion, and the location of that lesion would be different if there was or was not sensory involvement.

It would be impossible to document the diagnosis with each of the possibilities of these findings, but this chapter will discuss some general principles of how these data are used in diagnosis.

Upper Versus Lower Motor Neuron

The motor system is largely a two-neuron pathway, consisting of an upper motor neuron and a lower motor neuron. The upper motor neuron has its cell body in the cerebral cortex, located in the portion of the cortex according to the somatotopic organization (leg medial, arm superior, face lateral). The upper motor neuron projects through the corona radiata, which coalesces in the internal capsule (in the posterior limb), then continues its descent through the brainstem. Fibers destined for cranial nerves and the innervation of the muscles associated with them will exit this pathway within the brainstem. Fibers destined for the body continue descending in the most ventral aspect of each component of the brainstem—the crus cerebri of the midbrain, the basis pontis in the pons, and the pyramids in the medulla. In the pyramids, the corticospinal tracts decussate and continue descending to the spinal level responsible for their innervation. At that level, fibers exit the main corticospinal tract to then innervate lower motor neurons whose cell bodies reside in the ventral horn of the spinal cord. These neurons exit the spinal cord through ventral roots and end up innervating target muscles.

One key distinction in the localization of weakness is the distinction between damage to upper motor neurons and lower motor neurons. Lesions of upper motor neurons often affect groups of muscles, whereas lesions of lower motor neurons can affect single muscles. Lesions of upper motor neurons result in spasticity (i.e., velocity-dependent increase in tone), whereas lesions of lower motor neurons result in atrophy (decrease in muscle size) and fasciculations (spontaneous twitching of muscles). Deep tendon reflexes can also help distinguish between upper motor neurons and lower motor neurons lesions. With upper motor neuron lesions, reflexes are typically increased (along with the presence of the Babinski sign); with lower motor neuron lesions, reflexes are typically reduced.

Corticospinal Tract

Lesions of the corticospinal tract are, by definition, upper motor neuron lesions. Localization within the corticospinal tract is aided by additional signs and symptoms. Lesions of the cortex can be quite focal given the area over which motor information arises within the cortex; they often consist of the combination of motor and sensory deficits given that the primary motor and somatosensory cortices are adjacent. As the corticospinal tract descends through the corona radiata and into the internal capsule, more diffuse weakness is expected as a result of a lesion given the progressively small area into which fibers are compressed. As the corticospinal tract descends through the brainstem, lesions are often associated with cranial nerve deficits; a core principle of brainstem localization is that weakness and facial symptoms are crossed. That is, a patient with left-sided weakness due to a brainstem lesion will often have deficits of the right face. Lesions of the corticospinal tract in the spinal cord often cause sensory deficits and the combination of upper and lower motor neuron deficits.

Peripheral Components

Lesions of peripheral nerves typically cause a pattern of overlapping weakness and sensory loss in the distribution of named nerves (femoral, median). Lesions of the neuromuscular junction involve fluctuating weakness. Lesions of muscles (myopathies) typically present with symmetric, proximal weakness.

Generalized Weakness

Generalized weakness is a challenging localization. Much of the motor examination depends on comparison of a patient's age and state of health to what would be expected of a person of similar characteristics. Diagnosis depends on details of the presentation. If there is no lateralizing or proximal-distal difference in weakness, then the diagnosis is most commonly medical rather than neurologic. The differential diagnosis is broad and includes a host of metabolic, endocrine, nutritional, and infectious disorders. The weakness is typically mild to moderate and sometimes subjective.

When patients complain of diffuse or generalized weakness, they sometimes mean not asymmetric or not localized to an isolated muscle group or limbs. In those circumstances, the weakness is not really generalized.

Many neurologic disorders described as generalized are not really generalized. The demyelinating polyneuropathies, for example, do not present involving all regions, but rather they are typically distal-predominant. Amyotrophic lateral sclerosis (ALS) produces weakness that can ultimately involve most muscles; but on presentation, weakness is usually asymmetric, arm more than leg weakness, with a combination of corticospinal, and lower motor neuron findings. Most myopathies typically do not present with diffuse weakness in all muscle groups but rather proximal or otherwise in syndromic but symmetric distributions.

Localization of Findings

CENTRAL LESIONS

Hemiplegia is paralysis on one side of the body involving the arm and leg. The cause is corticospinal dysfunction descending from the contralateral cerebral cortex, although the lesion can be located anywhere from the cortex through the descending projections to and including the brainstem. Spinal hemisection (Brown-Séquard syndrome) is extremely rare and results in paralysis ipsilateral below the level of the lesion and pain and temperature loss contralateral below the level of the lesion. Stroke is the most common etiology of hemiplegia, but other causes are demyelinating disease and tumors.

Monoplegia is paralysis of one limb, the arm, or leg. Stroke can cause monoplegia with involvement of only the arm middle cerebral artery, (MCA) or leg anterior cerebral artery (ACA) distributions, however there are almost always other findings on examination that help with diagnosis (e.g., visual change, speech change, or subtle weakness or incoordination of the other extremity). Demyelinating disease is less likely to cause monoplegia than hemiplegia because of the lesser somatotopic organization of the white matter tracts than the cortex. Spinal lesions can produce monoplegia, including a small tumor or demyelinating lesion, but more common is cord compression, which can affect one an arm with lesser effect on descending pathways to the leg. Of course, it is easier for spinal lesions to produce leg weakness than arm weakness because of the traversing axons destined for the lower cord in the upper cord.

Paraplegia has a broad differential diagnosis. Among these are cord compression from a variety of causes and spinal cord infarction particularly from damage to the artery of Adamkiewicz, which is a prominent artery branched from the aorta that supplies the spinal cord at about T9, although there is significant variation in the level of arrival of the artery. Demyelinating disease can produce paraplegia, especially multiple sclerosis and neuromyelitis optica spectrum disorder.

Quadriplegia usually develops from high cervical spinal cord lesions. The most common cause is trauma with either transient or persistent cord compression. Spinal stroke in the cervical level is unexpected, although it has been reported in association with cervical spondylosis.

PERIPHERAL LESIONS

Lesions of the peripheral nerves and plexuses produce weakness in the distribution. Residents should keep charts and diagrams of the peripheral nerve anatomy handy as an aid to diagnosis.

The key to diagnosing motor deficit is accurate mapping of the deficit and knowledge of peripheral nerve anatomy. The presence or absence and distribution of associated sensory deficits also helps with diagnosis. Many of the potential peripheral nerve lesions are covered in other sections of this book, so this chapter will discuss how to approach deficits to localize the lesions.

Peripheral lesions are focal, multifocal, or generalized. When generalized, they can be proximal, distal, or both.

Spinal nerve root lesion is suggested when motor and sensory deficits fit within a single nerve root distribution. C6 is the most common cervical radiculopathy, followed by C7. In the lumbosacral region, L5 is by far the most common radiculopathy. These nerve root lesions are most likely due to osteophytes or disc disease. Osteophytes are seldom isolated, so dysfunction of more than one nerve root is common.

Plexus lesions deficits could be explained by involvement of two or more adjacent nerve roots. Knowledge of how the plexus is arranged makes this easier. For example, damage that fits within the distribution of the C5 and C6 roots may be in the upper brachial plexus. Common plexopathies in adults are trauma, neoplastic infiltration, radiation plexopathy, brachial plexitis, and thoracic outlet syndrome. In neonates, Erb palsy and Klumpke palsy are prominent.

Mononeuropathies are suggested by motor and sensory loss in the distribution of single nerves. These are fairly straightforward to diagnose; localization to a specific nerve but not involving a related nerve with more proximal association is diagnostic. The most common mononeuropathies coming to medical attention are median, ulnar, radial, and peroneal.

Polyneuropathies are suggested by sensory and often also motor involvement that spans neural and dermatomal distributions. The most common cause is diabetes, with more than half of patients with diabetes having some polyneuropathy. Other important causes are autoimmune disorders (e.g., Guillain-Barré syndrome, CIDP), hereditary disorders (e.g., Charcit-Marie-Tooth), cancers (e.g., myeloma), infections (e.g., viral such as HIV, bacterial such as leprosy), toxins (e.g., chemotherapy, alcohol), and nutritional deficits (e.g., thiamine, B12).

Mononeuropathy multiplex is a dysfunction of multiple mononeuropathies. This indicates pathology that has focal implications but produces multiple lesions. The most common causes are diabetes (which can produce polyneuropathy or mononeuropathy multiplex), vasculitis, leprosy, and tumors with multifocal involvement (especially lymphoma, leukemia, and paraneoplastic syndrome).

From this discussion, it is easy to see that most neurologists without photographic memories need to have access to charts of pathways and motor and sensory innervations. However, there are variations between individuals in motor supply to the muscles and the maps of sensory supply by nerve roots and peripheral nerves are not as precise or as consistent as they are assumed to be.

As neurologists localize a deficit to a possible lesion, they have potential causes in mind which correlate with the localization. Neurologist meld knowledge of localization and neuropathologic mechanisms to come to a differential diagnosis.

Sensory

Eli E. Zimmerman and Karl E. Misulis

Sensory Systems Localization

Two pathways, the dorsal columns and the spinothalamic tract, carry sensory information from the periphery to the brain, and they carry two distinct sets of information.

DORSAL COLUMNS

The dorsal columns pathway is responsible for fine touch and two-point discrimination, perception of vibration, and conscious proprioception (knowledge of where our joints, limbs, and bodies are in space). Because of its function, it is designed for speed of transmission and specificity of information. It accomplishes this through Meissner corpuscles (for fine touch), Pacinian corpuscles (for vibration), and muscle spindles and Golgi tendon organs (for proprioception). As this is a very fast-conducting pathway, it is not surprising that it uses highly myelinated fibers ($A\alpha$ and $A\beta$).

The first-order neuron in this pathway, which is pseudo-unipolar, starts in the periphery with its specialized receptor. Its axons run centrally and then through the cell body (which is connected via a short process, as it is pseudo-unipolar in structure). From the cell body, the central process moves medially and into the dorsal column of the spinal cord. This all occurs ipsilaterally to the initial stimulus.

There are two separate components of the dorsal column in the spinal cord. The fasciculus gracilis contains fibers from dermatomal levels T7 and below. The fasciculus cuneatus contains the ascending fibers from dermatomal levels T6 and above. This pathway is designed for speed. It minimizes synapses and crossing of fibers over others. So when incoming fibers enter the spinal cord, they take up the most medial location they can in order to be out of the way. Thus, the fasciculus gracilis is located medially (on each half of the spinal cord) and the fasciculus gracilis is located laterally within the dorsal column portion of each side of the spinal cord. From here, fibers ascend in their respective components of the dorsal column. These are still the first-order neurons, as there has not been a synapse. They remain ipsilateral to the stimulus. Fibers ascend to the brainstem, where they will have their first synapse in the caudal medulla.

The fasciculus gracilis and fasciculus cuneatus have corresponding nuclei (nucleus gracilis for fibers from T7 and below, and nucleus cuneatus for fibers from T6 and above) in the caudal medulla. These nuclei contain the cell bodies of the second-order neurons of the pathway. These second-order neurons immediately decussate as the internal arcuate fibers. Once the fibers have decussated, they end up in a collection of axons called the medial lemniscus, which continues to ascend. Information is now contralateral to the location of the initial synapse.

Fibers in the medial lemniscus continue to ascend in the brainstem until they reach the ventroposterolateral (VPL) nucleus of the thalamus, which is responsible for sensation (all modalities) from the body. The third-order neuron, whose cell body lies in VPL, then projects to the somatosensory cortex for conscious perception of the stimulus. Not surprisingly, there is a clear organization to the layout of the cortex. Medial portions of the cortex are responsible for the leg, whereas lateral portions of the cortex are responsible for sensation of face. The arm is between them.

SPINOTHALAMIC TRACT

The spinothalamic tract pathway is responsible for the perception of pain and temperature (both hot and cold). This is accomplished not through specialized receptors but rather through free nerve endings.

Whereas the dorsal columns pathway is designed for speed and specificity, this pathway is designed for sensitivity. This makes developmental and evolutionary sense. When a person steps on a nail, for example, it is much less important for them to know which exact millimeter of the foot has been affected than it is for them to know that there is a painful stimulus coming from the right foot and that they need to move it quickly. This is a slow-conducting pathway and uses lightly myelinated (Aδ) or unmyelinated (C) fibers.

The first-order neuron in this pathway, which is pseudo-unipolar, starts in the periphery (with its "receptor," free nerve endings). Its axons run centrally past the cell body (located in the dorsal root ganglion) and into the spinal cord via the dorsal root. Once the first-order neuron enters the spinal cord, it ascends two segments in the dorsolateral fasciculus of Lissauer. Once the axons have ascended to their eventual level, they dive into the grey matter of the spinal cord where they will synapse on the second-order neuron of the pathway in the dorsal horn of the spinal cord. The second-order neuron then decussates in the anterior white commissure of the spinal cord before taking its place in the anterolateral portion of the spinal cord. This is why this pathway is also called the anterolateral system. These fibers are now contralateral to the initial stimulus. As these fibers layer into this tract, laterally located fibers are responsible for the lower extremities, and those responsible for sensation from the trunk and then the upper extremity fill in medially. These second-order fibers ascend in the anterolateral portion of the spinal cord. As they run superiorly into the brainstem, the tract becomes known as the spinal lemniscus. Just as with the dorsal columns pathway, these ascend to the VPL nucleus of the thalamus. The remainder of the pathway is identical to the dorsal columns. The third-order neuron of the pathway has its cell body in the VPL nucleus of the thalamus. It projects rostrally to the cortex for conscious perception of pain and temperature sensation.

Cortical Lesions

Just as with lesions of the cortex causing motor deficits, lesions of the cortex can cause very isolated symptoms on the contralateral side of the body; similarly, when the primary somatosensory cortex is involved, motor deficits are also present given the proximities of these brain regions.

Thalamic Lesions

Thalamic lesions classically produce contralateral sensory deficit, but the thalamus is so complex that the results of lesions can be varied. Thalamic lesions can affect any portion of the structure, and thalamic infarction can be in one of a number of penetrating branches, so the symptomatology is diverse. In addition to sensory symptoms, the results of thalamic infarction and other types of damage include deficits in arousal, memory, speech, and contralateral ataxia. Ataxic hemiparesis can occur from thalamic infarct, although the cause is more commonly small-vessel infarction of the internal capsule or in the pons.

Brainstem Lesions

The two sensory pathways have slightly different trajectories as they ascend through the brainstem, so disorders of the brainstem can cause slightly different presentations of sensory loss depending on lesion location.

Spinal Cord Lesions

Lesions of the spinal cord can affect either sensory pathway, neither, or both, depending on the portion of the cord involved. In the example of cord hemisection, a patient will have ipsilateral loss of the information carried by the dorsal columns pathway (proprioception, vibration, fine touch) and contralateral loss of the information carried by the spinothalamic pathway (pain, temperature).

Peripheral Nerve Lesions

MONONEUROPATHIES

As the name implies, mononeuropathies occur with damage or compression to one single nerve, with deficits only in the distribution of that particular nerve. Common examples include a median neuropathy at the wrist (carpal tunnel syndrome) or compression of the lateral femoral cutaneous nerve (meralgia paresthetica).

POLYNEUROPATHIES

Polyneuropathies are typically caused by metabolic abnormalities, such as glucose intolerance, vitamin deficiencies, endocrinopathies, and heavy metal toxicity. These can be either axonal (more common) or demyelinating, depending on their effect on peripheral nerves. The common presentation of polyneuropathy is a length-dependent sensory loss, that is, longer nerves are affected before shorter ones. Additionally, sensory disturbances generally precede the onset of weakness.

MONONEUROPATHY MULTIPLEX

Mononeuropathy multiplex is suspected from involvement of multiple but not all nerves. This patchy involvement is most commonly caused by diabetes, but other important etiologies are leprosy, polyarteritis nodosa, and other vasculitides. Familial predisposition to pressure palsies may also present with findings of mononeuropathy multiplex, because of the multifocal yet independent nature of the compressive sites. The most common lesion seen in patients with diabetes is ulnar neuropathy.

Coordination

Karl E. Misulis and Martin A. Samuels

Localization of Coordination Control and Deficits

Coordination is a prominent part of the examination. Whereas coordination is typically considered to be a test of cerebellar function, coordination deficits can be produced by a wide range of lesions. Coordination depends on the integrity, not only of the brainstem and cerebellum but also of the sensory and motor afferent and efferent pathways and motor and premotor regions.

The location of the first thought of movement is not known. The premotor cortex of the frontal lobe is involved in planning movement and seems to do so by considering movement in the context of prior movements experienced and learned. Then this activates the motor cortex to drive the actual movements. For some movements, especially stabilizing movements, the supplementary motor cortex plays an additional role. The motor cortex projects to the subcortical nuclei, brainstem, and spinal cord. Along the way, there are sensory afferents that indicate how successful the attempts at movement were and aid in adjusting motor effort appropriately at both spinal and cerebral levels. Hence, deficits in coordination can be caused by dysfunction in a wide range of potential locations.

Cerebral cortex lesions usually produce lack of movement if severe and poorly controlled movement if not severe. Reasons for dysfunction include a wide range of pathologies that differ in acuity and hence differ in onset and physiologic compensation for the deficit. Stroke damage is acute, whereas a brain tumor produces slow onset and progression of symptoms.

The basal ganglia participate in control of motor function. The striatum receives afferents from the cortex, thalamus, and substantia nigra, among other regions. There is significant internal processing within the striatum, and output is chiefly to the globus pallidus and substantia nigra. Damage to the basal ganglia produces difficulty with coordination of movement rather than paralysis. This might include excess movement such as dyskinesias or dystonia or impaired movement with tremor and/or ataxia.

The cerebellum is a constellation of structures that serve to coordinate movement. The anatomy and functional physiology of the cerebellum and connections with other motor and sensory systems are complex, but simply, the cerebellar hemispheres coordinate movement of ipsilateral limbs. The cerebellar vermis is predominantly involved in coordination of gait and other midline functions. Cerebellar hemisphere lesions produce dysmetria during finger-nose-finger or heel-knee-shin testing on the side of the lesion. More midline cerebellar lesions produce gait ataxia with impairment in accurate foot placement. Note that vascular causes often affect the brainstem and the cerebellum, so cranial nerve deficits help with that localization.

Clinical Correlations

DIFFERENTIATING DEFICITS

Incoordination Versus Weakness

If patients are sufficiently weak, they will have difficulty with coordination testing. Many causes of weakness have most prominent symptoms distally, so that, for example, the fingers and hand are more affected than proximal muscles of the arm. Therefore, coordination of the hand may seem to be affected. Coordination testing is most accurate when strength is normal. If strength is impaired, then the neurologist must test coordination of muscles that do not depend on much power.

Limb Versus Gait Ataxia

The key to diagnosis is often the differentiation of the degree of limb ataxia versus gait ataxia. Cerebellar lesions that are midline produce gait ataxia. Cerebellar lesions that are in the hemispheres produce limb ataxia. Intermediate lesions of the cerebellum can cause gait difficulty and dysarthria. Not all ataxias are cerebellar. Lesions in multiple locations in the central nervous system (CNS), including brainstem, basal ganglia, thalamus, or cortex, can produce ataxia. There are differences in the ataxia associated with these lesions. Sensory ataxia will often produce a positive Romberg test (or its analogue in the upper extremity). The neurologist can assess the finger-nose-finger test in a patient with eyes open and closed as a Romberg analogue in the arms.

Brainstem Signs With Ataxia

Brainstem involvement with almost any disease process can affect not only brainstem nuclei but also tracts that are responsible for sensation and movement or afferents and efferents to the cerebellum. There are many ways in which damage to the brainstem can produce ataxia. Ataxia can be appendicular and/or gait and is usually associated with signs of cranial nerve defect, such as disorders of eye movements, facial motor or sensory function, or function of oropharyngeal muscles.

EXAMPLES

More examples are discussed elsewhere in this book, but here are some illustrative examples.

Cerebellar Stroke

Stroke affecting the cerebellum can produce purely cerebellar deficits, or it can affect the brainstem, in which case there will be signs of the brainstem damage. The cerebellar signs will include appendicular ataxia with Finger-Nose-Finger (FNF) and Heel-Knee-Shin (HKS) on the affected side. Cerebellar infarctions are often bilateral. Some cerebellar strokes are small, and the cerebellum is not so somatotopically organized that small lesions can be easily localized. In these small strokes, the symptoms of imbalance or ataxia may be subtle or not definitely abnormal.

Essential Tremor

Essential tremor (ET) is an action and postural tremor, without tremor at rest. This is a clinical diagnosis. There are no laboratory or imaging findings. The localization of the lesion is uncertain, although it is thought that it may be due to disordered influence of brainstem and cerebellar control over thalamocortical circuits, possibly by neuronal degeneration. ET is often familial and can be associated with development of gait ataxia in later years.

Parkinsonism

Parkinsonism includes Parkinson disease and a host of other disorders with a similar appearance. These are discussed in more detail in Chapter 5.7. Key features are increased tone, rigidity, resting tremor, and stooped posture. The different varieties of parkinsonism have differing proportions of some of these findings. Diagnosis is clinical, and there are no laboratory findings that make the diagnosis. In a dopamine transporter scan (DaTscan), a radiotracer binds to the dopamine transporter, showing less transporter in patients with Parkinson disease and some related conditions. DaTscan differentiates these parkinsonian conditions from patients who are normal or have ET, but it does not distinguish between Parkinson disease, multiple system atrophy, progressive supranuclear palsy, or Corticboasal Degeneration (CBD).

Gait

Karl E. Misulis and Howard S. Kirshner

Physiology and Localization of Gait

The bipedal gait is complex and depends on action of almost all parts of the nervous system. Gait is initiated in different ways depending on the purpose of the movement, whether intentional or reflexive. Gait generally originates in the cerebral cortex. Intentional initiation of gait is influenced by sensory inputs from multiple modalities. The resultant output of the sensory-motor cortex projects to the premotor and supplementary motor areas. These areas, in turn, generate the programmed movements for gait and feed those to corticobulbar and corticospinal centers for motor activation.

Cerebral output likely projects in part to the mesencephalic locomotor region that plays an important but poorly understood role in the coordination of gait, including walking and running. Output projects to motor systems especially for axial and proximal limb muscles. Although this is better understood for animals than humans, the function is thought to be related in human gait.

Gait is precise because of sensory feedback, both somatosensory and vestibular. These data are summed to modify the effort in a feedback manner. Did the intended movement occur, or is a correction needed? The cerebellum aids with this correction.

Types of Gait Abnormalities

Careful analysis of gait can identify the type of gait disorder. Here are some of the most important types of gait disorders.

SPASTIC GAIT

Bilateral corticospinal tract dysfunction at any level can produce a spastic gait. This is characterized by leg stiffness, narrow base, and often some circumduction on the forward swing to account for the difficulty with lifting the foot sufficiently.

HEMIPLEGIC GAIT

Features of the spastic gait are seen but are unilateral, usually due to cerebral or brainstem lesion, although spinal lesions can be seen. The patient often leans away from the hemiplegic side to allow for circumduction of the affected leg.

CEREBELLAR ATAXIA

Gait is usually broad-based with impaired placing that can put the patient at significant risk for falling. The absence of spasticity makes movements faster than with corticospinal tract dysfunction, so falling is more common. If the cerebellar damage involves the intermediate and lateral aspects, then limb ataxia is also present.

149

SENSORY ATAXIA

Deficit of sensory input can result in impaired feedback, thereby impairing gait. This can look similar to cerebellar ataxia, but a distinguishing feature is better performance when the patient's eyes are open and marked impairment when their eyes are closed.

PARKINSONIAN GAIT

Patients typically have narrow-based gait, stooped posture, reduced arm swing, and associated findings of resting tremor and cogwheel rigidity. These patients might not have Parkinson disease, but they may have any one of a number of other degenerative disorders with parkinsonian features.

FRONTAL LOBE ATAXIA

Patients present with small steps that can be mistaken for parkinsonian gait. There may even be some stiffness, although there should not be tremor or cogwheel rigidity; these are differentiating features.

FUNCTIONAL GAIT

Gait that is not due to organic abnormality has a variety of terms. We prefer "functional" for these disorders, because the defect is in performance or function of the process rather than in the neurologic systems. We do not routinely use the terms psychogenic or factitious, although these have been used. Differentiating some functional gaits from organic gait disorders can be difficult even for experienced clinicians. Clue to functional gait includes bizarre gait, which requires impressive coordination in order to be manifest. Astasia-abasia means inability to stand unassisted (astasia) and inability to walk (abasia). This is usually a conversion disorder, although some organic gait disorders can have a similar appearance. Some people can have both functional and organic findings.

Gait Disorders

STROKE

Stroke involving the cerebral hemispheres produces a hemiparetic gait, with stiffness of the contralateral leg and lifting of the pelvis on the contralateral side to aid the swing-through. Stroke involving the cerebellum can produce unilateral or bilateral difficulty with limb placement, resulting in a clumsy gait. The patient has to make corrections for the inaccurate placement. Stance is often wavering if the stroke was cerebellar.

MUSCULAR DYSTROPHY

There are multiple forms of muscular dystrophy. When there is proximal weakness, gait is characterized by accentuated pelvic tilt anteriorly and lifting of the knee with hip abduction.

PARKINSONISM

Stance is narrow-based, stooped, and may be associated with a paucity of spontaneous movements. The patient shows difficulty initiating gait and may have a few steps in place before moving on to a gait with short steps. The steps can become faster over time, with the patient leaning forward until losing balance (festinating gait).

NEUROPATHY

Gait is typically that of a sensory ataxia unless there is prominent motor deficit. Because there is a proprioceptive defect, patients often misjudge the surface so the foot lands imprecisely and often hard on the surface. If motor involvement has produced foot drop, there will be even higher steppage of the gait and more of a slapping of the landing.

Reflex Abnormalities

Karl E. Misulis and Martin A. Samuels

Reflex Physiology

Reflexes are used for examination purposes, but they demonstrate integral and sometimes complex functioning of the nervous system. Reflexes can be physiologic and pathologic. Physiologic reflexes use pathways that are normally functioning in a patient of the particular age and state. Pathologic reflexes are abnormalities that can be either errors within the reflex pathway or inappropriate responses for the age and state of the patient.

Tendon reflexes are elicited by using a combination of percussion and limb positioning to transiently lengthen a tendon. Contraction of the muscle is the normal response. Tendon reflexes are elicited with a certain character and strength in individuals with normal neurologic functioning. The reflex loops that serve these are used normally for precise control over movement.

If there is damage to the corticospinal tract innervating these fibers, then the affected tendon reflexes are reduced acutely because of loss of descending input and then become enhanced because of increased function of the segmental reflex pathways. This results in hyperreflexia with an enhanced response; if severe, clonus is elicited by the reflex. When reflexes are so enhanced, there is also activation of muscles not usually affected by the tendon reflex (i.e., generalization).

Damage to the sensory afferents serving the reflex will result in reduced reflex because of a reduction in the amplitude and synchrony of the afferent signal. Damage to the motor efferents will produce reduced reflex. Distinguishing motor versus sensory defect can be difficult. In general, with a sensory deficit, motor power should be normal; with a motor nerve defect, motor power will be reduced.

Frontal release signs are reflexes that are normally present in infants but are abolished in normal adults. In the presence of significant cerebral damage, especially frontal, they can recur and hence are sometimes termed frontal release signs. Glabellar, palmomental, snout, and grasp are the most common frontal release signs. Rooting is less common and less reliable but is discussed.

The Romberg test examines stability of stance and is essentially a test of proprioception. As such, it examines integrity of the dorsal columns. Cerebellar lesions will affect stance even when the patient has their eyes open.

Localization and Diagnosis of Reflex Findings

TENDON REFLEXES

Biceps Reflex

The biceps is supplied by the musculocutaneous nerve and mainly the C6 root. Biceps hyporeflexia in the absence of other abnormalities suggests a C6 nerve root lesion; a specific musculocutaneous nerve lesion is uncommon. Biceps hyperreflexia suggests a corticospinal tract lesion and is almost always associated with hyperactive triceps and brachioradialis reflex.

Triceps Reflex

Triceps reflex is served by the C7 nerve root and the radial nerve. Hyporeflexia can be due to damage to the C7 nerve root or the radial nerve. Hyperreflexia due to corticospinal tract dysfunction usually produces hyperreflexia of other arm reflexes.

Brachioradialis Reflex

Brachioradialis reflex is mediated by the C6 nerve root and the radial nerve. Hyporeflexia is usually due to damage to the C6 nerve root, but radial nerve damage can also produce it. Hyperreflexia from corticospinal tract damage also usually affects triceps and other upper extremity reflexes.

Patellar Reflex

Patellar reflex is also called the patellar reflex, but the examiner does not actually strike the patella, except for the occasional straight-leg knee reflex (e.g., trauma or other immobilized patient) where the reflex is elicited by percussion of the examiner's finger on the superior aspect of the patella. This reflex is served by the femoral nerve and L2 through L4 nerve roots. Hyporeflexia is usually produced by damage to the femoral nerve because single radiculopathy is unlikely to markedly reduce the reflex. Hyperreflexia due to corticospinal tract involvement produces increased ankle reflex.

Achilles Reflex

Achilles reflex is elicited by activation of the Achilles tendon of the gastrocnemius. The reflex is mediated by the sciatic nerve and mainly the S1 nerve root. Hyporeflexia is usually due to S1 nerve root damage. Hyperreflexia is common with stroke. The reflex may elicit clonus, and the knee reflex is usually enhanced.

FRONTAL RELEASE SIGNS

Frontal release signs are commonly used in evaluation of patients with dementia and encephalopathy, but their clinical utility is questioned. Despite the widespread use of these techniques, there is good supporting data only for the grasp.

Glabellar

Examiner taps between the patient's eyebrows, ensuring that their hand is not in the patient's line of sight so that there is no blink to visual threat. Abnormal response is blink that the patient cannot suppress.

Snout

Examiner taps the skin between the patient's upper lip and the nose. Abnormal response is pursing of the lips, which may resemble a snout. Alternative names have included orbicularis oris reflex, but that is a bit long, and oral reflex, but this term is used for the constellation of reflexes of infants.

Palmomental

Examiner strokes a finger across the palm of the patient's hand. An abnormal response is ipsilateral contraction of the perioral muscles.

Grasp

Examiner strokes the palm of the patient's hand, and the fingers curl as if to grasp the examiner's finger. Frank closure is not expected, and the curling may be subtle.

CORTICOSPINAL TRACT SIGNS

Plantar Reflex

Terminology can be confusing, and there are discrepancies in the literature. Hence, we use the term plantar reflex. Some authors use the term Babinski reflex to refer to performance of the test regardless of outcome and Babinski sign to be the abnormal response. Others use the Babinski reflex or Babinski response as the abnormal response. The examiner strokes the sole of the patient's foot from the midsole to the base of the toes, turning medially. A flexor (downward) response of the hallux and other toes is normal. An abnormal response is extension (upward) response of the hallux and fanning of the other toes. Data on validity of the plantar reflex are not as good as one would hope, but we believe that much of the fall-off in specificity of the plantar reflex is due to technique.

Finger and Foot Tapping

Repetitive finger tapping or foot tapping speed and consistency seems to be a fairly sensitive and specific assessment of corticospinal tract function. However, to be rigorous, multiple trials are needed, which cannot be performed during the routine neurologic examination. A brief one-trial test does not have the established documented validity that is needed for routine practice.

Hoffmann Sign

The examiner flicks the terminal phalanx of the patient's middle finger and watches for flexion of the thumb and index finger, which is the abnormal response. This is seen often enough in normal patients that it is not a helpful test of corticospinal tract dysfunction. If the test is abnormal in isolation, without other clinical evidence of corticospinal tract dysfunction, it should not be overinterpreted.

Clinical Correlations

Dementia from almost any cause, but especially frontotemporal dementia, can produce multiple frontal release signs, especially grasp, snout, and less likely palmomental.

Parkinsonism often produces positive glabellar response in the absence of other frontal release signs, unless significant dementia is associated.

Stroke produces hyperactive tendon reflexes in the affected limb(s). There is spread of the reflex to adjacent joints. If the leg is involved, there is an extensor plantar response.

Multiple sclerosis can affect almost any part of the body, so a clue to this diagnosis is abnormalities in reflex and other neurologic examination findings that cannot be explained by a single lesion. For example, hemiplegia with contralateral leg weakness would not be expected to be from a single lesion, if the contralateral arm has absolutely normal function and reflexes.

Spinal cord lesions when acute can cause spinal shock, where reflexes are suppressed. Reflexes below the level of the lesion quickly (hours to 2 days) become hyperactive with extensor plantar response bilaterally. Reflexes above the level of the lesion are normal unless they are affected by other pathology.

Pain

Karl E. Misulis and Martin A. Samuels

Pain is an important aspect of neurologic localization. It is also more difficult to localize than motor function. This is comparable to sensory examination where the determination of deficit is completely subjective. The first aspect of localization is the determination of whether it is a peripheral nerve, spinal, cranial nerve, or cerebral issue.

Pain is a presenting symptom in a minority of patients with neurologic conditions, unless those patients are being seen in a clinic or practice specifically targeting headache or neuropathic pain. In patients for whom pain is the predominant chief complaint, it is essential to localize and focus on that pain. For patients in whom the presenting issue is not pain related, asking questions about pain can help to localize the lesion. These questions are not only regarding sensory function but also regarding pain secondary to compensatory mechanisms due to of loss of function.

Knowing the anatomy of the central and peripheral nervous systems, the neurologist asks questions about the distribution of the pain to determine whether it is central or peripheral and its most likely distribution.

Determining the nature of the pain can help pinpoint the type of damage producing the pain, which again is an aid to diagnosis. Is the pain neuropathic, visceral, or musculoskeletal?

Pain classification differs, but in general pain is

- Neuropathic,
- Nociceptive,
- Inflammatory
- Functional.

Neuropathic pain is caused by irritation of the neural elements, either intraaxial or extraaxial. Trigeminal neuralgia and diabetic sensory neuropathy pain are examples of neuropathic pain.

Nociceptive pain is caused by damage to tissues, and it is typical of pain from trauma and other structural causes.

Inflammatory pain occurs when there is inflammation of select tissues. One example is inflammation around an abscess. There are also inflammatory components to many disorders, from giant cell arteritis to migraine and discusses some important pain syndromes.

This chapter presumes basic knowledge of pain mechanisms and pathways and discusses some important pain syndromes.

Headache

Headaches come in many types. The final common pathway to all pain is neural, but the foundation is either vascular, neuropathic, or inflammatory.

Migraine is described as a vascular headache, but the first changes are cortical with a spreading depression. This likely is responsible for the aura of migraine. Inflammatory changes develop, which then activate trigeminal via calcitonin gene-related peptide (CGRP) and produce the pain. Therefore, migraine appears to have neuropathic and vascular features with an inflammatory component. The aura, nausea, and character of the pain make the diagnosis of migraine, although not all migraines are preceded by an aura. Unilateral headache is associated particularly with migraine, though bilateral headaches are also seen. Throbbing pain, nausea, and photophobia and phonophobia are typically related. Patients want to lie down in a quiet, dark place.

Cluster headache has similarities to migraine in that there is activation of trigeminal nerves with an inflammatory response that may involve the cavernous sinus. Cluster headache is diagnosed by stereotypic attacks of unilateral periorbital and/or temporal pain that are brief and occur in clusters.

Occipital neuralgia is neuropathic pain in the distribution of usually one but sometimes both occipital nerves. Diagnosis is made on the basis of the episodic neuropathic nature of the pain and often elicited by the palpation of the greater or lesser occipital nerves.

Giant cell arteritis (GCA) is an inflammatory disorder that typically causes headache associated with tenderness in the region. Jaw claudication is helpful, but it is only present in about half of patient. The greatest risk of GCA is visual loss particularly when GCA is untreated, but it can occur even if GCA is treated. The etiology of GCA is not completely understood, but it involves inflammatory change in the arteries that can result in occlusion of affected vessels. GCA is also called temporal arteritis, but that name is not preferred because the pain is not always temporal. Diagnosis is suspected by the presence of unilateral temporal or regional headache and the coexistence of malaise, sometimes fever and recent weight loss, and tenderness over the affected area(s). Any visual loss is strongly supportive and should provoke expedited treatment.

Neuropathic Pain

In neuropathic pain, the origin of the pain is the nerves themselves as opposed to the nerves being the conduit of tissue pain to the nervous system.

Neuropathic pain can be central or peripheral. Central pain is generated by damage to central nervous system (CNS) structures, the most dramatic of which is the thalamus. Thalamic pain syndrome is a common, persisting, and very painful condition. Stroke, demyelinating disease, tumors, and almost any other condition with structural CNS damage can result in central pain.

Thalamic pain after stroke presents with unilateral sensory deficit with the initial stroke; then the pain develops as the sensory deficits are starting to recover, in approximately the same distribution. The pain can be spontaneous, but it can also be evoked by stimuli that would not normally be painful (allodynia).

Neuropathic pain has two major types, which can be described as large fiber or small fiber.

Clinical Syndromes

Sensory neuropathy from almost any cause can produce neuropathic pain, which is usually length dependent. Diabetic sensory neuropathy is a typical example. The diagnosis is suspected in patients with foot pain and history of diabetes. When the patient does not have diabetes, the differential diagnosis of sensory neuropathy is much larger and includes HIV, paraneoplastic syndromes, amyloidosis, and others.

Trigeminal neuralgia is typically characterized by severe lancinating pain in the distribution of the trigeminal nerve, particularly the lower divisions. Symptoms are almost always unilateral. Diagnosis is clinical, although imaging is performed to ensure that there is no other etiology.

Glossopharyngeal neuralgia is neuropathic pain with a stabbing or shooting character. The pain is in the back of the throat and often extends into the ear. The episodes are paroxysmal and brief. Diagnosis is clinical, although imaging is performed to rule out other pharyngeal and skull-base pathology.

Herpes zoster is reactivation of the varicella zoster virus (VZV). It presents with pain in a dermatomal distribution that often precedes development of a rash. The diagnosis is suspected when there is development of the rash. When the pain begins, other causes of radiculopathy are considered.

Multisystem Disorders

Karl E. Misulis and Eli E. Zimmerman

Overview

For multisystem disorders, the diagnosis often depends on identifying the combination of neurologic and nonneurologic manifestations. For example, neuropathy plus macrocytic anemia should raise concern for B12 or folate deficiency. Confusion, neuropathy, and gastrointestinal (GI) distress might raise concern for lead poisoning. Seizures with fasciculations and profuse salivation suggest cholinesterase toxicity (nerve agent).

This section discusses some important multisystem disorders. This is not a complete list, but it is illustrative of the types of presentations and the diagnoses they suggest.

Nutritional Deficiencies

B12 DEFICIENCY

Vitamin B12 deficiency is underdiagnosed. It can develop in the elderly, in vegetarians (especially vegans), and in people who have difficulty with absorption. The patient can present with cognitive, motor, and or sensory abnormalities. The term pernicious anemia is used when this occurs due to autoimmune causes. Macrocytic anemia is characteristic of B12 deficiency, and it looks very similar to what is seen with folate deficiency.

Neurologic complications can be in multiple locations, specifically the peripheral nerve, spinal cord, and brain. Common presentations of B12 deficiency are discussed here.

Cognitive Dysfunction memory disturbance and mood disturbance are the most common cognitive abnormalities. Psychosis can be seen (megaloblastic madness).

Neuropathy both motor and sensory disturbances are evident. The sensory changes are length dependent, so distal lower extremities are affected prior to proximal and upper extremities. The changes are sensory loss and paresthesias. Affected sensation is cutaneous and proprioceptive.

Myelopathy spinal cord involvement affects predominantly the dorsal columns and lateral tracts, resulting in loss of dorsal column sensation and corticospinal tract dysfunction with weakness and spasticity. Hence, there is a combination of upper and lower motor neuron dysfunction with B12 deficiency.

THIAMINE DEFICIENCY

Thiamine (B1) deficiency is most commonly seen in people who abuse alcohol, but it is also present in people with reduced intake because of low consumption of whole grains and meats that are high in thiamine. Patients with hyperemesis gravidarum or those who have undergone gastric bypass surgery can become deficient in thiamine as well. Neuropathy is the most common complication of B1 deficiency; Wernicke encephalopathy and Korsakoff syndrome are important complications. Cardiomyopathy can occur producing distal edema due to heart failure with capillary leak. This has been called *wet beriberi*.

Thiamine Deficiency Neuropathy

Neuropathy often presents with sensory symptoms ascending, which can resemble acute inflammatory demyelinating polyneuropathy (AIDP). The symptoms can be paresthesias and burning pain. Motor deficits then appear with weakness and often muscle cramps. Up to 25% of patients with thiamine-deficient neuropathy have concomitant Wernicke encephalopathy.

Wernicke Encephalopathy and Korsakoff Syndrome

These are considered together because they frequently coexist, and clinical differentiation is blurred. Classically, Wernicke encephalopathy presents with the triad of encephalopathy, ocular motor deficits, and gait ataxia. The complete triad is seldom seen. Encephalopathy is the most prevalent finding. Confusion, memory deficit, and inattention are typical. If untreated, prominent encephalopathy develops. Ocular motor abnormalities include any combination of nystagmus, gaze palsies, and CN VI palsy. Ataxia is a combination of central and peripheral deficits, including neuropathy and cerebellar ataxia. Korsakoff syndrome is on a continuum from Wernicke encephalopathy, and it usually follows one or more episodes of encephalopathy. Korsakoff syndrome presents with gait difficulty, more severe memory loss, and anterograde and retrograde amnesia. Confabulation is common although not universal. Wernicke encephalopathy is a medical emergency. If not identified and treated quickly, it can develop into Korsakoff syndrome, which is often irreversible.

FOLATE DEFICIENCY

Folate deficiency produces a similar presentation to B12 deficiency, with cognitive deficits being most common and peripheral nerve and spinal cord involvement occurring less commonly. Patients often have megaloblastic anemia. When a neurologist is considering a patient for possible B12 deficiency, they should also check folate levels.

Toxic and Metabolic Disorders

A host of toxic and metabolic disorders can present with neurologic complications. The most common manifestation is encephalopathy. When a patient is initially evaluated for unexplained mental status changes, toxic and metabolic disorders and concurrent infections are potential causes to consider. Almost any organ system can be involved. Patients may have hepatic or renal insufficiency that can develop insidiously. The combination of neurologic symptoms along with these organ abnormalities is the clue to this diagnosis.

Hepatic encephalopathy (HE) presents with encephalopathy, which is graded from mild behavioral change (grade I) to coma (grade IV). In the severe state, there are no distinguishing features. In milder encephalopathy, patients often present with confusion with asterixis. This suggests consideration of HE, but it is not specific for it. Reflexes may be brisk, and nystagmus is commonly seen. Encephalopathy is often provoked by concurrent illness (especially GI bleeding), medications including sedatives or ethanol, or high dietary protein intake. Elevated ammonia levels are not always seen in HE, and elevated levels can be seen in patients without HE.

Renal insufficiency produces cognitive deficits by direct uremic encephalopathy and by impaired clearance of some medications. Findings can be mild confusion to severe encephalopathy. Other than cognitive findings, asterixis can be seen, which may trigger concern for HE. Restless leg syndrome symptoms are often seen in patients with worsening renal insufficiency.

Nerve agents—Cholinesterase inhibitor intoxication nerve agents are an important although uncommon cause of multisystem toxicity with neurologic involvement. These are most commonly acetylcholinesterase inhibitors. As such, they can produce a constellation of central nervous, peripheral nervous, and autonomic abnormalities. Exposure is usually from overexposure to some insecticides. Nerve agents are also chemical weapons and have been used in terror attacks.

Autonomic stimulation produces early symptoms of salivation, lacrimation, and diaphoresis. Miosis or mydriasis and bradycardia or tachycardia can develop depending on the effects on the sympathetic ganglia. Respiratory failure is common with acute intoxication. Neurologic complications include weakness and fasciculations and can progress to seizures and coma.

Ethanol is one of the most common causes of toxic encephalopathy seen in the emergency department. The spectrum of symptoms can result in ethanol intoxication being mistaken for stroke, seizure, central nervous system (CNS) infection, or head injury. Common symptoms are confusion, behavioral disturbance, gait and appendicular ataxia, and nystagmus. Diagnosis is complicated by the coexistence of other conditions, such as a motor vehicle accident or fall accompanying the intoxication. How much of the presentation is due to ethanol versus head injury? Similarly, coexistent intoxication with other substances is common.

Lead exposure in adults is usually occupational, but there is also a risk in water supplies. Neurologic symptoms are often cognitive with deficits in concentration and memory, and affective disturbance with agitation or depression. Neuropathic involvement is predominantly motor and can produce wrist drop and/or foot drop. Acute intoxication can produce cerebral edema in addition to GI distress, and this combination is a clue to the diagnosis.

Mercury intoxication is rare but can produce weakness, tremor, confusion, and irritability. Exposure is usually industrial and is uncommon.

Autoimmune Disorders

Many autoimmune disorders affect different parts of the nervous system, resulting in potentially confusing localization. In addition, some are associated with nonneurologic involvement. These findings can be of additional help in diagnosis.

Systemic lupus erythematosus patients with systemic lupus erythematosus (SLE) can present with a host of neurologic complications. Among the most important are stroke, cognitive disturbance, and seizures. The pathology responsible for the vascular changes is diverse, but the incidence of almost all types of stroke, ischemic and hemorrhagic, is increased. Hypertension is a major cause, but occasionally anticardiolipin antibody or valvular abnormalities (Libman-Sachs endocarditis) are responsible. Encephalopathy can occur independently of stroke and symptoms can range from mild confusion to psychosis. The pathophysiology is incompletely understood and might be diverse. If the patient is on immunosuppressive agents for SLE, development of encephalopathy might also be due to opportunistic infection, so this must be considered. Lupus can cause cerebritis.

Sjogren Syndrome patients with Sjogren syndrome may present with neuropathy of various types. The spectrum of neurologic involvement is controversial. A wide range of polyneuropathies, mononeuropathies, mononeuropathy multiplex, and cranial neuropathies have been described. CNS involvement can include confusion but can also manifest symptoms of focal and multifocal demyelination with a recurring nature; this can appear similar to the presentation of multiple sclerosis (MS). In addition to brain involvement, optic nerve and spinal involvement can occur.

Sarcoidosis neurologic complications of sarcoidosis are common, and the disorder can present with neurologic symptoms from the onset. Multiple forms of neurologic involvement can occur, including granulomatous inflammation of the CNS, cranial neuropathies, or peripheral neuropathies. Diagnosis is usually established by identifying extraneural involvement, such as pulmonary or lymph nodes.

Genetic Disorders

Genetic disorders can have their root in several types of defects, including point mutations, changes in copy number, and changes in number of chromosomes. Point mutations can result in coding for the wrong amino acid in the target protein, termination of transcription, or alternation of regulation.

Rather than classifying neurogenetic disorders based on the type of mutation, they can be classified either on the basis of syndrome or on the pattern of genetic inheritance. For the purposes of localization and diagnosis, we will take the syndromic approach.

It is always important to ask about family history, but this is particularly important with diseases with strong genetic implications.

Dementia Alzheimer disease (AD) is the most common dementia and has strong heritability or predisposition based on genetic association. Three autosomal dominant mutations can lead to early-onset AD, but these are rare in the US population. Frontotemporal dementia (FTD) is less common than AD and earlier in onset. Several gene mutations relating to tau, progranulin, and *C9ORF 72* are associated with FTD, but over 50% of cases are sporadic.

Movement Disorder huntington disease is the most high-profile heritable movement disorder, but Parkinson disease also has a genetic predisposition. Essential tremor is often inherited as autosomal dominant.

Epilepsy a variety of epilepsies are strongly heritable with genetic predisposition, not only in patients with other physical and neurologic manifestations but also in patients in whom epilepsy is the only significant medical issue.

Multiple Sclerosis data are conflicting, but there appears to be a correlation between development of MS and having relatives with MS and other immune-mediated disorders.

Stroke genetics plays a role in risk of stroke but less so than other lifestyle and medical risk factors. Recent reports using genome-wide association studies (GWAS) have identified linkage between ischemic stroke, atrial fibrillation, and coronary artery disease, conditions that individually predispose to stroke.

Since the development of GWAS and related studies and the increasing availability of medical databanks that contain genetic information, an increasing genetic relationship is likely to be identified for many conditions with neurologic manifestations.

Psychiatric Disorders

Karl E. Misulis and Martin A. Samuels

Neurologists are often asked to assess patients with presentations that are thought to be possibly neurologic but that ultimately prove to be psychiatric. Some of these include:

- Catatonia,
- Psychosis,
- Psychogenic unresponsiveness,
- Nonepileptic events, and
- Psychogenic movement disorders.

Psychiatric Disorders With Neurologic Manifestations

Catatonia is manifested by the patient not moving and appearing unresponsive. Details of the presentation are varied, but typically there is increased tone with waxy flexibility where a limb holds a posture in which it is placed. The Bush-Francis Catatonia Rating Scale is often used to assess catatonia. Examination can help differentiate psychiatric catatonia from medical etiologies of catatonia. In psychiatric catatonia, there are totally intact reflexes, showing no signs of structural central nervous system damage or overdose of many agents that could cause unresponsiveness. The underlying psychiatric disorder can be depression, psychosis, bipolar, or other primary psychiatric disorder. Lorazepam challenge is sometimes helpful in diagnosing catatonia. Intravenous lorazepam 1 to 2 mg can produce restoration of responsiveness within 5 to 10 minutes. This test is only helpful if positive, as it does not exclude catatonia if negative. Catatonia associated with medical conditions can be related to a broad range of diagnoses, but autoimmune encephalitis is an important one to consider. Patients with anti–N-methyl-D-aspartate (anti-NMDA) receptor encephalitis can develop catatonia and can be difficult to treat.

Functional disorders are discussed in Chapter 5.12; these can be subtle or dramatic, with nonepileptic events and movement disorders such as astasia-abasia being quite prominent. Risk factors for functional movement disorders include psychologically traumatic events, physical injury or illness, and sexual abuse.

Parkinsonism can occur in patients with psychosis; it is often caused by neuroleptic agents. Newer atypical neuroleptics are less likely to produce parkinsonism, but this complication still occurs.

Mood disorders including anxiety and depression are more common in patients with epilepsy than in the general population.

Neurologic Complications in Patients with Psychiatric Disease

Substance use is more common in patients with psychiatric disorders. They can present to the neurologist in the acute care setting with overdose, cerebral hemorrhage, or ischemia related to cocaine use and similar exposures.

Drug-induced parkinsonism is most common with neuroleptics and less so with most of the newer antipsychotics.

Serotonin syndrome is an episode of marked increase in serotonin activity that can be due to selective serotonin reuptake inhibitors (SSRIs) and other serotoninergic drugs. The diagnosis is clinical and includes altered mental status, agitation, increased muscular activity such as tremor or myoclonus, or corticospinal tract signs such as restlessness, diaphoresis, tachycardia, hypertension, and hyperthermia. This combination of mental status and neuromotor and autonomic findings is typical.

Noncompliance is common in patients with psychiatric disorders. For example, patients with bipolar disorder may come on and off their medications; if they have seizures, this can be problematic. In a patient with breakthrough seizure, noncompliance is one cause to consider.

Neuroleptic malignant syndrome (NMS) is seen in patients who are given antipsychotics mainly for psychiatric disorders, but it can occur with administration of other related agents including some antiemetics. NMS symptoms can develop with abrupt withdrawal or reduction of some anti-parkinsonian medications, but many consider this to be a distinct although similar entity. NMS presents with altered mental status, fever, rigidity, and associated autonomic instability.

Hypoxic encephalopathy is one potential complication from a suicide attempt. Details depend on the mechanism, and there are findings on general medical examination that support hanging and intravenous drug use. With hanging, venous and arterial strokes can occur.

Diagnosis of Suspected Disorders

Disorders of Mental Status

Howard S. Kirshner and Karl E. Misulis

The disorders of mental status include focal syndromes, such as aphasia, apraxia, agnosia, and neglect, followed by more diffuse syndromes, such as delirium and dementia. The aphasias are discussed in Chapter 5.2.

Apraxia: Neurology of Learned Movement

Apraxia is a disorder of learned motor acts not caused by paralysis, incoordination, sensory deficit, or lack of understanding of the desired movement. In practical terms, apraxia is an inability to carry out skilled motor acts to respond to a command when the patient understands the command and can perform the same motor act in a different context. Liepmann, a German clinician, described three types of apraxia: ideomotor, ideational, and limb kinetic.

It is important to differentiate several diverse motor phenomena that are commonly confused with the principal varieties of apraxia. These are constructional, dressing, oculomotor, and gait apraxia.

Constructional apraxia, characterized by visuospatial difficulties, is associated with right hemispheric lesions. These patients may be unable to copy a drawing of a clock or a house. In most instances, this deficit is related to neglect of the left side of space or failure to appreciate the spatial relations of items rather than to a motor planning deficit, hence apraxia may not be the best name for it.

Dressing apraxia is also associated with right hemisphere lesions. The patients have difficulty relating the spatial aspects of a garment to the body. Again, this is a visuospatial deficit and not a true motor apraxic deficit.

Oculomotor apraxia refers to a difficulty with voluntary direction of the eyes in gaze and is associated with damage to the brainstem mechanism for control of eye movements.

Gait apraxia refers to an inability to walk that is not clearly explained by primary motor weakness, ataxia, or sensory loss. There is no easy way to demonstrate that the same sequential actions can be performed normally in a different context; therefore, it is unclear whether this gait disorder is a true apraxia.

A last example is **apraxia of speech**, discussed in Chapter 5.2. Whether apraxia of speech is a true apraxia is debated by aphasia experts.

IDEOMOTOR APRAXIA

Ideomotor apraxia refers to the failure to carry out a motor act in response to a verbal command, yet the patient understands the command and has the motor capacity to perform the same action in a different context. By Liepmann's model, the idea of the movement, decoded in Wernicke area, is disconnected from its execution in the premotor cortex of the frontal lobe. Ideomotor apraxia often accompanies aphasia in patients with left hemisphere lesions. Only a small percentage of patients with ideomotor apraxia have right-sided lesions. Patients with ideomotor aphasia typically fail to carry out the requested action to verbal command and perform only slightly better in imitation of the examiner, but they carry out the act much better when given the actual object.

A lesion in the left temporal lobe, which also causes aphasia, prevents information regarding the desired act from reaching the left premotor area. Ideomotor apraxia may be part of the deficit in Wernicke aphasia, but the impairment of comprehension makes it difficult to ascertain whether the patient has understood the command. In conduction aphasia and Broca aphasia, ideomotor apraxia may interfere with the patient following commands with limbs on either side of the body. Such apraxic deficits may create the mistaken impression that the patient has a comprehension deficit; asking the patient yes or no questions or giving simple pointing commands are tests to establish that auditory comprehension is intact. Finally, lesions of the corpus callosum can prevent motor information from reaching the right hemisphere motor area. This callosal apraxia affects movement of the left limbs only. The existence of callosal apraxia implies that the left hemisphere is dominant not only for speech but also for learned motor acts, because the right hemisphere cannot program the skilled movements independently.

This association of aphasia and apraxia may reflect the underlying symbolic nature of both speech and gestural expression, or it may simply reflect the anatomic contiguity of centers for speech–language function and those for learned motor acts. The association between apraxia and aphasia explains why most patients with aphasia cannot learn complex gestural languages such as American Sign Language.

IDEATIONAL APRAXIA

Ideational apraxia is a more complex phenomenon than ideomotor apraxia. Heilman proposed the term "conceptual apraxia" as a similar form of apraxia. There are two competing definitions of ideational apraxia. Some authors use it to mean apraxia for real objects. Ochipa and colleagues described a patient who could name objects but not demonstrate their use, as if he had lost the concept of their purpose (apraxia for tool use). The second definition of ideational apraxia is the loss of the ability to carry out a multistep activity, although each individual step may be performed appropriately. For example, a patient may not be able to fill, light, and smoke a pipe or assemble a coffee percolator and make coffee. Failure to carry out a series action may reflect a motor planning difficulty, as seen in frontal lobe lesions. It may be a more sensitive test for apraxia than single motor commands. By either definition, ideational apraxia is associated with left hemisphere lesions, often large temporoparietal lesions associated with severe aphasia. Both ideomotor and ideational apraxia also occur in Alzheimer disease (AD).

LIMB-KINETIC APRAXIA

The third of Liepmann's apraxia syndromes is limb-kinetic apraxia, a deficit of fine motor acts involving only one limb. Patients with mild pyramidal tract lesions may not be weak in gross limb movements but may have difficulty with rapid or fine movements of the fingers. Such apraxia may be a sign of a partial corticospinal tract lesion with mild weakness. Heilman and colleagues referred to this type of apraxia as a "loss of deftness." A left hemisphere lesion may be associated with limb-kinetic apraxia of both hands, whereas a right hemisphere lesion is usually associated with limb-kinetic apraxia of the left hand only.

Agnosias: Neurology of Recognition

Agnosias are disorders of recognition. Most affect a single sensory system (visual, auditory, or tactile agnosia), and others involve specific classes of items within a modality (prosopagnosia which is agnosia for faces and phonagnosia which is agnosia for familiar voices). In each case, the patient must be shown to have normal primary sensory perception, normal ability to name the item once it is recognized, and no general cognitive deterioration or dementia.

For example, a patient with visual agnosia may fail to recognize a bell by sight but can identify and name it by the sound of the bell ringing or by palpating it. Each sensory modality carries a somewhat arbitrary division between primary sensory cortical deficits and agnosia. Most agnosias require bilateral cortical lesions, cutting off input from the sensory modality in both hemispheres to the left hemisphere language centers.

In the visual system, bilateral occipital lesions may cause cortical blindness; partial lesions may permit primary visual perception of the elements of an object or picture, such that the patient can draw lines or angles representing the item but cannot identify the item. Shown a drawing of a pair of glasses, the patient may report two circles and identify it as a bicycle.

Prosopagnosia, or the inability to identify faces, is a subtype of visual agnosia in which patients cannot recognize family members or friends, although they can describe features, such as hair color, a mustache or beard, or accessories (e.g., hats or glasses). Frequently, the patient with prosopagnosia identifies the person by voice or gait pattern. Oliver Sacks described prosopagnosia, or perhaps a more profound visual agnosia, in *The Man Who Mistook His Wife for a Hat*.

Auditory agnosias also overlap with the syndrome of cortical deafness resulting from bilateral lesions of the temporal cortex. Some patients with bilateral temporal lobe lesions have preserved pure tone hearing but cannot understand spoken language. As discussed in Chapter 5.2, this deficit is referred to as pure word deafness. Geschwind suggested that pure word deafness results from a bilateral disconnection of the input from the primary auditory cortex (Heschl gyrus) to the left hemisphere Wernicke area. Rarely, patients show preserved auditory comprehension but impaired nonverbal auditory recognition, for example, identification of animal sounds or the characteristic sounds associated with an object such as a bell. This deficit is called auditory nonverbal agnosia. A last bitemporal syndrome is phonagnosia, the inability to recognize familiar voices.

In the tactile modality, parietal lesions often disrupt the identification of objects by feel, a deficit called astereognosis. A related deficit, agraphesthesia, involves the inability to recognize letters or numbers drawn on the hand. If the patient can describe the sensory characteristics of an object but not identify it, this can also qualify as tactile agnosia. In rare instances, patients with bilateral parietal lesions have no ability to recognize objects by touch on either side.

Delirium

No disorder in neurology is more striking or more distressing to patients, families, and medical personnel than delirium or acute encephalopathy. Delirium is second only to stroke as a cause for neurologic consultation Vanderbilt University Medical Center.

Delirium is defined as "a transient disorder of cognition and attention, one accompanied by disturbances of the sleep–wake cycle and psychomotor behavior." Multiple cognitive functions are affected in disparate areas of the brain.

Delirium typically involves alterations in the following features, although not all of them are seen in all patients or at once:
- Disturbed level of consciousness
  - Somnolence
  - Hypervigilance
  - Agitation
- Disturbed perception
  - Hallucinations
  - Illusions
  - Delusions

- Psychomotor abnormalities
  - Restlessness
  - Agitation
  - Disturbed sleep–wake cycle
- Autonomic nervous system hyperactivity
  - Tachycardia
  - Hypertension
  - Fever
  - Diaphoresis
  - Tremor

In current usage, the term delirium can be diagnosed when the patient is agitated, in a normal state of alertness, or somnolent.

Delirium is a common neurobehavioral syndrome, occurring in 30% to 50% of hospitalized patients over age 70. Because almost 50% of hospitalized patients are elderly, it is estimated that as many as 10% of hospitalized medical and surgical patients are encephalopathic at any given time. Though delirium often resolves over days to weeks, a substantial proportion of patients have ongoing cognitive deficits.

A number of specific risk factors for delirium have been identified:

- Preexisting cognitive deficits
- Age older than 80 years
- Prior brain disorder
- Hearing loss
- Vision loss
- Fracture on admission
- Symptomatic infection
- Stress
- Environmental changes
- Medications including
  - Neuroleptics
  - Narcotic analgesics
  - Sedatives
  - Anticholinergic drugs
- Medical procedures including
  - Use of restraints
  - Bladder catheterization
  - Surgery

DIFFERENTIAL DIAGNOSIS OF DELIRIUM

Differential diagnosis of delirium includes

- Psychosis,
- Dementia, and
- Focal brain syndromes.

Hallucinations are usually visual in delirium, but they are more typically auditory in psychiatric disorders. Delusional thinking can occur in delirium, but the delusions are more inconsistent and short-lived as compared to the chronic delusions of psychosis.

Dementia is typically gradual in onset and lacks the psychomotor agitation, sleep–wake abnormality, and autonomic hyperactivity seen in delirium.

Focal syndromes can occasionally overlap with delirium:

- Frontal lesions

- Left temporoparietal lesions with acute Wernicke aphasia
- Right temporoparietal lesions
- Bilateral medial temporal thalamic lesions
- Temporooccipital lesions with amnesia

Frontal lobe disorders can involve abulia or akinetic mutism, inappropriate humor, and the syndrome of approximate answers (Ganser syndrome). This can be seen in patients with frontal lobe damage and in psychosis and hysteria/malingering.

Wernicke aphasia, secondary to a left temporoparietal stroke or other lesion, may be mistaken for delirium.

Amnestic syndrome can mimic delirium and can manifest as loss of short-term memory resulting from bilateral posterior cerebral artery territory strokes, bilateral thalamic lesions, Wernicke-Korsakoff syndrome, or ruptured anterior communicating artery aneurysms.

Right temporoparietal lesions can cause a true delirium.

Prosopagnosia can be mistaken for delirium due to the defect in facial recognition.

Capgras syndrome, the patient fails to recognize relatives and friends and even calls them imposters. Whereas this condition may occur in psychotic disorders, it has been reported with bilateral temporal lobe damage.

CLINICAL FEATURES OF DELIRIUM

The clinical features of delirium are distinctive yet variable. Some patients manifest a prodrome of anxiety, restlessness, drowsiness or insomnia, and vivid dreams. There follows a cognitive/attentional disorder, disruption of the sleep–wake cycle, increased or decreased activity, and fluctuations in mental status, usually with nocturnal exacerbation (sundowning).

Cognitive disturbances involve perception, thinking, memory, orientation, and attention.

Misperceptions can take the form of hallucinations, such as mistaking intravenous tubing for a snake or seeing insects or animals on the wall.

Memory loss involves both immediate and short-term memory, which can be associated with disorientation to place and time but not usually to person. Loss of personal identity or claiming to be a famous person is usually a sign of psychosis.

Attention disorders are prominent in delirium. Patients are highly distractible and cannot pay attention to simple questions, let alone focus on which stimuli are important. Although language disorders are not usually emphasized in delirium, deficits in naming and in writing have been described.

Other clinical features of delirium include:

- Emotional changes (fear, anger);
- Disruption of the sleep–wake cycle with either hyper- or hyposomnolence;
- Psychomotor changes that can involve either agitation or lethargy; and
- Autonomic disturbances such as tachycardia and arrhythmias, hypertension, diaphoresis, flushing, dilated pupils, piloerection, and tremor.

These features distinguish delirium from dementia, in which only the negative cognitive symptoms are prominent.

ETIOLOGY OF DELIRIUM

The etiologies of delirium are legion, and a careful search must be made in each patient. Etiologies include the following:

- Metabolic
  - Hyponatremia
  - Hypercalcemia or hypocalcemia
  - Hyperglycemia or hypoglycemia

- Organ failure syndromes
  - Hepatic insufficiency
  - Renal insufficiency
  - Pulmonary insufficiency
  - Porphyria
- Endocrine disorders
  - Hypo- and hyperthyroidism
  - Hyperparathyroidism
  - Cushing syndrome
- Nutrition
  - Thiamine deficiency
  - Folate deficiency
  - Vitamin B12 deficiency
- Toxic causes
  - Alcohol
  - Drugs of abuse
    Amphetamines
    Cocaine
  - Chemical toxins such as lead
- Medications
  - Anticholinergic drugs
  - Excessive sedative medication
  - Withdrawal from many substances and medications
  - Polypharmacy, especially in older patients with dementia
- Infections affecting the nervous system
  - Encephalitis
  - Meningitis
  - Brain abscess
- Infections affecting systemic organs
  - Urinary tract infection
  - Pneumonia
- Structural causes
  - Hydrocephalus
  - Traumatic brain injury
- Autoimmune conditions
  - Autoimmune encephalitis
  - Lupus cerebritis
- Cancer related
  - Multiple metastases
  - Neoplastic meningitis
  - Paraneoplastic encephalitis
  - Radiation leukoencephalopathy
- Seizures (see later discussion)
- Stroke (see later discussion)
- Postoperative state (see later discussion)

Regarding seizures, marked disturbance of consciousness can occur with seizure activity without other overt signs. This can be during a subclinical seizure or as a postictal state.

Regarding stroke, patients usually show clinical findings of a stroke syndrome unless they have marked encephalopathy or unless the stroke damage is from multifocal ischemia or hemorrhage, which produces diffuse impairment in cerebral functioning. Cerebral venous sinus thrombosis can present as cognitive changes without noted focality, often in association with headache.

Postsurgical patients may develop delirium. Cardiac surgery involving cardiopulmonary bypass may be associated with microemboli to the brain, and such complications after surgery are frequent. Other factors such as hypotension and hypoxia during surgery likely also play a role. The intensive care unit, with its attendant stress and fear, sleep deprivation, environmental change, and constant extraneous stimulation, contributes to the development of delirium.

Dementias

Dementia is defined as a gradual deterioration of previously intact cognitive functions secondary to brain disease. Dementia may begin with one cortical deficit and then progress to multiple deficits. In Alzheimer disease, the most common dementing illness, memory loss is usually the first symptom, and other deficits follow.

Dementia can be caused by many disease processes, which can be classed into three major groups: systemic diseases, primarily involving organ systems outside the central nervous system; neurologic diseases, marked by degeneration of systems in addition to the higher cortical functions; and diseases presenting primarily with loss of cognitive faculties.

DEMENTIAS SECONDARY TO SYSTEMIC DISEASES

Most of the dementia-causing systemic diseases are treatable, and therefore their identification is of practical importance. For many metabolic disorders, such as disturbances of electrolytes (hyponatremia), failure of the liver or kidneys, and calcium disturbances, patients present with an acute confusional state or delirium rather than chronic dementia, but the two syndromes overlap.

Toxic disorders include the effects of chemicals, heavy metals, alcohol, and drugs. Chronic alcohol ingestion coupled with poor nutrition may cause symptoms of thiamine deficiency (Wernicke-Korsakoff syndrome). Technically, this syndrome involves pure memory loss rather than dementia, but there is evidence that chronic alcohol abusers may develop a true dementia as well. Among toxins, prescribed drugs are among the most common treatable causes of dementia. Sedative effects of multiple medications may combine to cause chronic mental impairment. A few drugs cause confusion directly, including anticholinergic drugs such as tricyclic antidepressants, antihistamines, and neuroleptics. A nutritional cause of dementia is vitamin B12 deficiency.

Infections are an infrequent but important cause of dementia. The most treatable cause is infectious meningitis. Viral encephalitis is a more acute syndrome that may leave dementia in its wake. Dementia is also an aspect of AIDS. Although some patients have secondary infections and tumors affecting the nervous system, HIV itself appears to cause chronic encephalitis, resulting in dementia (AIDS dementia complex). Multiple strokes can also cause dementia. Vascular cognitive impairment often is mixed with AD, representing the second most common cause of dementia after AD itself.

NEUROLOGIC DISEASES ASSOCIATED WITH DEMENTIA

The second group of dementias involves neurologic diseases that lead to cognitive deterioration. Normal pressure hydrocephalus and basal ganglia diseases are the most common examples.

Normal pressure hydrocephalus is characterized by the gradual onset of mental slowing and then frank dementia, gait difficulty, and urinary incontinence. Brain imaging studies show dilation of the cerebral ventricles out of proportion to the degree of brain atrophy. Some patients respond dramatically to shunting procedures, in which spinal fluid is rerouted from the cerebral ventricles into the abdomen, and experience return of mental function and improved gait and urinary continence.

Most other neurologic diseases associated with dementia fall under the heading of neurodegenerative diseases, in which specific populations of neurons deteriorate. Several diseases that affect the basal ganglia produce a pattern of subcortical dementia. The most common is Parkinson disease, which is characterized by bradykinesia (slowed movement), rigidity, resting tremor, masklike or expressionless face, and dysarthric speech. Patients exhibit slowed mental processes. A variant of Parkinson disease is Lewy body dementia, in which mental changes occur before or simultaneously with the motor manifestations of Parkinsonism. These patients have rapid cognitive fluctuations, prominent visual hallucinations, and a sleep disorder characterized by speaking or moving during sleep (REM sleep behavior disorder). At autopsy, the Lewy bodies may be present not only in the substantia nigra but also in the cortex. The family of Parkinson-plus disorders—corticobasal degeneration, progressive supranuclear palsy, and multisystem atrophy—is also associated with dementia. Other diseases that combine a movement disorder with a dementing illness are Huntington disease and Wilson disease. These will not be discussed here.

Another neurologic disease not considered primarily a dementia is multiple sclerosis (MS). Recent studies that have included neuropsychological test batteries have found that most patients with chronic MS have significant cognitive impairments. There is some suggestion that MS plaques in the deep periventricular white matter, seen frequently on brain magnetic resonance imaging (MRI) studies of these patients, may correlate better with cognitive and mood disturbances than with physical disability.

PRIMARY DEGENERATIVE DEMENTIAS

Alzheimer Disease

A few diseases primarily cause slowly progressive dementia. AD is the most common, accounting for 50% to 60% of most series of autopsied cases of dementia. The disease is defined by the presence of senile plaques in the neuropil of the cerebral cortex and neurofibrillary tangles (silver-staining strands) in the neurons of the cerebral cortex, hippocampus, and nucleus basalis. The disease is not truly diffuse but rather a multifocal disorder with a predilection for specific structures. The hippocampus and adjacent structures are critical for memory storage and retrieval. The nucleus basalis projects cholinergic fibers to wide areas of the cerebral cortex.

The pathological changes of AD are more quantitatively than qualitatively different from those of normal aging. Recent studies have found that nearly 50% of people who are older than 80 years meet the clinical criteria for dementia. Careful examination and testing for treatable factors, as discussed earlier, are therefore essential for diagnosing AD. Although many drug therapies are being tested in AD, the ultimate cause of the neuronal degeneration remains unclear. Deposition of beta-amyloid in plaques and neurofibrillary tangles within neuron nuclei are the main pathological changes. Gene mutations have been discovered in early onset, dominantly inherited cases, but these are the minority. Apolipoprotein E4 appears to be a risk factor for developing AD.

As mentioned previously, the most common presentation of AD is with short-term memory loss. Three variants of AD have been described. The frontal variant of AD presents with changes in personality and behavior, similar to those described previously under frontal lobe disorders and to frontotemporal dementia to be discussed later. The second variant is a progressive aphasia variant in which naming and repetition are affected early. This will be discussed later in the context of progressive aphasias. The third variant, posterior cortical atrophy, presents with visual disturbances. Patients go to eye doctors, who find nothing wrong; there is progressive difficulty with estimating distances, identifying objects visually, and the like.

Discussion of the management of AD is beyond the scope of this book, but there are medications that can improve memory and functioning of patients with AD. The degree of benefit is limited; within months to a year or two, patients are again declining. Approaches with antibodies against amyloid or tau proteins are under study. Probably the most effective ways of preventing dementia are healthy diet, exercise, avoidance of smoking or excessive alcohol intake, and treatment of vascular risk factors, such as hypertension and elevated lipids.

Frontotemporal Dementia

Another category of primary dementing diseases is called frontotemporal dementia (FTD), in which there is selective degeneration of the frontal and temporal lobes on one or both sides of the brain.

There are two basic presentations:
- Changes in personality and behavior
- Progressive aphasia, usually nonfluent

These two variants of FTD affect the frontal lobes. In the nonfluent primary progressive aphasia (PPA) variant, usually the left frontal lobe is affected, and this variant is often related to tau pathology.

Semantic dementia is another syndrome of progressive, fluent aphasia with anomia; it produces profound comprehension deficits, even for single words. This is not a tauopathy but is most commonly a progranulin mutation.

A logopenic variant of progressive aphasia has been described, with principal deficits of anomia and impaired repetition. This variety of PPA appears most often related to AD and amyloid accumulation in the brain.

Pick disease is a variant of FTD in which there are silver-staining intraneuronal inclusions called Pick bodies but few or none of the senile plaques and neurofibrillary tangles seen in AD. It is now usually subsumed under the FTD diagnosis.

Creutzfeldt-Jakob Disease

Creutzfeldt-Jakob disease is a rapidly progressive disease characterized by mood changes, dementia, seizures, myoclonus, and exaggerated startle responses. It is a degenerative process although the cause is an infectious agent. The course progresses from first symptoms to death in 6 to 12 months or less. The disease is rare, occurring in approximately one per one million people per year worldwide. It was found to be transmitted by inoculation of tissues via contaminated surgical instruments, corneal transplants, and pituitary extracts. It can also occur spontaneously or due to inherited conditions. A proteinaceous infectious particle (prion) is thought to be the cause of the disease, not a DNA-containing virus.

Early changes on MRI studies and specific spinal fluid tests (RT-QuIC, CSF tau levels, and the 14-3-3 protein) can be helpful in diagnosis. A variant of this disease is bovine spongiform encephalopathy (BSE), or mad cow disease, which has been transmitted by beef from infected cattle. There is no effective treatment for these prion diseases.

Traumatic Brain Injury

Traumatic brain injury (TBI) is a major cause of death and disability, particularly in young people. An acute blow to the head may cause instantaneous loss of consciousness and a brief period of retrograde amnesia, such that the patient does not remember the blow that caused the loss of consciousness.

MILD TBI

The term cerebral concussion implies a head injury with a brief loss of consciousness and brief retrograde amnesia but no other evidence of structural disruption of the brain. A great deal of research has concentrated on these minor head injuries and the resultant postconcussive syndrome.

Such patients often have normal brain imaging studies, including skull radiographs, computed tomography (CT) scans, MRI studies, and electroencephalograms.

Patients frequently complain of headaches, poor concentration and memory, insomnia, irritability, mood swings, and sometimes vertigo or dizziness. The damage caused by repeated concussions is a major concern in competitive athletics, and recent guidelines have been promoted to avoid such repetitive injuries.

SEVERE TBI

More severe brain injuries may initially cause coma and structural damage on MRI such as contusions or bruising of the brain, shear hemorrhages, and collections of blood in the subdural or epidural space. Such patients are more severely impaired than patients with concussive injuries, and they frequently have motor deficits and impaired cognition. These patients require prolonged rehabilitation.

Impaired memory and attention are common accompaniments, as are frontal lobe syndromes such as impulsive or agitated behavior. High-level language impairments are frequently found, especially in the organization of discourse. Occasionally, aphasias similar to those seen in stroke patients develop after TBI, especially in patients with localized traumatic injury to the left cerebral hemisphere.

CHRONIC TRAUMATIC ENCEPHALOPATHY

Patients with a history of multiple concussions or more serious brain injuries may develop a chronic dementing illness now called chronic traumatic encephalopathy (CTE). The pathology of this disorder has been clearly described, but the variety of clinical presentations is still being discovered.

Speech and Language Disorders

Howard S. Kirshner and Martin A. Samuels

Introduction

Speech and language are important to our human existence, and they affect our ability to communicate with other people. Speech involves the articulation of language sounds via the vocal apparatus. Language involves the manipulation of symbols in the production and comprehension of communication.

Aphasias are acquired disorders of language secondary to brain disease. The aphasias include specific syndromes in which language functions are affected by lesions of the left hemisphere. The syndromes are diagnosed by the bedside examination of speech and language presented in Chapter 1.3.

Evaluation of the Patient With Aphasia

The first task of the neurologist in evaluating a speech or language problem is to determine whether the patient is aphasic. The definition of aphasia distinguishes acquired language disorders from three other causes of abnormal communication:

- Developmental language disorders are excluded because aphasia is an acquired disorder in a patient with premorbid normal speech and language function.
- Motor speech disorders, such as dysarthria, disturb only spoken language output; written language expression and comprehension remain intact.
- Psychiatric disorders are excluded because the abnormal language content in psychiatric patients is due to a disturbed thought process rather than a language defect.

Paraphasic errors and neologisms (nonexistent words) characterize aphasia more than psychosis, except in a few untreated schizophrenic patients with "word salad speech" or in bipolar patients in a manic state who occasionally make "clang associations." A key difference between psychosis and aphasia is the patient's behavior; an aphasic patient usually behaves appropriately, although they are unable to communicate. The presence of other focal left hemisphere signs in aphasic patients also helps to indicate a neurologic rather than psychiatric disorder.

Motor Speech Disorders

Motor speech disorders refer to abnormalities of speech articulation in the absence of language dysfunction. On the bedside mental status examination, spontaneous speech, repetition, naming, and reading aloud may be abnormal, but auditory comprehension, reading comprehension, and writing should be intact. In general, if the examiner transcribes the speech output of a dysarthric patient and then reads it aloud, it should sound normal. Motor speech disorders are generally divided into dysarthria and apraxia of speech.

DYSARTHRIA

Dysarthria refers to a consistent misarticulation of phonemes, resulting from disturbances of muscular control over the speech mechanism due to damage of the central or peripheral nervous system. By definition, dysarthria is a neurologic disorder. It excludes local, structural disorders such as cleft lip or palate and laryngectomy. The type of dysarthria can aid in the diagnosis of disorders of the central and peripheral nervous systems.

Classification of Dysarthria

Dysarthria is divided into six subtypes based on neuroanatomic lesions, but it is distinguishable by auditory-perceptual characteristics that a clinician can learn to recognize at the bedside. Table 5.2.1 lists a summary of the Mayo Clinic classification of dysarthria. The six types of dysarthria are flaccid, spastic, ataxic, hypokinetic, hyperkinetic, and mixed. Subsequently, the Mayo Clinic group added a subtype of spastic dysarthria called unilateral upper motor neuron dysarthria.

Flaccid dysarthria results from bilateral, lower motor neuron lesions or bulbar palsy, involving cranial nerves, neuromuscular junctions, or muscles. The auditory characteristics include

- Breathy voice quality,
- Hypernasality, and
- Imprecise consonants (errors or distortions of consonant sounds).

Flaccid dysarthria may result from a brainstem stroke, traumatic brain injury, or neuromuscular disorders such as myasthenia gravis, bulbar polio, or Guillain-Barré syndrome.

Spastic dysarthria results from bilateral upper motor neuron lesions, also referred to as pseudobulbar palsy. The auditory characteristics are

- A strain-strangle, harsh voice quality;
- Slow rate; and
- Imprecisely articulated consonants, often with hypernasality.

TABLE 5.2.1 ■ **Classification of Dysarthrias**

Type	Localization	Auditory Signs	Diagnoses
Flaccid	Lower motor neuron	Breathy, nasal voice; imprecise consonants	Stroke; myasthenia gravis
Spastic	Bilateral upper motor neuron	Strain, strangle; harsh voice; slow rate; imprecise consonants	Bilateral strokes; tumors; primary lateral sclerosis
Unilateral upper motor neuron	Unilateral upper motor neuron	Consonant imprecision; slow rate; harsh voice quality	Stroke; tumor
Ataxia	Cerebellum	Irregular articulatory breakdowns; extensive and equal stress	Stroke; degenerative disease
Hypokinetic	Extrapyramidal	Rapid rate; reduced loudness; monopitch; monoloudness	Parkinson disease
Hyperkinetic	Extrapyramidal	Prolonged phonemes; variable rate; inappropriate silences; voice stoppages	Dystonia; Huntington disease
Spastic-flaccid	Upper and lower motor neuron	Hypernasality; strain-strangle; harsh voice; slow rate; imprecise consonants	Amyotrophic lateral sclerosis; multiple strokes

Darley FL, Aronson AE, Brown JR. Differential diagnostic patterns of dysarthria. J Speech Hear Res. 1969;12:246-269, and Duffy JR. Motor speech disorders. Substrates, differential diagnosis, and management. St. Louis:Mosby; 1995.

Causes of spastic dysarthria include bilateral strokes, tumors, and degenerative diseases such as primary lateral sclerosis.

Unilateral upper motor neuron (UUMN) dysarthria results from a UUMN lesion. The auditory signs are similar to the spastic type but are less severe. They include

- Harsh voice,
- Slow rate, and
- Imprecise consonants.

Common causes of UUMN dysarthria are a unilateral hemisphere stroke or brain tumor.

Ataxic dysarthria results from damage in the cerebellum or its connections. The auditory signs are

- Irregular articulatory breakdowns and
- Excessive and equal stress, also referred to as scanning speech.

Possible causes include cerebellar degenerations, strokes, and tumors. Multiple sclerosis frequently produces ataxic dysarthria, but it may be mixed with elements of flaccid, spastic, or UUMN dysarthria.

Hypokinetic dysarthria is associated with extrapyramidal or basal ganglia diseases. The auditory characteristics are

- Rapid rate,
- Reduced loudness,
- Monopitch (unvarying pitch level), and
- Monoloudness (unvarying loudness level).

The most common cause of hypokinetic dysarthria is Parkinson disease. Occasionally, strokes involving the basal ganglia can mimic this pattern.

Hyperkinetic dysarthria is associated with extrapyramidal disorders that have increased rather than decreased movement. The auditory signs include

- Prolonged phonemes (individual speech sounds become stretched out),
- Variable rate (sometimes too fast, sometimes too slow),
- Harsh voice quality,
- Inappropriate pauses or silences, and
- Voice stoppages (inappropriate absence of phonation).

Common causes of hyperkinetic dysarthria are dystonia (e.g., dystonia musculorum deformans), Joseph disease, and Huntington disease.

Mixed dysarthria has several subtypes. The auditory perceptual characteristics vary depending on which neurologic systems are involved.

Spastic-flaccid dysarthria results from involvement of both the upper and lower motor neuron systems. The auditory characteristics are

- Hypernasality,
- Strain-strangle, liquid sounding voice quality (phonation is accompanied by a gurgle),
- Extremely slow rate, and
- Severe consonant imprecision.

Spastic-flaccid dysarthria is typically caused by amyotrophic lateral sclerosis (ALS) but may be seen in multiple strokes.

Multiple sclerosis may produce a mixed ataxic-spastic-flaccid dysarthria resulting from cerebellar, upper motor neuron, and lower motor neuron involvement. The ataxic features (excessive and equal stress, slow rate) may be most prominent.

APRAXIA OF SPEECH

Apraxia of speech is a disorder intermediate between the dysarthrias and the aphasias. Apraxia of speech is a disorder of the programming of rapid sequences of phonemes. The patient does not have significant weakness, slowness, or incoordination of the speech apparatus. By this definition, apraxia of speech is a motor speech disorder, not a language disorder or aphasia.

Apraxia of speech is distinguished from dysarthria because the misarticulations are inconsistent; the patient may pronounce the same word differently, and sometimes normally, in different utterances. For example, a patient trying to repeat the word "catastrophe" might produce five different utterances, with one correct.

Apraxia of speech is distinguished from aphasia by the lack of language disorder. Apraxia of speech is rarely an isolated deficit and is often mixed with aphasia and sometimes with dysarthria.

The key features of apraxia of speech are

- Effortful, trial and error, groping articulatory movements, with attempts at self-correction;
- Dysprosodia, or disruptions in rhythm, stress (emphasis), and intonation of speech;
- Inconsistency, as in production of the word "catastrophe"; and
- Difficulty initiating speech.

Localization and Cause of Apraxia of Speech

The anatomic basis of the motor programming of speech sequences is likely the classical Broca area in the left inferior frontal gyrus because patients with Broca aphasia frequently have an associated apraxia of speech. The disorder can be seen with strokes, traumatic brain injury, degenerative disorders, tumors, and other causes.

Muteness

A patient with no speech output may have severe dysarthria (anarthria), severe apraxia of speech, a nonneurologic disorder such as a laryngeal obstruction, a frontal lobe syndrome with akinetic mutism, an extrapyramidal disorder such as severe Parkinson disease, a psychogenic state such as catatonia, simple uncooperativeness, or stupor.

- Muteness must be differentiated from aphasia:
- Some attempt at language output must be present to permit an examiner to diagnose aphasia.
- Normal writing and normal language comprehension make aphasia unlikely.
- Other signs of left hemisphere injury such as right hemiparesis and right hemianopia point to aphasia.
- In general, the aphasic patient tries to communicate by gesturing, grunting, or pointing; the patient is mute in speech but not in other behaviors.

Aphasias

Aphasias are divided into syndromes involving the primary language cortex and those involving other cortical and subcortical centers. The primary language cortex is arranged as a circuit of centers around the left sylvian fissure, involving the operculum (or roof of the sylvian fissure) in the frontal, parietal, and temporal lobes.

Since aphasia was first described, several clinical classifications of aphasia have been introduced. The aphasia syndrome diagnosis can be supported by standardized batteries such as the Boston Diagnostic Aphasia Examination (BDAE) or the Western Aphasia Battery (WAB).

There has been a tendency to classify aphasias into two groups: expressive versus receptive, motor versus sensory, fluent versus nonfluent, and anterior versus posterior aphasias. The problem with the expressive-receptive and motor-sensory dichotomies is that aphasias are rarely purely expressive or receptive. Virtually all persons with aphasia have abnormal language expression. The terms fluent versus nonfluent aphasia are at least descriptive and easily understood.

There are eight classical aphasia syndromes:

- Broca
- Wernicke

- Global
- Conduction
- Anomic
- Transcortical motor
- Transcortical sensory
- Mixed transcortical aphasia

Mixed transcortical aphasia is also called the syndrome of the isolation of the speech area. There are subsyndromes such as aphemia, pure word deafness, and the subcortical aphasia syndromes

BROCA APHASIA

Paul Broca described two patients who had a difficulty in articulation yet could comprehend spoken language. In modern descriptions, the typical patient with Broca aphasia speaks little or nonfluently. Broca aphasia can range from complete muteness to single word utterances or phrases and short sentences produced hesitantly. The disorder is an aphasia rather than a motor speech disorder because grammatical constructions are disturbed. Expressive speech is agrammatic; it reads like a telegram. For example, a patient with Broca aphasia who wanted to express that his wife would be coming to the hospital might say "wife...come ...hospital." See Table 5.2.2.

TABLE 5.2.2 ■ Broca, Wernicke, and Global Aphasias

Feature	Broca	Wernicke	Global
Spontaneous speech	Nonfluent, hesitant, from mute to agrammatic; often dysarthria	Fluent with paraphasic errors of both phonemic and verbal type	Nonfluent, mute or restricted to a stereotyped phrase
Naming	Impaired (tip-of-the-tongue)	Impaired, often paraphasic	Impaired
Auditory comprehension	Intact for simple material; impaired for complex syntactic constructions	Impaired, often for even simple questions	Impaired
Repetition	Impaired; hesitant	Impaired	Impaired
Reading	Difficulty reading aloud; often poorer reading than auditory comprehension	Usually impaired, with exceptions	Impaired
Writing	Difficulty writing, even with left hand	Well-formed but paragraphic	Impaired
Associated signs	Right hemiparesis; right hemisensory loss; apraxia of left limbs	With or without right hemianopia, usually no motor or sensory abnormalities	Most have right hemianopia, right hemiparesis, right hemisensory loss; often apraxia
Behavior	Frustrated, depressed, but appropriate	Often unaware of deficits; may be inappropriately happy; later sometimes angry, suspicious	Often depressed

Naming in Broca aphasia is impaired. Often the patient has some idea of the name and produces the initial letter or syllable, the so-called "tip of the tongue phenomenon." In some patients, naming of actions (verbs) is worse than naming of objects (nouns).

Repetition in Broca aphasia is usually only slightly better than spontaneous speech, showing the same articulatory difficulty and hesitancy.

Auditory comprehension is largely preserved, but sentences with complex grammar cause comprehension problems. For example, the sentence "the sculpture that Mary gave to Bill was beautiful" may cause confusion about who gave the sculpture and who received it. Modern evidence confirms that the Broca area is involved in both production and comprehension of phrases with complex syntax.

Reading is often more affected than auditory comprehension in Broca aphasia.

Writing is also affected. Most patients have weakness of the right arm, making it difficult for a right-handed patient to write with the dominant hand. The patient may refuse to write with the left hand, but if they attempt to write, only a few awkward letters emerge. Persons with injuries to the right arm can learn surprisingly quickly to write awkwardly but intelligibly with the left hand. The agraphia of Broca aphasia is thus not simply a motor disorder but is a central language disorder affecting writing.

Associated deficits with Broca aphasia include weakness of the right face, arm, and leg and often some sensory loss on the right side of the body. Visual fields are usually spared. Some studies have found an association between poststroke depression and infarctions of the anterior left hemisphere. Behaviorally, patients with Broca aphasia seem appropriately concerned about their stroke deficits; they are frustrated but fully aware. Some patients with Broca aphasia may show apraxia of the left limbs and fail to follow commands for use of the left limbs. The clinician should recognize this apraxia and not mistake it for lack of comprehension.

Lesions of Broca aphasia classically involve the posterior two-thirds of the inferior frontal convolution, the pars triangularis and pars opercularis. Precise lesion localization has significant clinical implications:

- Infarctions restricted to the cortical Broca area are associated with excellent recovery over a few weeks.
- Patients with lesions in areas 44 and 45 have primarily a deficit in initiation of speech without true aphasia.
- Patients with lesions only of the lower motor cortex have only dysarthria and speech hesitancy.
- Both areas 44 and 45 and the lower motor cortex have to be damaged to produce the full picture of Broca aphasia.

Fig. 5.2.1 shows a magnetic resonance imaging (MRI) scan from a patient with a transitory Broca aphasia and apraxia of speech. Patients with lasting Broca aphasia usually have larger lesions, involving not only Broca area but also much of the frontoparietal operculum.

Prognosis for recovery in Broca aphasia depends on how soon after the stroke that the patient is examined. Naeser and her colleagues reported that lesions associated with poor recovery of fluent speech always include two subcortical areas: (1) the subcallosal fasciculus deep to Broca area, and (2) the periventricular white matter along the body of the left lateral ventricle. The combined cortical-subcortical frontal lesion appears to be required for lasting nonfluency.

APHEMIA

Although Broca originally used the term "aphemie" to describe the aphasia that now bears his name, aphemia is now used to designate a more restricted syndrome of nonfluent speech, with normal comprehension and writing. Patients with aphemia are often mute initially, with hesitant speech emerging over a few days.

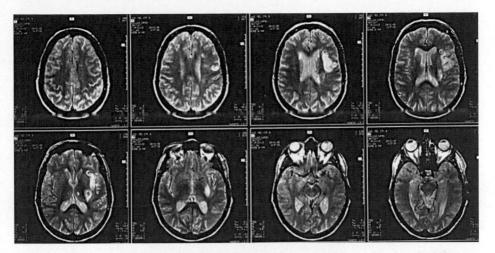

Fig. 5.2.1 Magnetic resonance image (MRI) of Broca aphasia and apraxia of speech. MRI of a patient with a stroke in the left frontal lobe, with Broca aphasia.

The deficits in aphemia are essentially those of isolated apraxia of speech. Both aphemia and pure apraxia of speech are uncommon syndromes; they are often associated with nearly complete recovery over a few weeks.

WERNICKE APHASIA

Wernicke aphasia can be thought of as the opposite of Broca aphasia. The patient with Wernicke aphasia speaks effortlessly and often with normal or even increased numbers of words (logorrhea). However, the content of the speech contains few meaningful nouns and verbs. There are many paraphasic errors of both literal (phonemic) and verbal (semantic) type. If the speech is filled with nonwords so that the meaning cannot be discerned, it is called jargon aphasia. In milder cases, sentences may begin normally, but the words then go awry. A listener unfamiliar with the native language of a person with Wernicke aphasia might not notice anything wrong, as the patient speaks fluently in a pattern that sounds like the speaker's native language. A native listener, however, hears few meaningful nouns and many speech errors. Comprehension is severely impaired.

The features of Wernicke aphasia are listed in Table 5.2.2 and in the following synopsis:
- Naming is impaired, often with utterances not resembling the target word or not words at all.
- Repetition is disrupted by paraphasic substitutions.
- Reading comprehension is often severely impaired, resembling auditory comprehension, but occasional patients may comprehend better in reading than in hearing or vice versa.

These differences may be important, as the use of a spared modality may facilitate communication with the patient. Patients with Wernicke aphasia with intact reading resemble the classic syndrome of pure word deafness (see later discussion), whereas those with spared auditory comprehension resemble patients with pure alexia with agraphia. Writing in Wernicke aphasia shows well-formed letters that are written effortlessly, but the writing is full of empty phrases, misspellings, and nonwords.

The associated deficits of Wernicke aphasia are often minimal. Patients may have right visual field deficits, but usually they have no significant weakness or sensory loss. Patients with Wernicke aphasia may be mistaken for psychotic or confused persons. They often seem unaware of their deficits, and they do not appear depressed initially. Later, they may become angry at not being

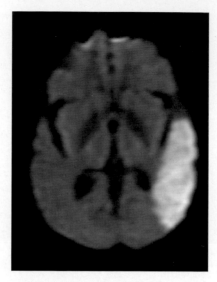

Fig. 5.2.2   Magnetic resonance image (MRI) of Wernicke aphasia and temporal lesion. MRI with diffusion weighted imaging of a patient with acute stroke, with Wernicke aphasia.

understood, and cases of agitation and even paranoid ideation and behavior have been reported with Wernicke aphasia.

The lesions of Wernicke aphasia classically involve the left superior temporal gyrus. Modern studies utilizing computed tomography (CT) and MRI scans have largely confirmed this localization, although some authors include the inferior parietal lobule (supramarginal and angular gyri, Brodmann areas 39 and 40) as part of Wernicke area.

Kirshner and colleagues found differences in the deficit profile of Wernicke aphasia, depending on whether the lesion was predominantly temporal or parietal. The temporal lesions were associated with more severe impairment of auditory comprehension than of reading, whereas the parietal lesions disturbed reading more than auditory comprehension.

Fig. 5.2.2 shows an MRI scan from a patient with a left temporal lesion and Wernicke aphasia but intact reading comprehension.

Incomplete lesions involving Wernicke area might be compatible with recovery, evolving toward deficit profiles of conduction or anomic aphasia (see later discussion) as comprehension improves.

PURE WORD DEAFNESS

Pure word deafness is selective deafness for auditory language. Expressive speech, writing, naming, and reading are typically normal, but the patient cannot understand spoken language and cannot repeat. The patient is deaf to words but not to other sounds, such as the bark of a dog. Many patients have mild language deficits, especially paraphasic speech and naming.

Most patients with pure word deafness have no other neurologic deficits and especially no weakness or visual deficits. Pure word deafness was classically explained as a disconnection between an intact Wernicke area and both auditory cortices. Cases of pure word deafness have been reported with bilateral, temporal lobe pathology such as herpes simplex encephalitis and bilateral strokes. Destructive lesions of both temporal lobes, involving the Heschl gyrus bilaterally, cause the syndrome of cortical deafness comprising loss of both word comprehension and identification of nonverbal sounds.

GLOBAL APHASIA

Global aphasia may be thought of as the sum of Broca plus Wernicke aphasia. The aphasia profile involves the loss of all elementary language functions (see Table 5.2.2); the patient speaks like a patient with Broca aphasia but comprehends like a patient with Wernicke aphasia, the worst of both worlds. Some patients speak only a verbal stereotyped phrase or stereotypy such as "wawawa." The syndrome is called mixed aphasia, if not all of the deficits are severe.

Most patients with global aphasia have severe associated deficits of right hemianopia, right hemiparesis, and right hemisensory loss, although there are exceptions. Most patients with global aphasia have extensive damage involving the left frontal, temporal, and parietal lobes. The most common etiologies are strokes caused by embolism to the middle cerebral artery and occlusion of the internal carotid artery. The syndrome also results from large tumors or large hemorrhages in the left basal ganglia and subcortical white matter.

Global aphasia often improves over time, with the deficit evolving toward another aphasia type. The evolution from global to Broca aphasia is the most common path for these patients, as comprehension gradually improves over weeks and months.

CONDUCTION APHASIA

Conduction aphasia is much less common than Broca, Wernicke, or global aphasia, comprising about 10% of aphasia cases. Conduction aphasia can be thought of as a disorder of repetition. A patient with conduction aphasia may not be able to repeat single words or phrases; one patient could not repeat the word "boy" but spontaneously said, "I like girls better."

Speech in conduction aphasia is typically fluent, although many patients make literal paraphasic errors. Their attempts to self-correct make their speech hesitant although still relatively fluent. Naming is variable. Auditory comprehension must be intact for conduction aphasia to be diagnosed. Reading for meaning is generally preserved, but reading aloud may produce errors. Writing is also variable. These features are summarized in Table 5.2.3.

Associated deficits in conduction aphasia are more variable than in the other aphasia syndromes. Many patients have combinations of right-sided motor and sensory deficits that usually are not severe, and many have apraxia.

The lesions of conduction aphasia involve the superior temporal lobe, without destruction of Wernicke area, or the inferior parietal region. As originally postulated by Wernicke, the lesions leave Broca and Wernicke areas intact but disrupt the connections between them.

ANOMIC APHASIA

Anomic aphasia is a syndrome in which naming difficulty is the primary abnormality. Spontaneous speech is fluent, with spontaneous word-searching pauses and circumlocutions. Naming is impaired out of proportion to other language functions, including auditory comprehension, repetition, reading, and writing (see Table 5.2.3). Associated deficits are variable or absent. Almost all patients with aphasia have some degree of anomia.

The lesions associated with anomic aphasia are variable. The sparing of repetition suggests that the perisylvian language circuit, from Heschl gyri to Wernicke area to Broca area, is intact. The lesions lie outside this circuit. In many patients who are recovering from aphasia, the mildest stage is anomic aphasia. Anomic aphasia may be the last stage in recovery in a variety of aphasic syndromes, including conduction, Wernicke, and even Broca aphasia. Anomia can be the

TABLE 5.2.3 ■ **Conduction and Anomic Aphasias**

Feature	Conduction Aphasia	Anomic Aphasia
Spontaneous speech	Fluent with literal paraphasic errors	Fluent with word-finding pauses and circumlocutions
Naming	Variably intact	Impaired
Auditory comprehension	Intact	Intact
Repetition	Poor	Intact
Reading	Variable aloud; comprehension intact	Intact
Writing	Variably intact	Intact except for word-finding difficulty
Associated deficits	Right hemiparesis; right hemisensory loss; visual field defect; apraxia all variable	Variable, often absent
Behavior	No characteristic feature	No characteristic features

TABLE 5.2.4 ■ **Transcortical Aphasias**

Feature	Transcortical Motor Aphasia	Transcortical Sensory Aphasia	Mixed Transcortical Aphasia
Speech	Nonfluent	Fluent	Nonfluent
Naming	Impaired	Impaired	Impaired
Repetition	Preserved	Echolalic	Echolalic
Comprehension	Preserved	Impaired	Impaired
Reading	Preserved	Impaired	Impaired
Reading	Preserved	Impaired	Impaired
Writing	Reduced	Paragraphic	Poor
Associated signs	Right leg weakness greater than arm weakness; abulia	Variable, often none	Right or bilateral hemiparesis

principal language deficit at early stages of Alzheimer disease (AD), and it also occurs in acute confusional states. Anomic aphasia is thus the least localizing of the aphasia syndromes.

TRANSCORTICAL APHASIAS

Three traditional syndromes of transcortical aphasia have been described to indicate the anatomic sparing of the perisylvian language circuit, with damage in other areas of the cerebral cortex. This explains why repetition is spared. Characteristics of the three transcortical aphasia syndromes are presented in Table 5.2.4.

Transcortical Motor Aphasia

Transcortical motor aphasia (TCMA) resembles Broca aphasia but with preserved repetition. The patient may speak little; sometimes they respond after a delay, or with just a word or two, but with normal repetition of sentences. Naming is variable, but auditory comprehension and reading are usually preserved. Patients may exhibit some of the same hesitancy in writing as in speaking. Most patients have at least a partial right hemiparesis.

TCMA is a frontal lobe syndrome affecting language. Frontal lobe disorders generally involve a lack of movement or a difficulty with the initiation of movement; in this case, a localized left frontal lesion causes reduced initiation of speech. The left frontal lesions are often within the territory of the anterior cerebral artery. The site of damage may be anterior to Broca area, deep in the subcortical frontal white matter, or on the medial surface of the frontal lobe in the vicinity of the supplementary motor area. In the anterior cerebral artery stroke syndrome, the right hemiparesis involves the arm more than the leg and the shoulder more than the hand; this is the opposite of the pattern of hemiparesis in the more common middle cerebral artery stroke. Some patients demonstrate an involuntary grasp response in the affected hand.

Transcortical Sensory Aphasia

The syndrome of transcortical sensory aphasia (TCSA) resembles Wernicke aphasia, except that repetition is spared. Speech is fluent and paraphasic; naming is also paraphasic. Auditory and reading comprehension are severely impaired. TCSA is uncommon as a stroke syndrome, although a few cases have been reported with lesions near the temporooccipital junction, classically sparing the Wernicke area itself. The syndrome has been described as a stage in the language deterioration of AD.

Mixed Transcortical Aphasia

Mixed transcortical aphasia (TCA) resembles global aphasia, except for the intact repetition; patients often repeat excessively or echolalically. Patients with less severe impairment of language modalities can have mixed transcortical aphasia. This syndrome, like TCSA, has been described as a late stage in the language deterioration of AD.

This eight-part classification is an oversimplification, but it is useful in the diagnosis of aphasia. These aphasia syndromes correlate not only with easily observed language behavior but also with well-established localizations of brain lesions.

SUBCORTICAL APHASIAS

Aphasia has been assumed to represent damage to the left hemisphere language cortex. In recent years, many cases of aphasia from subcortical lesions have been reported. As the name implies, subcortical aphasias are defined more by the location of the brain lesion than by specific language characteristics. Several patterns of language disorder have been described in patients with subcortical lesions.

Thalamic Aphasia

Thalamic aphasia was initially reported in patients with left thalamic hemorrhage. The aphasia pattern is fluent and often with paraphasic errors, but there is less loss of comprehension and repetition than in Wernicke aphasia.

Thalamic aphasia can reflect cerebral dominance. Hemorrhages in the right thalamus have produced aphasia in left-handed patients, indicating that language dominance in that hemisphere includes the thalamus.

Anterior Subcortical Aphasia Syndromes

Lesions of the caudate nucleus, putamen, and adjacent white matter have been associated with aphasia. The lateral basal ganglia region, including the putamen, globus pallidus, and internal capsule, is the most frequent site of hypertensive intracerebral hemorrhage. The aphasia characteristics in lateral basal ganglia hemorrhage vary with the location and size of the bleed; symptoms vary from dysarthria and minimal aphasia to severe, global aphasia. The most common subcortical aphasias are seen in ischemic stroke. The anterior subcortical aphasia syndrome is seen with ischemic strokes involving the head of the caudate nucleus, anterior limb of internal capsule, and anterior putamen in the territory of lenticulostriate branches of the middle cerebral artery.

Features of this syndrome include dysarthria and reduced fluency. Comprehension is mildly affected, and repetition is spared. Many patients have an associated right hemiparesis. Recovery of language function is usually good.

APHASIA IN LEFT-HANDED PATIENTS

More left-handed than right-handed people develop aphasia after a stroke, regardless of the side of the stroke. This suggests that left-handed patients have some language representation in both cerebral hemispheres. Although aphasia is more common in patients who are left-handed, their recovery may be better, suggesting that hemisphere dominance may be less rigid in left-handed individuals. Most left-handed patients with aphasia have left hemisphere lesions, a few have right hemisphere lesions. Occasional patients have atypical syndromes, such as a large right middle cerebral territory stroke with nonfluent speech but preserved comprehension, which suggests that comprehension is in the left hemisphere but expressive speech is in the right hemisphere. In general, left-handed people have similar aphasia syndromes after a stroke but with more variability in language characteristics and in recovery.

CROSSED APHASIA

Although more than 99% of right-handed patients with aphasia have left hemisphere lesions, some right-handed patients have aphasia secondary to right hemisphere lesions. As in left-handed people, most "crossed aphasia" cases resemble those of left hemisphere strokes in the analogous areas.

APHASIA IN SPEAKERS OF MORE THAN ONE LANGUAGE

Early theories of language in polyglots held that the patient's original, native language would fare better after a stroke than a newly acquired language, but a rival theory stated that the language most used before the stroke would recover better. Neither theory has held up consistently.

Patients who learn two languages together, as occurs in French Canada, or have equal facility in two languages have more similar aphasia patterns after stroke and similar patterns of brain activation in response to language tasks. The level of proficiency may be more important than the time of acquisition of the two languages.

Alexia and Agraphia
PURE ALEXIA WITHOUT AGRAPHIA

Alexia refers to an acquired inability to read. Patients can write but cannot read their own writing. On bedside examination, speech, auditory comprehension, and repetition are normal. Naming may be deficient, especially for colors.

Patients may be unable to read at first, but over time they learn to read letter by letter and spell out words one by one. They cannot read words at a glance, as normal readers do. By contrast, they understand words that are spelled aloud, and they can spell normally. Associated deficits include a right hemianopia or right upper quadrant visual field defect in most patients and often some short-term memory impairment. Most patients have no hemiparesis or sensory loss.

The causative lesion in pure alexia is a stroke in the territory of the left posterior cerebral artery, with infarction of the medial occipital lobe, often the splenium of the corpus callosum or the medial temporal lobe, and sometimes the thalamus.

ALEXIA WITH AGRAPHIA

Alexia with agraphia can be thought of as an acquired illiteracy in which a previously educated patient becomes unable to read or write. The oral language modalities of speech, naming, auditory comprehension, and repetition are largely intact, but many patients have fluent, paraphasic speech, and impaired naming.

This syndrome overlaps Wernicke aphasia, but it describes patients in whom reading is more impaired than auditory comprehension. Associated deficits include right hemianopia and elements of Gerstmann syndrome: agraphia, acalculia, right-left disorientation, and finger agnosia.

The lesions usually involve the inferior parietal lobule, especially the angular gyrus. Etiologies include strokes in the territory of the angular branch of the left middle cerebral artery, although mass lesions in the same region can produce the syndrome.

APHASIC ALEXIA

Many patients with aphasia have associated reading difficulties.

Four patterns of alexia have been recognized: letter-by-letter reading and deep, phonological, and surface alexia.

Pure alexia without agraphia is letter-by-letter reading, discussed previously.

Deep dyslexia is a severe reading disorder in which patients recognize and read aloud only familiar words, especially concrete, imageable nouns and verbs. They make errors in reading and cannot read nonsense syllables or nonwords. Word reading is not affected by word length or regularity of spelling; for example, a patient could read "ambulance" but not "am." Most patients with deep alexia and extensive left frontoparietal damage.

Phonological alexia is similar to deep alexia; the patient is not able to read nonwords but can read single nouns and verbs adequately.

Surface alexia involves spared ability to read by grapheme-phoneme conversion but inability to recognize long words at a glance or irregular words. These patients can read nonsense syllables but not words of irregular spelling, such as "colonel" or "yacht." Their errors tend to be phonological rather than semantic or visual (e.g., pronouncing "rough" and "though" alike).

AGRAPHIA

As with reading, writing may be affected either in isolation (pure agraphia) or in association with aphasia (aphasic agraphia). In addition, writing can be impaired by motor disorders, apraxia, and visuospatial deficits. Isolated agraphia has been described with left frontal or parietal lesions. Agraphias can be analyzed in the same way as the alexias.

Deep agraphia involves the inability to convert phonemes into graphemes or to write pronounceable nonsense syllables in the presence of the ability to write familiar words.

Phonological agraphia is similar, but the patient can write nouns and verbs better than articles, prepositions, adjectives, and adverbs.

With surface or lexical agraphia, patients can write regularly spelled words and pronounceable nonsense words but not irregularly spelled words. These patients have intact phoneme-grapheme conversion but cannot write by a "whole-word" or "lexical strategy".

Stroke and Other Vascular Disorders

Howard S. Kirshner and Eli E. Zimmerman

Introduction

Stroke is the most common serious neurologic disorder, the fifth leading cause of death in the United States and second in the world, and the most common cause of neurologic disability in adults. Over 800,000 strokes occur each year in the United States, which is more than one each minute. Many additional, small strokes, perhaps as many as 11 million per year in the United States, may be asymptomatic, but the accumulated effects can lead to vascular dementia.

A stroke is a focal abnormality of brain function, caused by either an obstruction in blood flow from occlusion of an artery (ischemic stroke) or hemorrhage from a ruptured blood vessel (hemorrhagic stroke). About 80% to 85% of strokes are ischemic, and 15% to 20% are hemorrhagic. The management of the stroke patient begins with diagnosis based on symptoms and signs. Stroke must be understood in terms of the risk factors for the condition, prior transient ischemic attacks (TIAs), prior strokes, and the developing symptoms and mode of evolution of the stroke itself. The neurologic examination serves to localize the lesion. The diagnosis is then confirmed by imaging studies. Treatment includes acute stroke management, including intravenous tissue plasminogen activator (tPA), mechanical thrombectomy, secondary prevention measures, and finally stroke rehabilitation.

Clinical Presentation: Symptoms and Signs

In general, stroke symptoms reflect dysfunction of focal areas of the brain that are affected by either ischemia or hemorrhage. This presentation of a focal deficit in a conscious patient, especially a patient of older age or with known risk factors, is instantly recognizable as a stroke to most people, including family members who are not medically trained.

TIAs involve temporary focal ischemia that resolves completely within minutes or hours. TIAs can be warning signs of stroke. Carotid distribution TIAs include transient obscuration of the vision of one eye (transient monocular blindness or amaurosis fugax) or symptoms of hemisphere ischemia, such as slurred speech or language difficulty and weakness or numbness of the contralateral side of the body. TIAs in the vertebrobasilar artery distribution are associated with combinations of dizziness, diplopia, slurred speech, numbness or weakness on one or both sides of the body, ataxia, and decreased level of consciousness. Symptoms of TIA resolve within 24 hours. A recent modification of the concept of TIA states that if transient symptoms are associated with an acute infarction on magnetic resonance imaging (MRI) scan, then the event is considered a stroke rather than a TIA. TIA is a major warning sign of stroke and is associated with a major risk of impending stroke.

The American Heart Association also lists sudden, severe headache as a warning sign of stroke. A sudden, severe headache, especially the worst headache of a patient's life, should raise the concern of a subarachnoid hemorrhage (SAH), which is usually caused by rupture of a cerebral aneurysm. Stiff neck makes the diagnosis of SAH even more likely. Although most headaches do not reflect SAH, this diagnosis is a medical emergency and one that clinicians should strive not to miss.

The symptoms of stroke are, in general, the same as those of TIAs. Patients presenting to an emergency department 1 to 2 hours after the onset of ischemic symptoms are very likely to have a stroke because most TIAs begin to resolve within minutes to a few hours.

In the case of a hemorrhage, the location of the bleed is of importance in determining the stroke syndrome. Intracranial hemorrhage (ICH) can occur into one of four separate spaces: the extradural, subdural, subarachnoid, and intracerebral spaces. Extradural hemorrhage usually occurs after head trauma in a young patient; the most common occurrence is a skull fracture that tears a dural artery such as the middle meningeal artery. This is a rapidly progressive, acute syndrome that often requires emergency neurosurgical evacuation. Sometimes a lucid interval occurs between the head injury and the development of symptoms, as the blood accumulates. Progression can then be rapid, and prompt diagnosis and neurosurgical consultation are critical.

Subdural hemorrhage (SDH) also occurs most often after trauma, but SDH may be either acute or chronic. Symptoms of a subacute or chronic SDH may develop gradually, sometimes without a clear history of trauma. Chronic SDH is more common in elderly patients in whom brain atrophy leaves a space between the brain and the skull, which is traversed by fragile bridging veins. Drowsiness and subtle neurologic symptoms and signs are the hallmark of SDH, and the clinician must have a high index of suspicion to send patients for diagnostic computed tomography (CT) or MRI scans.

SAH most commonly results from a ruptured aneurysm, although there are many patients with traumatic SAH. Headache and stiff neck are the most common symptoms of SAH, although a variety of other syndromes can occur.

The fourth type of hemorrhage, ICH, occurs directly into the substance of the brain. This is the type of hemorrhage that most closely mimics the presentation of an ischemic stroke. The most common cause of ICH, hypertension, tends to produce bleeds deep in the brain, in the putamen and basal ganglia most commonly and then the thalamus, brainstem, and cerebellum. Cerebellar hemorrhage is the most amenable to neurosurgical treatment and is therefore especially crucial to diagnose early. This hemorrhage syndrome often causes seemingly nonspecific symptoms such as dizziness, nausea, vomiting, and headache. The key to diagnosis is early gait ataxia. Patients who are dizzy from vestibular function can usually walk, but patients with cerebellar hemorrhage typically cannot. CT scan will then be diagnostic. Hemorrhage in the pons tends to cause bilateral hemiparesis and often coma. The prognosis is poor, unless the hemorrhage is small. Hemorrhage into the basal ganglia usually causes hemiparesis. Occasionally, hemorrhage in the caudate or thalamus breaks into the ventricular system and causes symptoms of increased intracranial pressure (ICP), without obvious focal symptoms and signs. Hemorrhage into the cortical-subcortical areas of the brain, termed lobar hemorrhage, may occur with hypertension but is more characteristic of a bleed related to coagulopathies (e.g., anticoagulation) or structural changes in small arteries that occur with aging (cerebral amyloid angiopathy).

Ischemic stroke, the result of an obstruction of blood flow to the brain, can have several mechanisms. The most common ones, by a widely used classification, are (1) large vessel, atherothrombotic strokes; (2) small vessel or lacunar thrombotic strokes; (3) cardioembolic strokes; (4) strokes caused by a variety of clinically definite, but less common mechanisms; and (5) cryptogenic strokes, or those for which a precise mechanism or cause is not discovered. In this last category, strokes that appear embolic, meaning sudden in onset, cortical-subcortical in distribution, and for which no source of embolus is found, are sometimes referred to as embolic strokes of unknown source or ESUS.

Localization of Specific Stroke Syndromes

The functional anatomy of the specific regions of the brain including cerebrum, basal ganglia, thalamus, brainstem, and cerebellum were discussed in previous chapters. This chapter presents the features that can help localize and diagnose specific stroke syndromes.

VASCULAR ANATOMY

In terms of vascular anatomy, the two internal carotid arteries (ICAs) supply most of the blood flow to the cerebral hemispheres. The carotid artery distribution is the anterior circulation, whereas the vertebrobasilar distribution is the posterior circulation.

The bifurcation of the common carotid artery into the ICA and external carotid artery (ECA) is a frequent site of lipid plaque accumulation in atherosclerosis, and disease at this location is often the cause of large vessel, thrombotic TIA, and stroke. Less commonly, stenosis of the ICA develops higher up in the intracranial portions of the ICA.

Intracranial large vessel disease develops with advanced atherosclerosis in patients with chronic risk factors such as hypertension, diabetes mellitus, hyperlipidemia, obstructive sleep apnea, and smoking. Intracranial atherosclerosis is more common in those of African and Asian descent. The ICA bifurcates into the anterior cerebral artery (ACA) and middle cerebral artery (MCA). Because the MCA takes a straighter course from the ICA, emboli more commonly travel there, although occasionally emboli involve the ACA or posterior cerebral artery (PCA) territories. In general, disease of the MCA is more commonly caused by emboli than by local atherosclerotic disease, whereas disease of the ACA is more equally distributed between embolic and local disease. MCA territory strokes are much more common than ACA territory strokes. The ICA also gives rise to a posterior communicating artery, joining the carotid circulation with the PCA, that arises from the basilar artery of the posterior circulation. Occasionally, the posterior communicating artery supplies most of the blood supply to the PCA on one or both sides; this is a normal variant sometimes referred to as a fetal PCA.

MIDDLE CEREBRAL ARTERY INFARCTION

The MCA bifurcates into an upper division and a lower division; the upper division of the left MCA supplies the motor speech area (Broca area), the motor strip in the precentral gyrus (face and arm areas), and the sensory strip in the postcentral gyrus, leading to the common syndrome of Broca aphasia and right hemiparesis in left MCA stroke. If only single branches are involved, more restricted deficits, such as Broca aphasia with only right facial weakness, may occur. Involvement of the inferior division branches causes a fluent, Wernicke aphasia (see Chapter 5.2), sometimes accompanied by a right upper quadrant visual field defect. Involvement of both upper and lower divisions of the left MCA, as in an embolus in the left MCA stem, produces global aphasia and right hemiplegia, which is a severe and disabling stroke syndrome. Visuospatial deficits and neglect behavior are commonly associated with right MCA. Involvement of deep branches of the MCA on either side also produces weakness of the leg and the arm because the descending fibers from the cortical leg area descend through the MCA territory and into the internal capsule, which is also largely supplied by deep branches of the MCA. Over time, however, the leg usually improves more than the arm after a left MCA stroke.

INTERNAL CAPSULE INFARCTION

Small vessel, lacunar infarctions in the territory of the deep, lenticulostriate branches of the MCA produce localized infarctions of the posterior limb of the internal capsule, resulting in the stroke syndrome of pure motor hemiparesis, without sensory signs, cortical behavioral or cognitive deficits, or visual field abnormalities. Larger infarctions in the lenticulostriate territory produce more complex syndromes including combined motor and sensory deficits, dysarthria, and even cognitive and language deficits.

THALAMIC INFARCTION

Lacunar infarctions in the thalamus which typically receives arterial supply from perforating vessels from the PCA, produce a pure sensory stroke with paresthesias and numbness on the contralateral side, sometimes followed by neuropathic pain (Dejerine-Roussy syndrome).

BASAL GANGLIA INFARCTION

The basal ganglia receives arterial supply predominately from the MCA lenticulostriate branches. Lacunes in the basal ganglia can produce contralateral weakness and clumsiness.

Small infarctions in the basal ganglia, sparing the internal capsule, may be relatively silent and are noted on brain imaging studies of patients without a clinical history of stroke.

VERTEBROBASILAR ANATOMY

The posterior circulation is comprised of the two vertebral arteries, arising from the subclavian artery on each side and merging within the skull to form the single, unpaired basilar artery. The vertebral arteries can be affected by atherosclerosis in their proximal portions, at the origin from the subclavian artery, or distally. The vertebral arteries are also a site of dissection, usually in more distal portions.

POSTERIOR INFERIOR CEREBELLAR ARTERY INFARCTION

The vertebral artery has one important branch intracranially, the posterior inferior cerebellar artery (PICA). The PICA supplies the lateral medulla and the inferior, lateral, posterior portion of the cerebellum. The stroke syndrome that results from occlusion of either the vertebral artery or the PICA is the lateral medullary syndrome of Wallenberg, the most common and therefore the most important of the named brainstem stroke syndromes.

The crossed sensory loss of the ipsilateral face and contralateral body is one of the hallmarks of the syndrome, along with ipsilateral Horner syndrome (ptosis and miosis), ipsilateral palate paralysis and dysphagia, ipsilateral ataxia, and ipsilateral lateral pulsion (a tendency to lean toward the side of the stroke when sitting or standing). Infarctions in the PICA territory can also involve isolated cerebellar infarction. The symptoms and signs of the Wallenberg syndrome are as follows:

- Ipsilateral signs
  - Numbness of face
  - Horner syndrome
  - Ataxia
  - Lateral pulsion
  - Dysphasia, palate weakness
- Contralateral signs
  - Numbness of arm, leg, trunk
- Unsided signs
  - Vertigo, nausea, hiccups

BASILAR ARTERY AND BRANCHES

At the level of the pontomedullary junction, the two vertebral arteries join to form the basilar artery. The basilar artery has two long, circumferential branches: the anterior inferior cerebellar artery (AICA) and the superior cerebellar artery (SCA).

The basilar artery terminates in the PCAs and gives off multiple penetrating branches along the way. A host of syndromes can be produced by occlusion of these branches. Most of these are discussed in Chapter 3.4.

Basilar Occlusion

Stroke due to basilar occlusion can produce a variety of syndromes depending on the level of involvement. Most common is occlusion in the pons. Damage is often asymmetric, but careful examination commonly shows bilateral corticospinal tract dysfunction. If strength allows testing of coordination, there is often appendicular ataxia as well. A major clue to brainstem damage rather than higher (cerebral) or lower (spinal) damage is bulbar symptoms of dysarthria and dysphagia. Oculomotor findings can include a variety of syndromes, including horizontal gaze palsy with relative preservation of vertical (especially upward) gaze, internuclear ophthalmoplegia (INO) that can be unilateral or bilateral, or an INO with a gaze palsy, which is the so-called "one-and-a-half syndrome."

Top-of-the-basilar syndrome produces relative sparing of the lower brainstem branches but often involves infarction of the midbrain and may produce Parinaud syndrome (see Chapter 3.4). Ocular motor abnormalities are common with a variety of manifestations. Occlusion of the PCAs without adequate collateral circulation can result in cortical blindness.

Anterior Inferior Cerebellar Artery

The AICA syndrome often involves ipsilateral cranial nerve (CN) VII (facial palsy) and VIII (deafness) abnormalities, ipsilateral ataxia, and contralateral motor and sensory deficits. The AICA syndrome has many variations, and many have traditional eponyms.

Superior Cerebellar Artery

The SCA syndrome involves ipsilateral ataxia and contralateral sensory loss. Other variably associated symptoms include dysarthria, nausea and vomiting, ipsilateral tremor, palatal myoclonus, and partial deafness.

Basilar Artery Penetrating Branches

The basilar artery gives rise to many, small penetrating branches that supply portions of the brainstem. The stroke syndromes of the brainstem are quite variable. Brainstem anatomy is discussed elsewhere in this text, and particular deficits are related to which perforating branch or branches are affected by ischemia.

Posterior Cerebral Artery

The PCA is a branch of the basilar in most people, although in some the PCA arises from the anterior circulation. The most common finding is a visual field defect that can be incomplete or complete in a hemifield depending on severity, location, and anatomy. Central vision is sometimes preserved because the corresponding occipital cortex is supplied by branches of the MCA.

INTRACRANIAL HEMORRHAGE

ICH is often due to hypertension, coagulopathy, trauma, or structural lesion predisposing to bleeding such as tumor, aneurysm, or other vascular malformation. A less common cause of ICH is cerebral venous thrombosis.

Clues to ICH include acute onset of headache or disturbance of consciousness early in the course or a known predisposing factor (e.g., brain metastasis, known aneurysm or vascular malformation, trauma, or anticoagulant therapy). Helpful for localization is also the development of deficits which do not fit into a defined ischemic stroke syndrome, that is, the deficits do not localize to occlusion of a single vessel.

Intraparenchymal hemorrhage (IPH) is most commonly due to uncontrolled hypertension, but trauma and coagulopathy often cause IPH. Patients present with focal deficits appropriate to the localization of the hemorrhage, along with somnolence. Nausea and vomiting are more frequent than in ischemic stroke.

SAH is often due to aneurysmal bleeding, but trauma is a common cause. Patients with aneurysmal hemorrhage often present with headache, neck pain, and somnolence or coma, and they often have marked hypertension that may be causative or reactive. Focal findings are uncommon other than ocular motor deficits.

Subdural hemorrhage is most commonly due to head injury, and it is often seen after fall or assault. Headache and confusion are common, and coma may be present if the hemorrhage is large. Diagnosis of SDH is considered especially if there are focal signs in addition to encephalopathy, such as one side with reduced tone and absent random movement when the other side does move.

Differential Diagnosis

Differential diagnosis must take place with TIA and stroke. TIA is an ominous symptom; TIA should be recognized as a medical emergency, and prompt diagnostic testing should be done to find the cause of the event and permit initiation of the proper preventive treatment. The differential diagnosis of TIA includes other causes of transient symptoms or spells, including migraine, seizures, and other transient alterations of consciousness.

The presentation of a focal deficit in an awake patient who has appropriate risk factors is so characteristic of stroke that, most of the time, the diagnosis is obvious. Occasionally, however, other brain pathologies mimic stroke. Migraine symptoms can be confused with symptoms of stroke and TIA, although most typically the focal symptoms of migraine occur during the aura and then improve as the severe headache ensues. Migraine with prolonged aura can more closely mimic a stroke, and occasionally a true infarction can follow the patient's typical migraine aura (migrainous stroke). Other focal brain pathologies such as tumors and abscesses or inflammatory disorders such as multiple sclerosis occasionally present in an acute fashion. SDH in elderly patients is also frequently mistaken for stroke. A clear history of abrupt onset of symptoms usually favors stroke; the less clear the history, as in the patient "found down" at home, the more likely another diagnosis will emerge. About 15% of initial stroke diagnoses made by emergency medical technicians turn out to be incorrect (stroke mimics).

Several rapid screening tools for the diagnosis of stroke have been developed. One of the easiest to remember is the Think FAST paradigm developed at the University of Cincinnati. The "F" stands for facial weakness, the "A" for arm drift or weakness, the "S" for slurred speech or inability to speak or understand language, and the "T" for time, emphasizing the emergent nature of stroke treatment. A more recent modification of the "FAST" procedure is BE FAST, which adds balance issues and eye signs, either visual field loss or abnormalities of the extraocular movements, usually occurring in posterior circulation strokes.

Laboratory and Radiological Investigation

The first aspect of stroke diagnosis, after clinical diagnosis, is a brain imaging study.

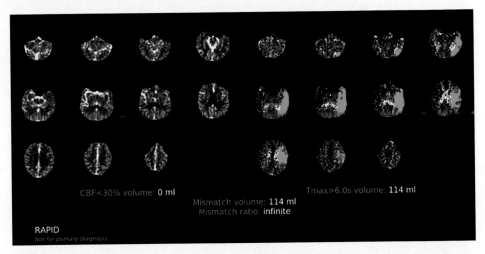

Fig. 5.3.1 Computed tomography (CT) perfusion image of a stroke. This shows a perfusion brain map. On the left side are areas of reduced cerebral blood flow (none); on the right side are areas (*green*) of delayed blood transit time. This indicates a large penumbra of tissue at risk, with no visible infarction. The images are from the RAPID perfusion method.

COMPUTED TOMOGRAPHY

The CT scan has traditionally served as the primary diagnostic test. CT has the capability to detect hemorrhage early and to delineate the location and extent of an ischemic lesion, but it may take 2 to 3 days before a cerebral infarction becomes clearly visible on CT. Occasionally, CT can image the thrombus in an occluded MCA (hyperacute MCA sign), and an experienced interpreter can detect subtle, early signs of ischemia in stroke. In general, however, CT is less sensitive for the detection of early infarct changes than MRI.

CT ANGIOGRAM

Additions to the CT armamentarium include CT angiography (CTA), imaging the cerebral and neck vessels with contrast infusion, and CT perfusion studies, mapping areas of cerebral blood flow after contrast infusion such that areas of extremely low blood flow can be assumed to be associated with irreversible infarction. If the area of core damage is small and the area of hypoperfusion is larger (the ischemic penumbra), then potential stroke damage can be avoided with interventional treatments such as mechanical thrombectomy. Fig. 5.3.1 shows a CT perfusion imaging study of a penumbra of ischemic but not infarcted tissue.

This shows a CT perfusion brain map. On the left side are areas of reduced cerebral blood flow (none), on the right side an area (in green) of delayed blood transit time. This indicates a large "penumbra" of tissue at risk, with no visible infarction. The images are from the Rapid Processing of Perfusion and Diffusion (RAPID) perfusion method. This evidence is important for planning mechanical thrombectomy procedures.

CT VENOGRAM

CT venogram is performed in a fashion similar to CTA with injection of iodinated dye followed by a CT scan, but the timing of acquisition differs from CTA so that the veins are revealed. This is most commonly used when there is concern for intracranial venous sinus thrombosis.

MAGNETIC RESONANCE IMAGING

A few centers use acute MRI scanning, which can delineate areas of ischemia very early in ischemic stroke (within minutes to an hour) via the diffusion weighted imaging (DWI) modality. If a timed contrast infusion is added, a perfusion weighted image (PWI) can identify areas of ischemia that have not yet become infarcted, similarly to the CT perfusion method. Finally, magnetic resonance angiography (MRA) can image the cerebral arteries, much like CTA. MRI can also reveal intracerebral hemorrhage with a T2* or gradient echo sequence, which shows both acute and chronic blood products as a black signal.

PET AND SPECT

Other brain imaging techniques such as single photon emission computed tomography (SPECT) and positron emission tomography (PET) scanning are used primarily as investigational procedures for stroke. The SPECT scan, with and without a vasodilator such as acetazolamide, can show whether brain perfusion is compromised by a vasodilator, suggesting decreased cerebrovascular reserve. New MRI techniques such as MR spectroscopy can also detect biochemical changes associated with ischemia.

Two other techniques permit visualization of cerebral vessels. Doppler ultrasound technology permits real-time ultrasound imaging of the carotid bifurcations and Doppler signal analysis of blood flow. This relatively inexpensive, noninvasive vascular imaging technology detects stenosis in the carotid vessels almost as accurately as MRA and CTA, although the imaging of the vertebral arteries is difficult. MR vessel wall imaging can also be used to differentiate atherosclerotic changes in intracranial arteries from vasculitis. This technique is still somewhat experimental.

Transcranial Doppler (TCD) can visualize flow in the major intracranial arteries.

CATHETER ANGIOGRAPHY

The traditional catheter arteriogram is the gold standard of vascular diagnosis; iodinated contrast can be injected directly into cerebral vessels, usually via femoral artery catheterization, and the arteries of the neck and brain can be imaged by standard radiographic technology. Arteriography is superior for detecting very small lesions such as aneurysms or changes in small arteries as is seen in cerebral vasculitis, but it has the disadvantages of being invasive, with complications possible from injury to vessels (dissection; thrombus or plaque material breaking off and embolizing to the brain) and from effects of the iodinated contrast agent.

CARDIAC IMAGING

Complete evaluation of the source of a stroke also involves investigation of the heart, looking for a source of embolism to the brain. Electrocardiography (ECG) and heart rhythm monitoring are useful in stroke patients because arrhythmias such as atrial fibrillation can occur intermittently, yet they pose a serious risk of embolic stroke. Echocardiography images the heart to look for thrombus within the left atrium or ventricle, poor contractility of the ventricle, valvular pathology, or an abnormal shunt between the right and left sides of the heart. Atrial septal defects or the more common patent foramen ovale occur in as many as 25% of the population. These shunts provide a conduit whereby clots from the venous circulation can cross from the right to left side of the heart and then embolize to the brain (paradoxical embolization). The echocardiogram is augmented by injection of agitated saline, and the bubbles can be visualized crossing from the right to left atrium. Transesophageal echocardiography (TEE), in which the ultrasound probe is placed in the esophagus directly behind the heart, has permitted more accurate diagnosis of cardiac conditions.

TCD can also be combined with intravenous injection of agitated saline, and microemboli to the brain can be detected.

LABORATORY STUDIES

Another important area of clinical testing in stroke patients involves blood tests. A complete blood count (CBC) is always indicated in stroke patients. Rarely, thrombocytosis or increased red blood cell counts can be a cause of stroke, as can severe anemia. Elevated platelet counts (thrombocytosis) can also lead to clotting in cerebral vessels, whereas thrombocytopenia can lead to bleeding. Tests of clotting such as the prothrombin time (PT) and partial thromboplastin time (PTT) can detect clotting defects that lead to cerebral hemorrhage. A host of blood tests have been developed to detect an increased clotting tendency or hypercoagulable states. The lupus anticoagulant or anticardiolipin antibody can be associated with arterial clotting and stroke syndromes. Most of the other tests for hypercoagulability are more related to venous thrombosis and pulmonary embolism; these include protein C and S, antithrombin III, factor V Leiden, prothrombin gene mutation, and others. These are associated with stroke mainly in the presence of a patent foramen ovale. Elevated homocysteine levels are also associated with a higher risk of stroke. Finally, blood tests for endocrine (especially diabetes mellitus), metabolic, and organ function can be important in stroke. Plasma lipids are important to gauge risk of both myocardial infarction (MI) and stroke; fasting total cholesterol, high-density lipoprotein (HDL), low-density lipoprotein (LDL), and triglycerides should be tested in virtually all stroke patients.

Overview of Treatment

Treatment of stroke is not a focus of this book. Suffice it to say that for all of the advances in diagnostics for stroke, advances in treatment have been equally impressive. This chapter gives a brief overview.

The treatment of stroke is divided into acute interventions and chronic, preventive therapies. Acute treatment of acute ischemic stroke includes thrombolytic therapy. Intravenous tPA is a clot dissolver. The odds ratio of a favorable outcome in stroke patients treated with intranvenous tPA is 1.7:1. The number needed to treat (NNT) is the number of patients who need to be treated to see one response. For tPA the NNT is approximately 5; it seems as if more people should respond, but this is actually a good number. For comparison, the NNT for aspirin preventing recurrent acute ischemic stroke was found to be approximately 79. Currently, tPA is being replaced by another thrombolytic agent, tenecteplase, which has the advantage of being a single bolus dose.

Mechanical thrombectomy has been increasingly used, and the NNT for that is approximately 2. There are a variety of techniques, but they are constantly improving. This involves threading a catheter into the occluded or stenosed artery and using mechanical and thrombolytic therapy to improve perfusion. If done early enough on patients who meet criteria for treatment, both intravenous thrombolytic therapy and endovascular therapy are the best treatments for acute ischemic at the time of this writing.

After acute treatment of stroke, the next task is prevention; because this is started after a stroke, it is termed secondary stroke prevention. The strategies used involve a combination of medications including antiplatelet agents or anticoagulants and best management of other risk factors including hypertension, hyperlipidemia, cardiac arrhythmia, smoking, sleep apnea, and other factors.

Recent updated guidelines for acute stroke treatment have been published by the American Heart Association / American Stroke Association. Guidelines for secondary prevention (after stroke or TIA) have also been published by the American Stroke Association. Because this is a rapidly moving field, latest literature and expert opinion should be consulted for current best practices.

Seizure Disorders

Karl E. Misulis and Eli E. Zimmerman

Classification of Seizures and Epilepsy

A seizure is a set of clinical symptoms due to abnormal electrical activity of the brain. Epilepsy is a syndrome where there have been recurrent unprovoked seizures or a single unprovoked seizure with findings to indicate that there is a comparable risk of subsequent seizure as would be seen in a patient with two unprovoked seizures. Therefore, all patients with epilepsy have seizures, whereas not all patients with seizures have epilepsy.

Seizures come in a variety of types with different clinical features. The classification scheme has evolved, and some authors and practitioners adhere to now-obsolete schemes. Because of this, neurologists need to be aware of the new accepted schemes and the parallels in prior terminology.

Seizures are first classified into generalized or focal onset. Generalized seizures are those that have a generalized onset, that is, the seizures did not start in a specific focus and then spread. These are subdivided into motor onset and nonmotor onset. Motor onset seizures would include the generalized tonic-clonic (GTC) seizures. Nonmotor onset seizures would include absence seizures.

Classification of epilepsies is complex, but for the purposes of localization and diagnosis it is appropriate to introduce it here. The seizure classification is first and most important.

Epilepsies are classified as focal, generalized, combination of focal and generalized, and unknown. This classification is based on the origin of the discharges that comprise the seizures. There are also classification strata based on whether the seizures are structural, genetic, metabolic, infectious, immune, or unknown, which are not pivotal for localization.

Classification of seizures is as follows:

- Focal onset
  - Awareness
    - Aware
    - Impaired awareness
  - Onset
    - Motor onset
    - Nonmotor onset
  - Focal to bilateral tonic-clonic seizures
- Generalized
  - Motor onset
  - Nonmotor onset (absence)
- Unknown onset
  - Motor onset
    - Tonic-clonic
    - Epileptic spasms

- Nonmotor onset
- Unclassified

Classification of epilepsies is as follows:

- Epilepsy types
  - Focal
  - Generalized
  - Combination of focal and generalized
  - Unknown
- Etiologies
  - Structural
  - Genetic
  - Infectious
  - Metabolic
  - Immune
  - Unknown
- Epilepsy syndromes
  - Idiopathic generalized epilepsies
    - Childhood absence
    - Juvenile absence
    - Juvenile myoclonic
    - Generalized tonic-clonic
  - Self-limited focal epilepsies
    - With centrotemporal spikes
    - Self-limited occipital epilepsies
    - Other self-limited frontal, temporal, or parietal epilepsies

Clinical Features of Seizure Types

GENERALIZED TONIC-CLONIC SEIZURE

GTC seizures usually begin abruptly with loss of consciousness that is followed by generalized tonic and then clonic activity. If the GTC arises in a patient with juvenile myoclonic epilepsy (JME), myoclonic jerks may precede the GTC phase. The patient's eyes are usually partly open, and their mouth is often open. Their head may turn to either side, without the seizure being considered a focal onset type. Postictal sleepiness and confusion are expected.

ABSENCE SEIZURE

Absence seizure begins with a cessation of activity without the patient falling to the ground. There is loss of awareness and responsiveness despite maintenance of posture. Automatisms may occur; the patient may move the mouth, lick the lips, or fumble with an object in the hand. Duration is usually less than 15 seconds. There is no postictal state.

FOCAL AWARE SEIZURE

Focal aware seizures have a focal onset and produce symptoms that do not affect consciousness. Most common are focal motor activity and/or sensory symptoms, but emotional and cognitive changes can occur as long as the patient retains awareness during the event. Otherwise, the seizure would be considered a focal impaired awareness seizure.

FOCAL IMPAIRED AWARENESS SEIZURE

Focal impaired awareness seizures are focal onset seizures that can either start with impaired aware-ness or start with a focal aware phase. With impaired awareness, the patient often has complete loss of contact with the world and is not responsive. For some, the altered awareness may be less dramatic, sometimes just with confusion.

FOCAL TO BILATERAL TONIC-CLONIC SEIZURE

Focal to bilateral tonic-clonic seizures are focal onset seizures that spread to both hemispheres pro-ducing tonic-clonic seizures. They may develop from focal aware or focal impaired awareness seizures.

Localization and Diagnosis of Epilepsy

Generalized onset seizures do not have a focal localization. For diagnosis, specific entities are characterized by clinical findings and by electroencephalogram (EEG) findings.

Focal onset seizures do have a localization, and they are classified based on clinical character-istics and location of the focus.

FOCAL EPILEPSY SYNDROMES

Temporal lobe epilepsy (TLE) usually starts with an aura that is often epigastric, but a more psychic aura such as déjà vu can occur. Impaired awareness occurs with staring. Automatisms are sometimes seen, such as lip smacking. These are the most common symptoms, but the range of manifestations is wide. TLE is the most common of the focal onset epilepsies.

Frontal lobe epilepsy can begin with an aura, although this is less common than with TLE. Sometimes there is a vague sensation in the head that is hard to describe. Epigastric sensations re-sembling TLE can occur. Contralateral focal motor activity can be clonic or tonic. Specifics of the activity help with localization; for example, arm involvement suggests lateral activation of the mo-tor cortex, whereas more leg involvement suggests medial involvement. An often misdiagnosed seizure of frontal lobe origin is from the supplementary sensorimotor area that can present with posturing and tonic activity. This activity can be bilateral yet typically does not affect conscious-ness; hence, these are often misdiagnosed as nonepileptic events.

Parietal lobe epilepsy can begin with a sensory aura that can march. It can manifest as tingling, numbness, or various types of pain and discomfort. Rare auras can be distortion of perception of body position. The sensory symptoms often march; although they are usually contralateral to the focus, they are occasionally bilateral or even ipsilateral. Vertigo is sometimes seen. On the other hand, most patients with focal epilepsy of parietal localization have symptoms that spread to the frontal or tem-poral lobes or even occipital lobe. Frontal spread may produce focal tonic or clonic activity, posturing, and head and eye deviation. Temporal spread can produce staring and oroalimentary automatisms.

Occipital lobe epilepsy often begins with a visual aura. The aura can be simple or complex. Lights can be persistent or flashing, and they may be moving. Some patients may see complex images such as a scene, especially with spread toward the temporal lobes. Motor activity can be blinking, nystagmus, or eye deviation, usually to the contralateral side.

GENERALIZED EPILEPSY SYNDROMES

Epilepsy with generalized tonic-clonic seizures alone usually begins in the second decade with GTC seizures. These often occur on awakening but can occur at any time. They are worse with sleep deprivation.

Childhood absence epilepsy starts in the first decade, between 4 and 10 years of age. Absence seizures can occur multiple times per day. Initially they might not be noticed by others. Seizures may remit by the third decade, but this is not invariable. Childhood absence epilepsy may evolve into JME.

Juvenile absence epilepsy starts in the second decade, but otherwise it is similar to the childhood presentation. A higher proportion of patients with juvenile absence epilepsy have GTC seizures in addition to the absence seizures. Remission can occur, but this variety is more likely to persist into adult life.

JME has onset in the second decade, usually between 12 and 18 years of age. Myoclonic seizures develop and are most often noticed on awakening. They are exacerbated by sleep deprivation. Most patients develop GTC seizures as well. The clue to the origin is the myoclonus, which may have been unnoticed until the GTC seizure occurs. Seizures may be triggered by startle.

NONEPILEPTIC EVENTS

Nonepileptic events are not seizures, so they are not called seizures. These are events that resemble seizures but are not due to abnormal neuronal discharge. Nonepileptic events is the preferred term, and the terms pseudoseizures and nonepileptic seizures are not preferred terms.

Diagnostic Approach to Patients With Seizures

Most patients with seizures have a normal neurologic examination, although some seizures can be associated with focal findings that may correlate with a focal structural lesion or cognitive delay or decline, which is evidence of an underlying cause. The key to diagnosis is the clinical presentation that includes the history and description from the patient and description from observers, because the patient usually cannot observe and describe their own seizures.

EEG is performed in almost all patients with an initial presentation of possible seizures. Table 5.4.1 shows clinical and EEG findings seen with some important epilepsy syndromes. Caution is needed; an interictal EEG is often normal in patients with epilepsy, so a normal EEG does not rule out epilepsy. On the other hand, focal sharp waves do not make the diagnosis of epilepsy. A small but nonnegligible proportion of the population shows sharp waves or spikes yet does not manifest seizures. In the absence of seizures, neurologists do not treat these waves. When EEG abnormalities are seen in patients with epilepsy, they can be focal, generalized, focal and generalized, or multifocal. There are a host of specific findings that can be diagnostic of a certain type of epilepsy, such as absence or JME.

TABLE 5.4.1 ■ Electroencephalogram (EEG) and Epilepsies

Epilepsy	Clinical	EEG
Absence epilepsy	Episodes of unresponsiveness, sometimes with automatisms	3/sec spike-wave pattern
Generalized tonic-clonic epilepsy	Episodes of generalized stiffness and shaking with unresponsiveness	5 to 6/sec poly-spike-wave pattern
Focal epilepsy	Episodes of clonic or tonic focal motor activity	Focal discharges contralateral to the motor symptoms
Nonepileptic events	Clinical seizure of various presentations: staring spells, focal or bilateral shaking	Normal cerebral activity; muscle and movement artifact on the EEG

Computed tomography imaging is often done emergently when a patient presents with seizure and has persistent postictal phase or focal signs. A structural lesion is considered, such as tumor, hemorrhage, or infarction.

Magnetic resonance imaging is a better test for looking for structural lesions in a nonemergent situation. This is performed on most patients with focal onset seizures, but it is often not needed in patients with generalized onset seizures who fit into one of the epilepsy syndromes not usually associated with a focal structural abnormality, such as childhood absence or JME.

Advanced diagnostic studies such as positron emission tomography are not typically needed unless epilepsy surgery is being considered for medically refractory epilepsy; this should be the province of the epileptologists.

Neuromuscular Disorders

Karl E. Misulis and Eli E. Zimmerman

Clinical Presentations of Neuromuscular Disorders

Neuromuscular conditions produce motor and/or sensory disturbance, but the key to suspicion of this localization is the history and examination. To illustrate, the findings in the following scenarios direct the search to a neuromuscular process.

Scenario 1: Weakness of the legs knowing nothing else about the presentation, weakness of the legs could be due to a midline cerebral lesion, a thoracic spinal cord lesion, neuropathy affecting predominately the legs, or myopathy. If the weakness is mainly distal and there is sensory loss distally on the legs with reduced ankle reflexes, the diagnosis is most likely peripheral neuropathy, which often affects legs before becoming symptomatic in the arms. Alternatively, if there is weakness that is most prominent proximally without sensory deficit, the diagnosis is more likely myopathy.

Scenario 2: Weakness of the hand without additional information, the localization could be cerebral cortex, subcortical structures, cervical spine, nerve root, plexus, or peripheral nerve affecting one or more nerves. When the examination shows that the deficits are in wrist and finger extension and elbow extension, the diagnosis of radial neuropathy is more evident.

Scenario 3: Weakness of arms and legs spasticity on one side without sensory symptoms suggests a focal cerebral lesion. Spasticity of all extremities without sensory symptoms suggests degeneration of the descending corticospinal tract neurons; a high spinal lesion sufficient to produce bilateral motor involvement would not leave sensory function unaffected.

Findings that trigger consideration of neuromuscular causes include

- Neurologic deficit that fits into the distribution of a single neuromuscular structure, or
- Deficit that cannot be explained by a central lesion.

Approach to Suspected Neuromuscular Disorders

HISTORY AND EXAMINATION

History focuses on primary and associated symptoms. The primary symptoms are those that bring the patient to medical attention; these are usually weakness, sensory loss, or pain. Associated symptoms are elements that the patient might or might not mention, so the examiner has to ask specifically about these. The link to the patient's chief complaints might not be evident. For example, if a patient reports weakness without sensory symptoms and mentions that they fatigue more easily, the examiner might ask about eyelid droop, double vision, or dysphagia; these symptoms might be mild enough to not be offered as complaints, yet are supportive of a diagnosis of myasthenia. On the other hand, the examiner might ask about muscle twitching and cramps, which if present would raise concern for motor neuron disease.

History components and some suggested conditional elements may include sensory and motor deficits.

- Sensory deficit: Neurologist asks about distribution, tempo on onset and progression, and association with pain and/or weakness.
- Motor deficit: Neurologist asks about location(s), rate and pattern of progression, association with sensory symptoms, fasciculations or cramps, and bulbar symptoms.

Examination components and some suggested conditional elements that apply to patients with either or both motor and sensory complaints may include the following:

- Motor examination
  - Test of strength of select muscles includes those involved in the complaint and at least one proximal and distal muscle group from each limb.
  - Patient is observed for fasciculations or cramps.
- Sensory examination
  - Examiner maps the deficit of the complaint to multiple modalities, often including light touch, sharp, vibration, proprioception, and temperature; less commonly used is two-point discrimination.
  - Examiner screens the asymptomatic portions of the limbs and face with light touch and expands the examination in specific regions as needed.
  - If a sensory level is detected (e.g., with a suspected spinal cord lesion), then marching up and down by dermatomes is appropriate.
- Reflex examination
  - Tendon reflexes are performed for ankle, knee, biceps, triceps, and brachioradialis as part of the basic neurologic examination. If there is indication of corticospinal tract involvement, additional tendon reflexes might be tested, including pectoral, crossed adductor, and others.
  - Plantar response is routinely tested. This is combined with examination for ankle clonus.
  - Pathological reflexes such as glabellar, snout, and others are not routinely part of the neuromuscular examination.
- Cranial nerve examination
  - Ocular motor function including eye movements and lid function are routinely tested.
  - Patient is observed and examined for facial (cranial nerve [CN] VII) function.
  - Testing light touch of the face, including all three divisions of the trigeminal nerve.
  - Examiner conducts detailed examination of speech motor function: linguals ("ta ta ta"; CN XII), labials ("pa pa pa"; CN VII), and palatal ("ka ka ka"; CN X).

Note that the sensory examination has to be efficient and goal-directed. Patients can become easily fatigued from answering the many questions of the sensory examination, and findings often become unreliable.

DIAGNOSTIC STUDIES

Nerve conduction studies (NCS), electromyography (EMG), muscle biopsy, nerve biopsy, and laboratory tests are discussed in Table 3.6.1.

NCS and EMG are performed in almost all patients with neuromuscular disease. These tests are a precise extension of the physical examination and can usually classify the disorder.

Muscle biopsy is performed when the diagnosis is muscular dystrophy, inflammatory myopathy, or other myopathy.

Nerve biopsy is not routinely performed on patients with neuropathy because it is invasive and destructive. Nerve biopsy is only performed if the results would change the management of the patient. This test is used for multifocal neuropathy where there is not a known cause and where the consideration is vasculitis.

Laboratory studies are tailored to the suspected diagnosis. If neuropathy is identified and the cause is not known, laboratory tests for metabolic, nutritional, and immune parameters are more likely to be performed. If neuromuscular transmission disorder is suspected, then laboratory tests for myasthenia and Lambert-Eaton myasthenic syndrome are considered. If myopathy is suspected, the muscle enzymes, creatine phosphokinase (CK) and aldolase are tested.

Specific Disorders

NEUROPATHIES

Diabetic Neuropathy

Common types of diabetic neuropathy include the following:
- Sensorimotor axonal neuropathy
- Mononeuropathy
- Mononeuropathy multiplex
- Diabetic polyradiculopathy
- Sensory neuropathy
- Autonomic neuropathy

Mononeuropathies due to diabetes mellitus include cranial nerve palsies, especially of CN III and CN VI. These are discussed in Chapter 3.4.

Sensorimotor neuropathy with diabetes is an axonal degeneration that is clinically indistinguishable from the multitude of other axonal sensorimotor neuropathies. Diabetes is the most common cause of axonal neuropathy in the United States. Distal numbness in a stocking and glove distribution is present early in the course. Weakness develops later and involves distal muscles, especially the intrinsic muscles of the feet, tibialis anterior, and hands.

Mononeuropathy Multiplex. Diabetes is the most common cause of mononeuropathy multiplex. The ulnar nerve is commonly affected, producing wasting of ulnar-innervated intrinsic muscles of the hand and numbness of digit 5 and the ulnar half of digit 4. Median and peroneal nerves are also commonly affected. Cranial neuropathies include oculomotor palsy (see Chapters 3.4 and 4.2).

Diabetic sensory neuropathy affects predominantly unmyelinated C fibers and small myelinated fibers, which serve pain and temperature sensation and, to a lesser extent, light touch. Symptoms include a burning pain distally. Feet are affected first; the pain later ascends, and the hands may be affected. Patients notice the pain especially at night when trying to sleep. Examination shows increased threshold for touch stimuli; stimuli, when perceived, are often painful. Vibration and proprioception are unaffected early in the course, but they are eventually lost. NCV testing shows preserved motor and sensory NCVs early in the course, but the size of the sensory nerve action potential (SNAP) is reduced. Later, the sensory NCV is slowed, and the SNAP ultimately disappears. Motor NCV eventually slows because the diabetic sensory neuropathy is really a sensorimotor axonal neuropathy with predominantly sensory features.

Diabetic Polyradiculopathy. Patients experience pain, sensory loss, and muscle weakness appropriate to the level of involvement. In the cervical region, this is termed Parsonage-Turner syndrome. When involvement is in the upper lumbar region, the clinical syndrome of diabetic amyotrophy (Brun-Garland syndrome) is produced. Pain is in the low back and upper legs, and there is weakness of the quadriceps and psoas with a reduced quadriceps reflex. Sensory loss is in the L2-L4 distribution, although the dysesthetic pain may overshadow the heightened sensory threshold. Direct involvement of the femoral nerve has been implicated by some clinicians.

Diabetic radiculopathy may occur in the thoracic dermatomes, often triggering extensive evaluation for spinal lesions. Because of the important differential diagnoses of herniated disk, spinal tumor, and degenerative disease, magnetic resonance imaging of the affected area often has to be performed.

Guillain-Barré Syndrome

Guillain-Barré syndrome (GBS) is a group of autoimmune neuropathies, the most common of which is acute inflammatory demyelinating polyneuropathy (AIDP). It affects Schwann cells, producing demyelination of peripheral nerves. Proximal myelin segments are affected first. Patients present with generalized weakness, which usually spares the extraocular muscles. Facial weakness may be prominent. Sensory symptoms include numbness that spans sensory modalities and is most prominent distally. Reflexes are almost always absent, even early in the course.

Motor and sensory NCVs are slow, and the waveforms have a dispersed appearance. The waveforms have a lower amplitude and longer duration, indicating that there is increased variance in conduction velocity. However, in patients with very early disease, NCVs may be normal. F waves are absent or markedly delayed in almost all patients, and they are abnormal before distal peripheral nerve conduction is affected. EMG shows reduced motor unit recruitment; subsequent axonal degeneration produces fibrillation potentials, although this is uncommon early in the course. Cerebrospinal fluid (CSF) in GBS has high protein with few or no white blood cells (WBCs) This pattern is called cytoalbuminologic dissociation.

The axonal variety of GBS is a rare condition that presents with similar symptoms and signs, but neurophysiological studies show mostly axonal degeneration with less impressive demyelination.

Differential diagnosis of GBS includes other causes of subacute weakness, such as tick paralysis, acute porphyria, botulism, hypophosphatemia, hypokalemia, and rare toxic neuropathies (caused by, for instance, organophosphate insecticides, N-hexane, or arsenic). HIV-associated GBS is of increasing concern.

The term polyradiculoneuropathy is used by many experts for the "P" in AIDP and in chronic inflammatory demyelinating polyneuropathy (CIDP), and it is probably a more accurate term than polyneuropathy. This chapter uses the more common and shorter term.

Chronic Inflammatory Demyelinating Polyneuropathy

CIDP is an autoimmune disorder of peripheral nerves. Although CIDP is sometimes considered a chronic form of GBS, the immunology may be very different. Patients present with proximal and distal weakness, absent reflexes, and distal sensory loss. CSF shows high protein with few or no WBCs. NCV testing shows multifocal slowing with increased latencies of the compound motor action potentials (CMAPs) and SNAPs. EMG shows reduced motor unit recruitment early in the course. With secondary axonal degeneration, denervation is seen in the muscles. The differential diagnosis of CIDP includes the hereditary demyelinating neuropathies, paraneoplastic neuropathy, HIV neuropathy, and demyelinating neuropathy with monoclonal gammopathy.

Acute Motor Axonal Neuropathy

Acute motor axonal neuropathy (AMAN) is a rare subtype of GBS that is mainly seen in China and Japan. As opposed to AIDP, it is axonal rather than demyelinating; it is purely motor and does not involve sensory nerves.

Patients present with rapidly progressive flaccid paralysis. Diagnosis is suspected when NCVs show reduced motor action potential amplitude and normal sensory conductions. Prognosis and treatment are similar to AIDP, with most patients having good recovery.

Acute Motor Sensory Axonal Neuropathy

Acute motor sensory axonal neuropathy (AMSAN) is a subtype of GBS where both motor and sensory nerves are affected, but it is axonal rather than demyelinating. This is rapidly progressive; unlike AIDP and AMAN, it has a poorer prognosis for recovery. The diagnosis is suspected when nerve conductions show reduced action potential amplitude without the marked slowing and dispersion of the waves seen in AIDP.

Hereditary Neuropathies

Classification of hereditary neuropathies has evolved. The most prominent is a collection of disorders with the name Charcot-Marie-Tooth (CMT) disease. Presentation is foot drop and pes cavus (high arch due to imbalance of foot muscles), hammer toes, and ankle twisting. Pes cavus without other aspects of the syndrome are present in up to 10% of normal people, although a subset is thought to have undiagnosed neuromuscular disorder. Pes cavus is not specific for CMT disorders; other neuropathies can produce the deformity. There are many types of CMT, but this chapter will only consider the most common and emblematic of the group. Inheritance for them is usually autosomal dominant with variable penetrance, but there are autosomal recessive variants. Most of what were classified as hereditary sensorimotor neuropathies are now classified as CMTs; however, they are increasingly being classified by gene defect in authoritative publications. Because neurologists do not know the gene defect when they are localizing and diagnosing a neuropathy, this chapter will stick to a syndromic classification.

- CMT 1 has demyelination predominating.
- CMT 2 has axonal damage predominating.
- CMT 3 is early-onset demyelinating neuropathy including Dejerine-Sottas and congenital hypomyelinating neuropathy.
- CMT 4 is a group of autosomal recessive sensorimotor demyelinating disorders.

CMT type 1 is an autosomal dominant disorder with demyelination predominating. NCVs are slow. EMG often shows distal denervation, but the demyelinating findings predominant. This was termed the hypertrophic form of CMT.

CMT type 2 is also an autosomal dominant disorder but with axonal dysfunction predominating. Distal weakness is prominent with little sensory symptomatology. NCVs are near normal, but EMG shows prominent denervation.

Hereditary neuropathy with liability to pressure palsies (HNPP) presents with episodes of compressive neuropathies. This is due to a deletion in the same *PMP22* gene that is duplicated in CMT type 1. Deficits usually resolve, but static lesions can develop.

Hereditary sensory and autonomic neuropathy is a family of disorders including five entities, all of which are characterized by sensory loss and autonomic manifestations without motor symptoms. Type I is autosomal dominant, and the remainder are recessive or of uncertain inheritance. Sensory NCVs are slow with reduction in amplitude of the SNAP; SNAP may be unrecordable in many patients. Motor NCVs and CMAPs are normal in most patients, although motor NCVs may be slightly slowed in type 3 (familial dysautonomia or Riley-Day syndrome), indicating that type 3 is a predominantly, though not purely, sensory neuropathy. Many of the sensory neuropathies have autonomic involvement that manifests as anhidrosis, orthostatic blood pressure, and fluctuating body temperature. Type 4 is congenital insensitivity to pain with anhidrosis.

Mononeuropathies

Cervical Radiculopathy. Most cervical radiculopathies are due to lateral prolapse of the intervertebral disk. Occasionally, osteophytes or spondylitic bars may produce the same effect.

C5 radiculopathy is uncommon but presents with sensory loss in the radial forearm. Motor deficit if present is in deltoid and biceps. Biceps reflex can be reduced. NCS is usually normal. EMG can show denervation of deltoid, biceps, and relevant paraspinal muscles.

C6 radiculopathy produces sensory deficit in digits 1 and 2 and can produce weakness of biceps and brachioradialis. Brachioradialis reflex is often diminished. NCS is usually normal. EMG can show denervation in the biceps and paraspinal muscles.

C7 radiculopathy is the most common of the cervical radiculopathies. Patients present with sensory deficits on digits 3 and 4. Weakness can be seen in wrist extensors and triceps. Triceps reflex is often diminished. NCS is usually normal. EMG can show denervation in the extensor digitorum communis, triceps, and paraspinals.

C8 radiculopathy can present with sensory deficit on digit 5 and weakness of intrinsic hand muscles. NCS is usually normal. EMG can show denervation of intrinsic muscles of the hand, triceps, and paraspinals.

Brachial Plexopathy. The most common brachial plexopathies are brachial plexitis, neoplastic infiltration, radiation plexopathy, and trauma. The brachial plexus is illustrated in Figure 2.6.2 (see Chapter 2.6).

Brachial plexitis is a syndrome of pain in the shoulder and upper arm that develops into dysfunction of a portion of the brachial plexus, usually upper plexus C5–6, although lower plexus can be predominantly involved. As pain abates, weakness progresses.

Trauma is the most common cause. It usually affects the upper plexus, C5–6, because of downward pressure on the shoulder relative to the neck. Lower plexus injuries can occur especially with the arm hyperextended over the head. Trauma can result in stretch injury, which has a fairly good prognosis for recovery, or root avulsion, which has generally a poor prognosis for recovery.

Neoplastic infiltration is most commonly from lung or breast cancer, and it most often affects the lower plexus. Patients have significant pain as infiltration develops, which is one helpful differentiating feature from radiation plexitis to which cancer patients are often susceptible. Neoplastic infiltration usually affects the lower plexus, supplied by roots C8 and T1. Horner syndrome can occur.

Radiation plexitis occurs in cancer patients who have received treatment to the area. This involves the upper plexus more than the lower plexus; this is a helpful differentiating feature from neoplastic infiltration. There are also some electrophysiological changes that help with this differentiation.

Neonatal brachial plexus palsy (NBPP) is presumably related to traction, although there is conflicting pathophysiological data and opinion. This includes Erb palsy involving the upper trunk affecting nerve roots C5 and C6, and Klumpke palsy of the lower plexus affecting C8 and T1 nerve roots.

Median Neuropathy. The most common median neuropathy is carpal tunnel syndrome, followed by anterior interosseus syndrome, pronator teres syndrome, and the ligament of Struthers syndrome.

Carpal tunnel syndrome is entrapment of the median nerve at the wrist. Patients present with pain at the wrist and sensory loss on the thenar side of the palm. With severe cases, there can be weakness of the abductor pollicis brevis and opponens pollicis. NCS shows increased motor distal latency through the wrist and slow sensory NCV through the wrist. With severe cases, there may be denervation in the abductor pollicis brevis.

Anterior interosseus syndrome is damage to the nerve of the same name as it leaves the main trunk of the median nerve in the forearm. Patients present with forearm pain and often with weakness of thumb and index finger movement. NCS shows increased distal latency of the pronator quadratus. EMG shows denervation in the pronator quadratus, flexor pollicis longus, and the median-innervated portion of the flexor digitorum profundus.

Pronator teres syndrome is compression of the median nerve as it passes through the pronator teres in the proximal forearm. Patients present with tenderness over the muscle and weakness of distal median-innervated muscles. NCV shows slow conduction through the proximal forearm and denervation in distal median-innervated muscles including abductor pollicis brevis, flexor digitorum superficialis, and the median side of the flexor digitorum profundus but no denervation of the pronator teres itself. The pronator teres is innervated proximal to the site of damage, although it is often tender.

Ligament of Struthers syndrome is compression of the median nerve by the ligament that is a fibrous band above the medial epicondyle. Clinically, this resembles pronator teres syndrome, except that the pronator teres itself is denervated.

Ulnar Neuropathy. The ulnar nerve is most commonly injured at the elbow, across the ulnar groove and extending into the cubital tunnel. Distal damage to the ulnar nerve can produce varying symptoms and signs; the combination of weakness of the interossei with sparing of the abductor digiti minimi and of sensory function suggests a deep branch lesion in the palm. This injury can be seen in bicycle riders. Compression of the superficial sensory branch may produce sensory symptoms over digit 5 without motor findings.

Ulnar nerve entrapment at the elbow is usually due to mechanical damage at the elbow; it is more likely if there are other predisposing causes of neuropathy. This presents with numbness over digits 4 and 5, often with significant pain at the elbow that is worse with flexion. NCS shows slow motor NCV across the elbow. EMG show denervation in the abductor digiti minimi and ulnar half of the flexor digitorum profundus.

Ulnar nerve entrapment at Guyon canal is where the ulnar nerve passes from the forearm to the hand. Patients often have pain in the region with sensory loss on the ulnar side of the hand but not the forearm. Weakness of the abductor digiti minimi is expected but not weakness of the more proximal forearm muscles. NCS shows slowed ulnar conduction across the wrist. EMG shows denervation in the abductor digiti minimi and first dorsal interosseus.

Radial Neuropathy. The most common radial neuropathy is Saturday night palsy, which is compression of the radial nerve at the spiral groove of the humerus. It received this name because it typically occurs in patients who rest their arm over a bed or chair when they are deeply asleep, especially when intoxicated. All of the distal radial-innervated muscles in the arm may be affected. The triceps may also be affected if the compression is proximal to its innervation. Patients present with wrist drop and preserved finger flexors and intrinsic muscle strength in the hand. Wrist and finger flexors may appear to be weak if the hand is allowed to fall into a flexed position; the examiner must forcibly extend the wrist to at least the neutral position to accurately test these muscles.

Posterior interosseus nerve damage occurs as the radial nerve enters for forearm. The superficial sensory branch has left by this time, so sensation is typically intact. EMG shows denervation of wrist and finger extensors but sparing of supinator and extensor carpi radialis longus, which are innervated from branches above the level of the lesion.

Lumbosacral Radiculopathy. Lumbosacral radiculopathy typically produces back pain radiating down the leg in a distribution appropriate to the involved nerve root.

S1 radiculopathy is the most common lumbosacral radiculopathy. There is usually sensory loss at the lateral foot, digits 4 and 5, and outside of the sole. Weakness may be present in gastrocnemius and gluteus maximus, but these are so strong that weakness may be difficult to detect. Ankle (Achilles) reflex is usually diminished. NCS is usually normal. EMG shows denervation in affected muscles.

L5 radiculopathy is the second most common lumbar radiculopathy. There are no reflex abnormalities. Weakness of the peroneus longus and tibialis anterior muscles is very helpful for this diagnosis. Examination of the tibialis posterior action can differentiate between L5 radiculopathy and peroneal neuropathy because this muscle is innervated by a branch of the tibial nerve.

L2, L3, and L4 radiculopathies are much less common than L5 and S1. They produce sensory loss in the associated regions of the thigh extending into the lower leg. NCS is usually normal. EMG can show denervation in quadriceps and paraspinal muscles.

Lumbosacral Plexopathy. The most common causes of lumbosacral plexopathy are neoplastic infiltration from paravertebral metastases and local extension of abdominal tumors such as gastrointestinal and renal tumors.

Lumbar plexitis is rare, and its course and presentation parallel those of brachial plexitis. Patients with lumbar plexopathy present with weakness spanning single dermatomal or neural distributions, such as quadriceps and adductors. NCVs are usually normal. EMG can show denervation, but it is frequently normal if performed early in the course. The lumbosacral plexus is illustrated in Figure 2.6.3 (see Chapter 2.6).

Neoplastic lumbar plexopathy usually occurs from direct compression and invasion by tumor, either primary site or metastatic. Lung and breast cancers are common primary tumors. Intraabdominal and pelvic tumors of various types also damage the lumbosacral plexus. Presentation is usually with severe neuropathic pain, especially shooting pain and with a positional nature.

Radiation lumbosacral plexopathy usually presents with little pain and more weakness and sensory loss in the appropriate distribution.

Traumatic lumbosacral plexopathy occurs usually with severe body injury and sometimes secondary to regional bony injury. Many of the patients who sustain prominent traumatic lumbosacral plexus damage do not survive their injuries.

Peripartum lumbosacral plexopathy is due to mechanical effects of the fetus and uterus. The plexus is further susceptible to damage during descent and delivery, which can result in weakness and sensory loss in the leg with proximal and distal manifestations.

Sciatic Neuropathy. Injury to the sciatic nerve usually occurs where it exits the pelvis. Typical causes include intramuscular injections, pelvic fractures, blunt trauma to the buttock or posterior thigh, and stretch from trauma or surgery.

The peroneal division is more susceptible to traumatic injury than the tibial division; therefore, some sciatic neuropathies are misinterpreted as peroneal nerve palsies. Patients present with weakness of the tibialis anterior. Weakness of the gastrocnemius is difficult to assess because of the tremendous strength of this muscle even in small individuals; the proportionate weakness required for the deficit to be detectable is large.

Peroneal Neuropathy. Peroneal neuropathy is most often due to compression of the nerve at the fibular neck. Damage to the peroneal division of the sciatic nerve may produce similar symptoms. Patients present with weakness of the tibialis anterior and peronei, producing impaired dorsiflexion and eversion of the foot. NCV is slowed across the fibular neck. EMG shows denervation in the tibialis anterior and peroneus longus. Differentiation of peroneal neuropathy across the fibular neck from a more proximal peroneal lesion is accomplished by EMG of the short head of the biceps femoris. This muscle is innervated by a branch of the peroneal division after it has separated from the tibial division but before it has passed through the popliteal fossa.

Tibial Neuropathy. Tibial neuropathy is uncommon and usually is a result of traumatic injury; gunshot wounds, needle injections, and motor vehicle accidents with leg fractures are frequent causes. Most patients with proximal tibial neuropathy also have dysfunction of the peroneal division. Patients present with weakness of the gastrocnemius and soleus muscles, which manifests as an inability to stand on the toes or, minimally, relative weakness of plantar flexion.

Tarsal tunnel syndrome is an uncommon problem; it occurs due to entrapment of a distal branch of the tibial nerve as it passes behind the medial malleolus. Patients present with pain and dysesthesias in the foot and with tenderness in the region of entrapment. NCV shows slowing of conduction in the medial and lateral plantar nerves, which are the terminal branches of the tibial nerve. EMG may show denervation in the abductor hallucis and abductor digiti minimi with entrapment of the medial and lateral plantar nerves, respectively.

Femoral Neuropathy. The femoral nerve is injured in the pelvis as it crosses under the inguinal ligament or in the leg. Weakness is most easily detected in the psoas because the quadriceps is so strong. Absent patellar reflex is common. Sensory loss is over the anterior thigh and medial aspect of the calf; this loss in a saphenous nerve distribution is helpful in differentiating femoral neuropathy from lumbar radiculopathy. NCV of the femoral nerve can be done easily in trim individuals but may be impossible in heavier patients. EMG shows denervation of the quadriceps with sparing of adductors (which are innervated by the obturator nerve).

Lateral Femoral Cutaneous Neuropathy. Entrapment of the lateral femoral cutaneous nerve occurs as it crosses beneath the inguinal ligament. Obesity and pregnancy predispose to this lesion. Patients present with numbness and often pain on the lateral aspect of the thigh. The deficit does not extend below the knee. Lateral femoral cutaneous neuropathy is differentiated from femoral neuropathy by the presence of a lateral sensory deficit and absence of a motor deficit. NCV of this nerve can be reliably performed in trim individuals but may be technically difficult in heavier patients, who are especially prone to lateral femoral cutaneous nerve entrapment. This disorder is termed Meralgia paresthetica.

Obturator Neuropathy. This very rare condition is usually due to obturator hernia or pelvic fracture. Patients present with weak hip adductors. NCVs are not performed on this nerve. EMG shows denervation in the adductors with preservation of femoral-innervated muscles.

MOTOR NEURON DISEASE

Motor neuron diseases spare sensory nerves and must be distinguished from myopathies, which also only produce motor symptoms. The three most important motor neuron diseases are discussed in the following sections.

Amyotrophic Lateral Sclerosis

In amyotrophic lateral sclerosis (ALS), degeneration of the upper and lower motor neurons develops in midlife or later. Patients present with weakness without sensory loss but with upper motor neuron signs, including hyperreflexia and upward plantar responses. EMG shows widespread fasciculations and denervation.

Spinal Muscular Atrophy

In spinal muscular atrophy (SMA), degeneration of lower motor neurons without effect on upper motor neurons begins in utero. Patients present with weakness and hypotonia without sensory or upper motor neuron signs. Late onset cases of SMA must be distinguished from ALS and muscular dystrophies.

Poliomyelitis

In poliomyelitis, an enterovirus affects the lower motor neuron during an acute illness characterized by malaise, fever, and asymmetric paralysis. The presentation is classic and distinct from that of other motor neuron diseases, but poliomyelitis must be differentiated from GBS and postinfectious encephalomyelitis. EMG shows denervation without sensory nerve involvement and with only mildly slowed motor NCVs in contrast to findings in GBS (see earlier discussion).

Multifocal motor neuropathy is easily confused with other motor neuron diseases. Rather than neuronal degeneration, the pathology is multifocal demyelination affecting motor axons. Laboratory tests may show high titers of antibodies to gangliosides. Multifocal motor neuropathy is differentiated from other motor neuron degenerations by NCV and EMG.

MYOPATHIES

Dystrophies

Muscular dystrophies are characterized by degeneration of muscle fibers associated with infiltration of connective tissue. Patients generally present with weakness with a distribution determined by the specific entity. EMG shows myopathic pattern. NCS is usually normal. Diagnosis is made by clinical syndrome and is confirmed by EMG as a myopathy. Muscle biopsy or gene analysis usually confirms the exact type.

Duchenne muscular dystrophy (DMD) is an X-linked recessive disorder that presents as weakness predominant in the legs. Pseudohypertrophy of the calves is often seen. Gower sign, the patient having to climb up their own legs to stand, is common.

Becker dystrophy is chemically and genetically related to DMD and is also X-linked recessive. Clinical presentation is similar to DMD but is less severe.

Facioscapulohumeral dystrophy (FSH) is an autosomal dominant disorder with facial weakness followed by subsequent development of arm weakness.

Limb-girdle dystrophy is a family of disorders that generally present with arm and shoulder weakness. Inheritance of this condition varies.

Myotonic dystrophy is an autosomal dominant disorder with weakness and muscle wasting and signs of myotonia on clinical examination and EMG. Clinically, this is often elicited by tapping the thenar muscles with a reflex hammer and observing sustained contraction. Associated findings can include cataracts, glucose intolerance, and a characteristic pattern of muscle wasting giving a recognizable facial appearance.

Emery-Dreifuss dystrophy is family of disorders with any inheritance. Commonality is presentation of humeroperoneal weakness and contractions, including proximal arms and distal legs. Cardiomyopathy is classically associated with this dystrophy.

Oculopharyngeal dystrophy is an autosomal dominant disorder that presents with ptosis, which can be severe enough to obscure vision. Facial weakness is typical. Dysphagia can also be severe.

Scapuloperoneal dystrophy is a family of autosomal dominant disorders related to FSH but with different genetic loci. Patients present with weakness of shoulder muscles and foot drop.

Distal muscular dystrophy (DD) is a family of disorders with autosomal dominant or recessive inheritance, with the commonality being weakness that begins distally in arms and legs and then progresses proximally.

Inflammatory Myopathies

Inflammatory myopathies may be autoimmune or infectious. Autoimmune myopathies include polymyositis and dermatomyositis. Polymyositis is classified by whether it is associated with skin changes (dermatomyositis) or associated systemic disorders, such as neoplasm or connective tissue disease. Infectious myopathies include a wide range of parasitic, bacterial, and viral infections.

Polymyositis (PM) presents as progressive proximal weakness that is symmetric in the upper and lower extremities. Although this is an immune-mediated inflammatory myopathy, it is not typically painful. Creatine kinase (CK) is elevated. Muscle biopsy shows inflammatory infiltrate.

PM can be associated with cancer although less so than with dermatomyositis. Criteria for the diagnosis of PM have been established. Most of the following features must be present for diagnosis:

- Myopathic pattern on EMG
- Perifascicular atrophy, mononuclear infiltration, and degenerating and regenerating muscle fibers on muscle biopsy
- Elevated CK

Dermatomyositis (DM) is an immune-mediated myopathy that presents similarly to PM but differs in that there are skin manifestations with discoloration of the eyelids and rash on the dorsum of fingers. Association with cancer is about twice that of PM. Bohan and Peter devised a classification scheme for PM and DM, as follows:

- Type I: idiopathic PM
- Type II: idiopathic DM
- Type III: PM or DM associated with cancer
- Type IV: childhood PM or DM associated with vasculitis
- Type V: PM or DM associated with collagen vascular disease

Inclusion body myositis (IBM) is an inflammatory myopathy that presents as distal weakness of the arms and legs and is often diagnosed after treatment for presumed polymyositis has failed. The diagnosis is ultimately made on muscle biopsy by finding characteristic vacuoles.

Polymyalgia rheumatica (PMR) presents with muscle pain and stiffness, especially in the proximal arm and shoulder girdle. This is often suspected when erythrocyte sedimentation rate (ESR) is found to be high. As such, it is often associated with giant cell arteritis (GCA).

Viral myositis presents with muscle pain that can be associated with fever and symptoms of nonneurologic infection. Myositis can progress to rhabdomyolysis. Causes are varied, but enteroviruses and influenza viruses are common. Diagnosis is typically clinical and easy if there are symptoms of a recent viral illness. Biopsy is not usually needed.

Bacterial myositis presents with hot, swollen, and tender muscles. This is a diffuse process, but *Staphylococcus aureus* can occasionally present with focal or multifocal muscle infections.

Parasitic myositis presents as muscle pain and fever or malaise. In diagnosing, the neurologist should consider toxoplasmosis, cysticercosis, and trichinosis. History of travel or other exposure is important. Muscle biopsy may be needed to determine the precise diagnosis.

Viral myositis frequently presents in children with diffuse myalgias. CK is increased but less so than in some other disorders of skeletal muscle.

Metabolic Myopathies

Metabolic myopathies result in muscle damage through impairment in energy metabolism or abnormal storage of metabolic products that secondarily interfere with muscle metabolism. These disorders are suspected especially with

- Myoglobinuria;
- Cramps with exercise; and
- Exercise intolerance, sometimes with second-wind phenomenon.

There are so many metabolic myopathies that detailing them is beyond the scope of this book. The following paragraphs discuss some of the most important from the standpoint of incidence and educational importance.

Myophosphorylase deficiency is also known as McArdle disease. This is an autosomal recessive glycogen storage disease that presents with cramps on exercise and myoglobinuria. Patients often exhibit a second-wind phenomenon, regaining strength if they persist in the present effort. Diagnosis is made by muscle biopsy showing deficiency of phosphorylase plus excess glycogen storage.

Phosphofructokinase (PFK) deficiency presents similarly to myophosphorylase deficiency, is autosomal recessive, and includes cramps with exercise, but there is no second-wind phenomenon. Diagnosis is made by muscle biopsy.

Phosphoglycerate kinase deficiency is an X-linked recessive disorder that presents with cramps on exercise. Cerebral developmental disorder can also occur. Muscle biopsy shows the enzyme deficiency.

Phosphoglycerate mutase deficiency is a glycogen storage disease that presents with cramps, exercise intolerance, and myoglobinuria. Diagnosis is made on muscle biopsy. Inheritance is autosomal recessive.

Alpha-glucosidase (acid maltase) deficiency (Pompe) is a glycogen storage disease that presents with progressive proximal weakness that can progress to the point of affecting respirations. There are multiple types of mutations that can be responsible for the condition, so presentation is variable. When an infantile form, the presentation is rapid and severe. In older patients, the presentation is with a limb-girdle pattern that progresses more slowly than the infantile form. Diagnosis is confirmed with enzyme analysis of blood or muscle biopsy.

Periodic Paralysis

Periodic paralysis includes a group of disorders characterized by episodic weakness. The exact symptoms and chemistry differ between individual disorders.

Hypokalemic periodic paralysis is characterized by attacks of weakness that begin in proximal muscles and spread to distal muscles. An attack can be provoked by rest following intense exercise or by a high-carbohydrate meal and can last up to several hours. Familial hypokalemic periodic paralysis is inherited as autosomal dominant. Diagnosis is confirmed by the presence of low potassium levels during an attack. Provocative testing can be performed with an oral glucose load. Muscle biopsy is often not needed but can show myopathic findings. NCVs are normal between attacks.

Hyperkalemic periodic paralysis presents with attacks of weakness, but the potassium is usually elevated. This paralysis is also inherited as autosomal dominant. Normokalemic periodic paralysis has also been described. Hyper- and hypokalemic periodic paralyses can also be associated with other metabolic disorders, including thyrotoxicosis and renal failure, and with use of some drugs.

Endocrine Myopathies

Hyperthyroidism is associated with multiple symptoms including tremor, irritability, heat intolerance, weight loss, and weakness. Neuromuscular disorders associated with thyrotoxicosis include myasthenia gravis (MG), periodic paralysis. and myopathy.

Hypothyroidism is associated with lethargy, weakness, and cold intolerance. Neuromuscular findings may be proximal weakness and percussion myotonia, with associated delayed relaxation of tendon reflexes.

NEUROMUSCULAR JUNCTION ABNORMALITIES

Neuromuscular junction (NMJ) disorders are characterized by defective transmission from motor neurons to muscle fibers. The deficit can be prejunctional or postjunctional. NMJ disorders are suspected when there is weakness that fatigues, and there is no sensory involvement. Involvement of ocular as well as axonal and appendicular muscles is supportive; most myopathies do not involve ocular muscles prominently, whereas ptosis or ocular motor deficit can be a prominent initial symptom.

Myasthenia Gravis

MG is an autoimmune disorder due to antibodies that bind to the ACh receptors (AChRs), causing increased turnover; therefore, fewer receptors are available for binding with ACh. Most patients present with ocular motor weakness, characterized by diplopia and/or ptosis. The extraocular muscle weakness spans nerve distributions, which differentiates MG from single or multiple cranial nerve palsies. Patients with ocular MG have no axial or appendicular weakness, whereas patients with systemic MG present with proximal weakness that tends to be better in the morning.

NCVs are usually normal with single stimuli. EMG is usually normal. Repetitive stimulation of peripheral nerve at low rates (two to five stimulations per second) produces a decrement in the amplitude of the CMAP. Single-fiber EMG shows increased jitter and blocking.

Botulism

Botulism is due to impaired release of ACh from the presynaptic terminal, resulting in less activation of the AChR. Patients present with autonomic symptoms, including abdominal cramps, diarrhea, and constipation, that are followed by generalized weakness including prominent ocular motor and bulbar involvement. Pupil constriction is impaired. CMAP amplitude is reduced. Repetitive stimulation at low rates (two to five stimulations per second) causes no decrement, but the amplitude of the response is increased after exercise. Repetitive stimulation at high rates (20 to 50 stimulations per second) reveals an incremental response to successive stimuli in the train. The response seen is often patchy, with some muscles being normal.

Myasthenic (Lambert-Eaton) Syndrome

Myasthenic syndrome is an autoimmune disorder in which antibodies act at the presynaptic terminal to impair the release of ACh. Most patients with this syndrome have cancer, so it is usually a paraneoplastic disorder. Myasthenic syndrome is also associated with other autoimmune diseases, including systemic lupus erythematous and polymyositis.

Myasthenic syndrome presents with proximal or generalized weakness. Autonomic symptoms, including dry mouth and impotence, often develop, although they are less severe than those seen with botulism. Ophthalmoplegia or ptosis is unusual.

Motor NCV is normal, but the CMAP is of low amplitude. Sensory NCV and SNAP amplitude are normal. Repetitive stimulation shows a decremental response at low rates of stimulation; after exercise, CMAP amplitude is markedly increased, but the decremental response persists. High rates of stimulation produce an incremental response.

Headache

Eli E. Zimmerman and Howard S. Kirshner

The diagnosis of headache depends on the report of head pain and on a specific classification of the headache depending on details of the history and examination. Headache is classified as primary or secondary.

Principles

The brain itself has no pain sensation. Headaches are caused by irritation, disruption, inflammation, or compression of other structures within the head and skull:
- Skin, subcutaneous tissues, muscle
- Eyes, ears, teeth, sinuses
- Meninges
- Blood vessels, including arteries and venous sinuses
- Epineurium of cranial nerves
- Headaches are first classified as primary or secondary.

Primary Headaches

Primary headaches are defined as head pain resulting from pathophysiological mechanisms that are not the result of another medical condition. This section will discuss several of the most common primary headaches, including migraines, tension-type headaches, cluster headaches, and trigeminal neuralgia.

Migraines are very common; they affect over 10% of the population, occur with or without aura, and often run in families. They are two to three times more common in women than men.

The following lists are based on the International Classification of Headache Disorders (ICHD) criteria.

Migraine without aura consists of the following indications:
- At least five lifetime attacks, lasting 4 to 72 hours
- At least two of:
  - Unilateral location
  - Pulsating/throbbing quality
  - Moderate/severe pain intensity
  - Aggravation by or causing avoidance of routine physical activity
- At least one of:
  - Nausea and/or vomiting
  - Photophobia
  - Phonophobia

Migraine with aura consists of the following indications:
- Two attacks with both:
  - One or more of the following fully reversible aura symptoms:
    - Visual
    - Sensory
    - Speech/language
    - Motor
    - Brainstem
    - Retinal
  - At least three of these indications:
    - At least one aura symptom spreads over $\geq$5 minutes.
    - Two or more aura symptoms occur in succession.
    - Each aura symptom lasts 5 to 60 minutes.
    - At least one aura symptom is unilateral.
    - At least one aura symptom is positive.
    - The aura is accompanied, or followed within 60 minutes, by headache.

Tension-type headaches, which are probably the most common headache type, are defined by the ICHD as having:
- Episodes lasting from 30 minutes to 7 days.
- At least two of:
  - Bilateral location,
  - Pressing or tightening (nonpulsating) quality,
  - Mild or moderate intensity, or
  - Not aggravated by routine physical activity.
- Both of:
  - No nausea or vomiting and
  - No more than one of photophobia or phonophobia.

Cluster headaches, which are one of the trigeminal autonomic cephalalgias, are named for their periodicity. They occur nightly, over days to weeks, and then remit, or there are multiple attacks per day. These are defined as having:
- At least five attacks, with severe or very severe unilateral orbital, supraorbital, or temporal pain lasting 15 to 180 minutes.
- Either or both of:
  - At least one indication, ipsilateral to the headache, of:
    - Conjunctival injection and/or lacrimation,
    - Nasal congestion and/or rhinorrhea,
    - Eyelid edema,
    - Forehead and facial sweating, or
    - Miosis and/or ptosis.
  - A sense of restlessness or agitation:
    - Occurrence between every other day and eight per day.

Finally, **Trigeminal neuralgia** consists of recurrent paroxysms of unilateral facial pain in the distribution of one or more divisions of the trigeminal nerve, precipitated by innocuous stimuli within the affected trigeminal distribution. Trigeminal neuralgia exhibits all of the following features:
- Lasting from a fraction of a second to 2 minutes
- Severe intensity
- Electric shocklike, shooting, stabbing, or sharp in quality

Secondary Headaches

Secondary headaches are secondary to an underlying medical condition.

A few examples of secondary headaches include the following:

- Meningeal irritation due to blood (subarachnoid hemorrhage), infection (bacterial or viral or fungal meningitis), or medications (nonsteroidal antiinflammatory drugs, intravenous immunoglobulin)
- Vascular causes, such as vasculitis, subarachnoid hemorrhage, posterior reversible encephalopathy, or hypertensive emergency
- Intracranial hypertension due to space-occupying lesions, hydrocephalus, or idiopathic intracranial hypertension (pseudotumor cerebri)
- Intracranial hypotension, which can be spontaneous or due to cerebrospinal fluid leak

There are multiple causes of secondary headaches not due to brain dysfunction, such as glaucoma, optic neuritis, otitis media, sinusitis, skull-based lesions, temporomandibular joint dysfunction.

Headache Red Flags

The red flags for headaches are remembered with the mnemonic SNOOP:

- Systemic illness: fever, weight loss, cancer, advanced HIV
- Neurologic symptoms: confusion, impairment of consciousness, focal findings
- Onset: sudden, abrupt, "thunderclap"
- Older age: new or progressive in adults older than 50 years
- Prior headache history: first headache or different frequency, severity, or manifestations

In general, the first or the worst headache of the patient's life causes the clinician to take the headache seriously. These qualities should prompt the search for secondary causes for headache.

Movement Disorders

Karl E. Misulis, Martin A. Samuels, and Howard S. Kirshner

Movement disorders are impairments of movement not due to corticospinal tract dysfunction, although some movement disorders can be associated with corticospinal findings as a component (e.g., multiple system atrophy; MSA). Movement disorders may involve increased (hyperkinetic) or decreased (hypokinetic) movement. The key to diagnosis for most of these is clinical presentation, history, and examination. There are no scans for many of these disorders that are diagnostic.

Movement disorders are separated into the following categories, although not all disorders neatly fit into each category:

- Akinetic-rigid syndromes
- Tremor
- Dystonia and dyskinesia

This chapter considers some of the most common movement disorders and some disorders that are uncommon but illustrative from the standpoint of clinical diagnosis.

Akinetic-Rigid Syndromes

PARKINSON DISEASE

Parkinson disease (PD) is characterized by rigidity, bradykinesia, and tremor; however, not all of these may be present, especially early in the course. Gait is stooped with decreased arm swing. Steps are small and slow when the patient begins to walk but accelerate with distance (festination), predisposing the patient to falling down. Facial expression is reduced. Writing becomes smaller. The tremor is most prominent in the position of repose, most prominent in the arms, and averages 4 to 5 hertz. Rigidity and tremor are often asymmetric early in the course. Late in the course, abnormalities in postural reflexes make ambulation hazardous.

At least 50% of people with PD develop dementia. In patients followed for more than 10 years, the proportion may be as high as 75%.

Tremor of PD is often confused with ET. Distinguishing features are discussed in the section on ET in this chapter.

The differential diagnosis of idiopathic PD includes all of the other akinetic-rigid syndromes discussed in this section plus frontal lobe damage, which can result in a shuffling gait and lack of initiative; these symptoms may be mistaken for parkinsonism. All patients with parkinsonism must be asked specifically about neuroleptic and antiemetic exposure. Examination should detail the severity and distribution of the tremor, rigidity, bradykinesia, and gait and postural instability to aid with diagnosis and to facilitate future comparisons during treatment. DaTscan can be helpful in differentiating PD from ET, although it is used only in difficult cases. It will be similarly abnormal in all of the Parkinson-like syndromes.

VASCULAR PARKINSONISM

Vascular disease is second to Parkinson disease as a cause for parkinsonism. Clinical presentation has significant overlap, but a distinguishing feature is the predilection for involvement of the lower half of the body. In addition to Parkinson features, there are often corticospinal defect findings because of the multifocal ischemic changes. Tremor is often absent in vascular parkinsonism. However, ischemic changes on brain imaging do not make the diagnosis of vascular parkinsonism because chronic cerebrovascular disease is common in patients of the age of many of those who present with parkinsonism.

From the standpoint of localization, the finding of parkinsonism in association with corticospinal tract dysfunction or aphasia supports the diagnosis of vascular etiology.

DIFFUSE LEWY BODY DISEASE

Some patients with parkinsonian features will manifest dementia early in the course. Aphasia and apraxia are common. Pathologically, Lewy bodies are distributed diffusely through the cortex rather than having a restricted distribution in the substantia nigra. Other associated features include rapid fluctuations in mental status, with lucid periods and confused periods, REM sleep behavior disorder (movements or speech during sleep), and early visual hallucinations.

MULTIPLE SYSTEM ATROPHY WITH PREDOMINANT PARKINSONISM

Multiple system atrophy with predominant parkinsonism (MSA-P) was formerly termed striatonigral degeneration, and it is characterized by rigidity and bradykinesia with less tremor than seen in idiopathic PD. The diagnosis is often suspected when the patient does not respond to dopaminergic agents. No clinical features can clearly distinguish MSA-P from more typical PD, and the diagnosis is only confirmed at autopsy.

PROGRESSIVE SUPRANUCLEAR PALSY

Progressive supranuclear palsy (PSP) is characterized by rigidity, gait difficulty with a tendency to fall, and prominent oculomotor abnormalities. The ocular motor abnormalities are supranuclear in that the patient has impaired voluntarily gaze, but doll's head maneuvers (i.e., passive movement of the head from side to side) reveal preserved eye movement with passive turning of the head, at least early in the course. Vertical gaze, particularly downward, is most prominently affected, with involvement of horizontal gaze late in the course. The supranuclear deficit extends not only to ocular movement but also to other brainstem functions. Patients frequently have dysarthria and dysphagia. Eventually, degeneration of the brainstem results in deficits that cannot be overcome by reflexive maneuvers. Dementia is common, although it is usually mild.

The degeneration is not confined to the deep nuclei. Areas affected include substantia nigra, globus pallidus, subthalamic nuclei, periaqueductal gray, superior colliculus, and pretectal nuclei. Neuroanatomic localization is less important than recognition of the clinical syndrome for diagnosis.

CORTICOBASAL DEGENERATION

Corticobasal degeneration (CBD) is a neurodegenerative disease that has core features of akinesia and rigidity plus other variable features that can include alien hand syndrome, myoclonus, dystonia, and apraxia, usually asymmetric, with involvement of an upper limb. Alien hand syndrome is considered iconic for CBD but is not present in all patients and perhaps not even in the majority. Alien limb syndrome involves a patient's impression that the limb does not belong to them and that it is not under their voluntary control.

DRUG-INDUCED PARKINSONISM

Drug-induced parkinsonism differs from classic PD because of its lesser degree of tremor, but clinical differentiation may be impossible. A history of drug use, especially neuroleptics, is present in patients with drug-induced parkinsonism. Parkinsonism can develop from people who abuse illicit drugs. Drugs that have antidopamine action (e.g., metoclopramide) may be prescribed for gastrointestinal symptoms and can produce parkinsonism.

Tremor

The most common types of tremor are ET, Parkinson tremor, and enhanced physiologic tremor. ET is most prominent with action, Parkinson tremor is most prominent at rest, and enhanced physiologic tremor is noted by patients during episodes of anxiety or anger. Anxiety may exacerbate ET.

An action tremor can develop with cerebellar damage; it is accompanied by a characteristic incoordination of movement, often referred to as intention tremor. Cerebellar damage is seldom confused with PD or ET.

ESSENTIAL TREMOR

ET is most prominent with action or in the outstretched arm (postural) and is less apparent at rest. Stress exacerbates the tremor, leading some patients and clinicians to call it nervous tremor. Ethanol suppresses the tremor, and some patients develop alcohol-use disorder as a result. The tremor is most prominent in the hands, although the head is frequently affected, producing titubation. Voice tremor may occur. ET is strongly inherited, and at least half of cases have a genetic foundation.

Misdiagnosis of ET as parkinsonism by nonneurologists is among the most common errors in clinical practice, although some patients with parkinsonism can develop an ET type of tremor. The two are generally differentiated by the effect of action on the tremor: ET is most prominent with movement or posture of the arms, whereas Parkinson tremor is most prominent in repose. The frequency of ET is 5 to 8 hertz, which is faster than the 4-5 hertz of PD. Other findings of parkinsonism, such as rigidity, bradykinesia, and loss of postural reflexes, are typically not found in ET. One of the purposes of the DaTscan is to differentiate PD and related conditions from ET.

PARKINSON TREMOR

Tremor associated with PD is most prominent at rest and has a frequency of 4 to 5 hertz. The tremor is damped by action, but it is often still present. Associated neurologic findings of parkinsonism include bradykinesia, rigidity, positive glabellar reflexes, and impaired postural reflexes.

ENHANCED PHYSIOLOGIC TREMOR

Enhanced physiologic tremor is a high-frequency tremor that is most prominent with posture and action. It is exacerbated by anxiety, fatigue, and many drugs. Some of the most important provocative drugs and toxins are valproic acid, lithium, beta-agonists, theophylline, heavy metals, caffeine, cocaine, and neuroleptics. Tremor associated with alcohol withdrawal is also enhanced physiological tremor.

Disorders With Dystonia and/or Dyskinesia

EARLY-ONSET DYSTONIA

There are a host of genetic mutations that are associated with dystonia. This is the category that has replaced the term dystonia musculorum deformans. They are labeled by their mutations. They may be inherited or sporadic.

This is a generalized dystonia, but it often begins in one extremity, such as turning of the foot. Over time, other muscles are affected; eventually, most body muscles are involved. Dystonia affecting proximal muscles, including those of the trunk, interferes with gait and produces body postures during walking that can resemble those seen in adults with cerebral palsy. The gait may be so bizarre that the cause is mistakenly believed to be psychogenic. Progression is expected.

Onset is typically in childhood; the problem is often thought to be a focal dystonia until more generalized signs develop. Focal dystonias are much less likely to progress to generalized dystonia in adults.

ADULT-ONSET DYSTONIAS

There are a range of dystonias that appear in adults, and these are named for their manifestations rather than their genetics. For most, the genetics is not well characterized. These include cervical dystonia, blepharospasm, upper limb dystonia, and others. Most are idiopathic, but some limb dystonias have been correlated with a variety of structural lesions and are not confined to the basal ganglia.

DOPA-RESPONSIVE DYSTONIA

Dopa-responsive dystonia begins in childhood, with progressive dystonia first affecting the legs. There is a 2:1 female predominance. Average age of onset is 6 years. The dystonia is worse late in the day and better after sleep.

Identification of patients with dopa-responsive dystonias is important because they respond to low doses of levodopa (L-dopa). This disorder may be present in up to 10% of children who present with idiopathic dystonia; therefore, it is reasonable to try L-dopa in all such patients.

FOCAL DYSTONIAS

Spasmodic torticollis is the most common focal dystonia. Patients present with involuntary head turning or tilting. Initially, the movements are intermittent, but they subsequently become persistent. Patients often learn that a light touch on the face can cause the head to turn back to the primary position (sensory trick). Pain from sustained muscle contraction is common. The exact lesion responsible for torticollis is not known, but basal ganglia dysfunction has been implicated.

Blepharospasm is characterized by forced eye closure with depression of the eyebrows. It begins with frequent blinking and is only recognized by patients when sustained eyelid closure impairs vision.

Oromandibular dystonia can take a variety of forms, including forced tongue protrusion and jaw opening or closing, often with dysarthria and dysphagia. Spasmodic dysphonia is due to involuntary contraction of laryngeal muscles. Meige syndrome is blepharospasm with oromandibular dystonia.

Writer's cramp is one of the task-specific focal dystonias. It is characterized by muscular contraction of intrinsic muscles of the hand, and it is exacerbated by writing and other fine movements.

HUNTINGTON DISEASE

Huntington disease (HD) is characterized by choreiform movements, most prominent in the hands, that are exacerbated by movement, including walking. The chorea becomes generalized later in the course of the disease. Associated neurologic findings include ocular motor dysfunctions such as saccadic pursuit, gaze impersistence, and convergence paresis. Tongue protrusion is common. Psychiatric abnormalities include personality change, psychosis, and ultimately dementia.

The diagnosis is supported by positive family history, computed tomography (CT) and magnetic resonance imaging (MRI) scans showing atrophy of the caudate nucleus, and genetic testing. Counseling is performed prior to genetic testing to ensure that the patient understands the implications of the diagnosis.

Degeneration is widespread in HD, with cortical and subcortical atrophy; therefore, HD cannot be thought of as having a focal anatomic localization. The gene is localized to chromosome 4. HD is inherited as autosomal dominant with absolute penetrance; the frequency of new mutations is much lower than the frequency of uncertain parentage. HD shows anticipation, that is, clinical manifestations appear earlier in successive generations. Patients with HD at a young age commonly present with rigidity rather than chorea. The age at which symptoms develop is partially determined by the number of abnormal repeats in the gene.

SYDENHAM CHOREA

Sydenham chorea presents with typical choreiform movements that last for a week or weeks then abate. Occasional patients will have recurrent bouts of chorea. Most patients are children between 5 and 15 years of age. Most but not all patients will have a prior history of rheumatic fever. This disorder has become rare with the increasing use of antibiotics effective against group A streptococcal infections.

WILSON DISEASE

Wilson disease is a defect in copper metabolism with autosomal recessive inheritance. Copper accumulates in the liver, brain, cornea, and other organs, and the resultant liver disease produces nausea, vomiting, anorexia, malaise, and weight loss. Neurologic involvement causes personality change, affective disturbance, dystonia, tremor, rigidity, dysarthria, and gait difficulties.

Wilson disease should be considered in young individuals with a movement disorder, unexplained liver disease, and personality change. Diagnosis is supported by a Kayser-Fleischer ring in the cornea on slit-lamp examination. Serum ceruloplasmin concentration is usually low, but occasional patients may have levels in the normal range. Liver biopsy can confirm copper accumulation but is usually not necessary. Brain imaging shows degeneration of the basal ganglia plus cortical atrophy with compensatory ventricular dilatation.

DYSKINETIC CEREBRAL PALSY

Many patients with cerebral palsy present with prominent developmental disability and spasticity. In contrast, patients with dyskinetic cerebral palsy present with choreoathetosis, dystonia, and myoclonus and with less intellectual dysfunction than is seen in patients with prominent cortical involvement.

CHRONIC BILIRUBIN ENCEPHALOPATHY

Chronic bilirubin encephalopathy (CBE; previously termed kernicterus due to bilirubin staining of the basal ganglia) is characterized by choreoathetosis with dystonia, often accompanied by mental retardation, oculomotor abnormalities, and spasticity. Kernicterus closely resembles athetoid cerebral palsy.

NEURODEGENERATION WITH BRAIN IRON ACCUMULATION

Neurodegeneration with brain iron accumulation (NDBIA; formerly known as Hallervorden-Spatz disease) appears in childhood with progressive choreoathetosis or parkinsonism. Dystonia is common early in the course. Adult-onset NDBIA disease often manifests as parkinsonism. Iron is deposited in the globus pallidus, the pars reticularis of the substantia nigra, and the red nucleus.

The diagnosis is considered in children with progressive choreoathetosis, parkinsonism, or dystonia. MRI shows abnormal areas of low signal, most prominently in the globus pallidus, on T2-weighted images. CT is usually not helpful.

PAROXYSMAL CHOREOATHETOSIS

Paroxysmal choreoathetosis begins in childhood and is characterized by episodic chorea or dystonia that has a defined beginning and end. The disorder can be divided into two subsets, depending on whether the paroxysms are kinesigenic (i.e., triggered by movement): paroxysmal kinesigenic choreoathetosis and paroxysmal nonkinesigenic choreoathetosis. Both often show autosomal recessive inheritance and mostly affect males.

Paroxysmal kinesigenic choreoathetosis starts in childhood and is characterized by movement-induced paroxysms that usually last 5 minutes or less. Paroxysmal nonkinesigenic choreoathetosis starts in infancy and is not triggered by movement. Paroxysms can last for hours.

No clear-cut pathologic localization has been identified with these disorders. Identification of the paroxysmal dyskinesias is important because of their occasional response to benzodiazepines and anticonvulsants.

TARDIVE DYSKINESIA

Tardive dyskinesia (TD) is characterized by repetitive orolingual movements including lip smacking, tongue protrusion, and chewing movements. Limb muscles may be involved, which gives the appearance of chorea.

TD develops after prolonged neuroleptic exposure. Unlike other neuroleptic-induced syndromes, such as parkinsonism and malignant neuroleptic syndrome, TD may persist following discontinuation of the neuroleptic; it may appear to worsen shortly after discontinuation of the drug.

The location of the lesion producing TD is not completely known. One hypothesis suggests that there is supersensitivity of the dopamine receptors in the striatum, an example of postdenervation supersensitivity.

HEMIBALLISMUS

Damage to the subthalamic nucleus is thought to be the cause of hemiballismus, which is characterized by violent movements of the contralateral limbs, mainly through the proximal muscles. The limbs have a flinging appearance. Smaller distal movements are common as well, creating a continuum between ballism and chorea. The distal movements have more of the appearance of chorea.

The most common cause of hemiballismus is infarction. Other primary causes include tumor, hemorrhage, and demyelinating plaque from multiple sclerosis.

Visual Disorders

Eli E. Zimmerman and Karl E. Misulis

Approach to Differential Diagnosis

ASSESSMENT OF THE VISUAL DISTURBANCE

Visual disturbance usually falls into one of several categories but sometimes it is in more than one category, depending on whether visual loss is accompanied by other deficits.

Types of visual loss include

- Monocular loss,
- Binocular loss,
- Hemianopia,
- Diplopia, and
- Positive visual disturbance.

MONOCULAR VISUAL LOSS

Monocular visual loss is due to a lesion of the eye or of the optic nerve.

Pupillary response can help to distinguish between these locations, although imperfectly. If there is an afferent pupillary defect (APD), then optic neuropathy is more likely than ocular etiology, although severe ocular damage can produce APD.

Disc appearance varies depending on etiology. If the disc shows swelling or especially if there is hemorrhage, the neurologist should consider Giant cell arteritis (GCA), nonarteritic ischemic optic neuropathy, infections, and other etiologies with inflammatory or infiltrative features (e.g., tumor). If the disc is normal or shows mild swelling, optic neuritis or neuromyelitis optica (NMO) are possible causes. If the disc is absolutely normal, the neurologist should consider posterior ischemic optic neuropathy.

If there is no APD, or even mild relative defect, then the neurologist should consider retinal arterial or venous ischemia, although those should have fundus findings. The neurologist should also consider central serous maculopathy.

BINOCULAR VISUAL LOSS

Subacute to acute binocular visual loss has a broad differential diagnosis with some differences from monocular.

Full-field binocular visual loss of recent onset can be due to bilateral occipital ischemia, bilateral retinal dysfunction, or bilateral optic nerve dysfunction. Cortical blindness from occipital ischemia should result in preservation of pupillary responses; if there is bilateral retinal or optic nerve pathology, then there should be apparent bilateral APD. Papilledema suggests idiopathic intracranial hypertension (IIH) as a cause, but bilateral optic neuritis should be considered. Methanol poisoning can produce bilateral visual blurring and blindness.

Hemifield binocular visual loss is most commonly due to stroke and often is incomplete because of the complex vascular supply to the optic radiations and cortex. In a transient ischemic attack (TIA), this loss would not be persistent. Migraine can produce hemifield visual loss, although often there are also associated visual phenomena. Similarly, seizure can produce hemifield visual loss and can be associated with transient positive visual symptoms. Related, posterior reversible encephalopathy syndrome (PRES) presents with similar symptoms.

In macular sparing with a hemianopia, there is damage to the occipital primary visual (calcarine) cortex around the calcarine sulcus. If stroke or other structural lesion spares the most posterior/occipital portion of this sulcus, which serves the macula, then the hemianopia is macular sparing. This is most common with posterior cerebral artery (PCA) stroke because the posterior macular region of the cortex receives at least some supply from the middle cerebral artery (MCA).

Binocular superior quadrant visual loss (quadrantanopia) is typically due to damage to the optic radiations as they pass through the temporal lobes.

Binocular inferior quadrantanopia is usually due to damage in the contralateral parietal region, affecting visual projections to the super side of the visual cortex.

The deficits affecting the quadrants are not exact because the optic tract projections are not perfectly organized.

DIPLOPIA

Diplopia is discussed in more depth in the chapters concerning brainstem and cranial nerve function, but a few important clinical scenarios are discussed here.

Oculomotor (CN III) palsy presents with ptosis, diplopia, and the unopposed CN IV and CN VI result in the affected eye being abducted and depressed, so-called "down and out." The pupil usually is dilated and nonreactive. Common causes are diabetic oculomotor palsy, compression from intracranial aneurysm, trauma, and tumors. Impending herniation can also cause oculomotor palsy, but this would not be a finding in isolation.

Abducens (CN VI) palsy presents with diplopia with failure to abduct one eye. If both eyes are affected, then abduction bilaterally is deficient. CN VI palsy is often due to diabetes with the pathway being vascular. Increased intracranial pressure (ICP) from any etiology, trauma, or tumor can also cause this.

Trochlear (CN IV) palsy presets with diplopia with a torsional component because of the complex mechanics of the superior oblique. To compensate, head tilt to the side opposite the CN IV palsy can resolve the diplopia.

Internuclear ophthalmoplegia (INO) is due to damage to the medial longitudinal fasciculus and results in failure of adduction of one eye with gaze to the opposite side. In the primary position, there might be no diplopia. The opposite eye abducts but has nystagmus because of the failure of the affected eye to adduct. The most common cause in younger patients is multiple sclerosis (MS). The most common cause in older individuals is stroke.

One-and-a-half syndrome is an INO with a gaze palsy. For example, when the right gaze is tested, the right eye may be able to look right, abduct, but the left eye cannot adduct. On the other hand, neither eye can look left with left gaze. This finding indicates a left gaze palsy with an INO affecting the opposite gaze. The most common causes are stroke and MS.

Ptosis is drooping of the eyelid. There are many potential causes. This chapter is referring to ptosis without oculomotor palsy. Among the causes to be considered are Horner syndrome, trauma, congenital ptosis, myasthenia, and a host of rarer conditions.

Prechiasmal Lesions

RETINA

Diseases of the retina are varied in etiology and are often distinguished by ophthalmologic examination; they typically cause monocular vision loss. Some retinal causes of acute vision loss include central retinal artery or vein occlusion, retinal detachment, and vitreous hemorrhage, whereas processes such as diabetic retinopathy and macular degeneration tend to progress over years.

OPTIC NERVE

The classic disease affecting the optic nerve is optic neuritis, which can occur as part of a larger syndrome (MS or neuromyelitis optica) or can occur in isolation. The hallmarks of optic neuritis are monocular vision loss that is painful, particularly with eye movements. It typically progresses over the course of hours to days. Diagnosis of optic neuritis relies on clinical history, funduscopic examination, and imaging.

Certain tumor syndromes, such as neurofibromatosis type 1, can cause tumors of the optic pathway, including the optic nerves. As typically happens with tumors, disease (and thus monocular vision changes) takes place over the course of months to years.

Lesions of the Optic Chiasm

The most classic disease affecting the optic chiasm is a tumor of the pituitary gland, which sits just inferior to the optic chiasm. Given that the nasal fibers within the optic nerves carry information from the temporal visual field, and that these are the ones crossing via the optic chiasm, these lesions typically cause bitemporal hemianopsia.

Retrochiasmal Lesions

OPTIC TRACT

Lesions of the optic tract are relatively uncommon, although they can occur in tumor syndromes such as neurofibromatosis type 1.

OPTIC RADIATIONS

Lesions affecting the pathway from the lateral geniculate nucleus to the occipital lobe are common, such as ischemic and hemorrhagic stroke, tumors, and demyelinating disease, although these lesions rarely cause vision loss in isolation.

PRIMARY VISUAL CORTEX

Lesions of the occipital lobe are similarly diverse (stroke, tumor, demyelination, PRES), although they are much more likely to cause vision loss in isolation. For example, a stroke of the PCA territory can often have a homonymous hemianopsia as its only manifestation.

HIGHER ORDER VISUAL CORTEX

Given the wide range of visual processing the brain must accomplish to interpret visual input, there are many disorders of the higher order visual cortex. Some of these include achromatopsia, which is the impairment of color vision; prosopagnosia, which is the impairment of face recognition; or other visual agnosias, which limit the ability to name or recognize items by only visual cues.

Autoimmune Disorders

Karl E. Misulis, Martin A. Samuels, and Eli E. Zimmerman

Overview of Autoimmune Disorders

Autoimmune disorders rely on clinical diagnosis including localization. However, there is no specific examination finding that indicates autoimmune pathogenesis. The diagnosis of most autoimmune disorders is syndromic and is supported by careful examination, laboratory studies, and usually imaging. In general, most autoimmune disorders have localization that is in either not confined to a singular neurologic localization or is not confined to neurologic localization at all but rather spans organ systems.

The list of autoimmune disorders is large, so this chapter will focus on a few select disorders for which history and examination can suggest the diagnosis:

- Optic neuritis
- Multiple sclerosis
- Neuromyelitis optica
- Autoimmune encephalitis

Optic Neuritis

Optic neuritis (ON) is characterized by inflammation and demyelination of the optic nerve. This finding is usually idiopathic, although approximately 50% of patients with ON subsequently develop multiple sclerosis (MS). Clinical features cannot clearly differentiate isolated ON from MS-associated ON.

History is typically visual loss in one eye, although near-simultaneous bilateral involvement can occur. Pain with eye movement suggests optic nerve inflammation. Visual field defect is usually central as opposed to hemifield or quadrant defect that is seen with brain lesions. Color vision is lost more than visual acuity. Expert examination of the eye is important to rule out ocular causes that can be confused clinically with ON. With ON, the eye usually shows papilledema, although over time optic atrophy develops.

ON is suspected when patients report subacute onset of monocular or binocular visual loss, especially when there is pain with eye movement. Pain of the eye itself raises concern for a primary globe issue. Abrupt loss of vision suggests a vascular etiology. History of other transient neurologic deficits suggests MS.

Multiple Sclerosis

MS is characterized by numerous regions of demyelination with relative preservations of axons. Initial symptoms are related to focal central nervous system (CNS) damage and can occur almost anywhere. The most important lesions are of the optic nerve and spinal cord. Patients may appear with ON or transverse myelitis; however, only a subset of patients with these isolated conditions develop MS.

Common early symptoms include visual disturbance, hemiparesis or hemisensory loss, myelopathy, dizziness, ataxia, and trigeminal neuralgia. Symptoms may be mild enough to escape the attention of patients or clinicians for years. When a patient complains of a neurologic deficit that might be a presentation of MS, the clinician must specifically ask about previous neurologic deficits.

The lesions are in the white matter and are easily seen on T2-weighted magnetic resonance imaging (MRI) in most patients. Enhanced T1-weighted images may show plaques and may be more sensitive for acute lesions. It has become apparent that MS also may manifest as a progressive gray matter degenerative process with smoothly progressive symptomatology, as opposed or in addition to episodes or attacks. Progressive MS may be superimposed on the episodic form of the disease. Patterns of MS include primary progressive, relapsing-remitting, and secondary progressive stages of the illness. The diagnosis of MS requires multiple attacks in space and time, diagnosed by clinical findings and/or MRI.

Diagnosis is made by findings on history and examination of more than one CNS lesion. MRI may show plaques, but in the absence of clinical findings of multiple lesions, the diagnosis of MS is not made. A single attack is named clinically isolated syndrome (CIS) or radiologically isolated syndrome (RIS). Cerebral spinal fluid (CSF) analysis may show oligoclonal immunoglobulin G (IgG) in the CSF but not in the serum, an abnormal IgG to albumin ratio, myelin basic protein, and/or antibodies to myelin basic protein. None of these findings is diagnostic, and none is 100% specific for MS. However, in the appropriate clinical setting, these CSF abnormalities can support the diagnosis. Evoked potentials (EPs) can provide supportive evidence of MS by showing clinically silent lesions. For example, in a patient with ON, an abnormal visual EP is expected, but an abnormal somatosensory EP may suggest a spinal or cerebral lesion; therefore, MS becomes more likely.

Diagnosis of clinically definite MS requires two attacks and clinical signs of two separate neurologic lesions. Laboratory-supported definite MS requires two attacks and clinical signs of one lesion plus MRI or EP evidence of an additional lesion or a single attack with associated clinical findings plus clinical or MRI or EP evidence of another lesion. Laboratory evidence includes oligoclonal bands or increased IgG in the CSF.

A diagnosis of clinically probable MS requires two attacks with clinical signs of one lesion or one attack with associated clinical findings with clinical, MRI, or EP evidence of another lesion. Laboratory-supported probable MS requires two attacks with CSF abnormalities.

On the basis of clinical and laboratory data, patients may be classified as

- Clinically isolated syndrome,
- Relapsing-remitting MS,
- Primary progressive MS, or
- Secondary progressive MS.

CIS is diagnosed when a patient has a first episode of focal or multifocal deficits consistent with demyelination without other provocation but without previous events. Some but not all of these patients will go on to develop relapsing-remitting MS (RRMS).

RRMS is diagnosed when a patient has had two or more separate events of unprovoked demyelination in different locations. The two events can be evidenced by two separate clinical events or one event plus MRI evidence of other lesions.

Primary progressive MS (PPMS) is diagnosed when there is continuous progression from disease onset, although there can be superimposed flares and improvements. The key is the progressive trajectory from the onset.

Secondary progressive MS (SPMS) is diagnosed when there is occurrence of a one or more demyelinating events and then steady progression with or without superimposed flares. Patients typically carry the diagnosis of RRMS before transitioning to SPMS.

Neuromyelitis Optica Spectrum Disorder

Neuromyelitis optica (NMO) is now renamed as NMO spectrum disorder (NMOSD). Demyelination is prominent in the optic nerves and spinal cord, hence the origin of the name.

A history suggesting the diagnosis of NMOSD includes episodes of visual loss involving either both eyes or one shortly after the other. Patients often develop myelopathy consistent with transverse myelitis and when present with ON, the combination strongly suggests the diagnosis of NMOSD.

Clinical involvement is not confined to the spinal cord and optic nerves; some caudal brainstem involvement can also occur. MRI supports the diagnosis if there is spinal cord and optic nerve involvement without other brain involvement, but half or more patients may have brain abnormalities on MRI, which might suggest MS. The diagnosis is more specifically supported by positive aquaporin-4 (AQP4) antibody in the serum, especially during an attack.

Autoimmune Encephalitis

Autoimmune encephalitis (AIE) is brain inflammatory change with an immune-mediated etiology as opposed to infectious etiology. AIE is caused by antineuronal antibodies. The prototypic disorder is anti-NMDA receptor encephalitis. The presentation often involves symptoms of encephalitis such as fever, headache, confusion, and seizures, but it has differentiating features including psychosis or hallucinations. There are no specific findings on CSF and MRI, although CSF pleocytosis is expected, and MRI may show FLAIR changes. For anti-NMDA receptor encephalitis, a specific CSF antibody can make the diagnosis, but often treatment should begin before the result of the testing is completed.

Lambert-Eaton Myasthenic Syndrome

Lambert-Eaton myasthenic syndrome (LEMS) is discussed in Chapter 5.5. This is an autoimmune disorder that is suspected when a patient has weakness suggestive of myasthenia but with prominent autonomic signs, including dry mouth, and often without ophthalmoplegia or ptosis that would suggest myasthenia gravis.

Infectious Diseases

Karl E. Misulis and Martin A. Samuels

Overview of Infectious Disease

Neuroinfectious diseases are a prominent aspect of acute care neurology. For many patients, there is not a specific localization but rather a mode of presentation that raises suspicion for infections of the nervous system.

Effects of systemic infections on the nervous system are even more common than direct infections, and neurologists are often asked to diagnose neurologic symptoms in patients with systemic infection.

The diagnostic approach begins with suspicion. There are several clinical scenarios that raise concern for neuroinfectious disease.

Headache with neck stiffness with an otherwise normal examination suggests meningeal inflammation. If there is a fever or mental status changes, then bacterial meningitis is considered, as are viral encephalitides, especially Herpex Simplex Virus (HSV).

Confusion and fever have a broad differential diagnosis, and they are often due to delirium from a systemic infection rather than primary central nervous system (CNS) infection. However, meningitis or encephalitis is certainly possible, and empiric treatment is often needed even before diagnosis is confirmed.

Confusion and focal findings suggest encephalitis or brain abscess. Meningitis can produce focal signs if there is secondary vascular change.

Headache, fever, and seizure suggest abscess or encephalitis. If there are focal signs, then abscess is suggested; if there is seizure without focal signs, then encephalitis is more likely. Note that febrile seizures are not expected in adults, so CNS infection is considered.

Infections of the Nervous System

ABSCESS

Abscesses can be single or multiple; when multiple, they cause multifocal signs and symptoms. Brain abscesses develop due to extension of infection from structures near the brain or from hematogenous dissemination. Spread of infection from the mastoid or other sinuses usually produces solitary abscesses. Hematogenous dissemination has a predilection for multiple abscesses. Multiple abscesses are prevalent with infective endocarditis, HIV, congenital heart disease, and lung abscesses. The clinician should consider nonneurologic involvement, sources of emboli, and immune deficiency. Evaluation may include echocardiogram, blood cultures, urine culture, complete blood count, HIV test, and chest radiograph.

Brain abscess is suspected when a patient has the triad of headache, focal neurologic signs, and fever, but these symptoms are present in a minority of patients. Therefore, the absence of any of the triad features does not exclude brain abscess. When a patient has a presentation that raises concern for meningitis, brain imaging should be done, if available, prior to lumbar puncture (LP). When bacterial infection is suspected, antibiotics and antiviral agents are begun as soon as the diagnosis is given reasonable suspicion, even before imaging is performed. If LP is not practical, antibiotics and antivirals are started and blood cultures are initiated.

MENINGITIS

Meningitis can be bacterial, viral, or fungal. There is overlap, but generally, bacterial meningitis is more fulminant than the other two. The most common presentation of bacterial meningitis is headache, fever, neck stiffness, and often nausea with or without confusion.

LP is the definitive test for meningitis, but brain imaging should be performed prior to LP if there is altered mental status or focal neurologic signs. The most dangerous lesions with regard to deterioration from LP are lesions near the midline, in the posterior fossa, and intraspinal/extramedullary processes. If the LP is delayed, then laboratory tests and blood cultures are performed and antimicrobial therapy is begun immediately.

Fungal meningitis, particularly cryptococcal meningitis, is seen most often in patients with HIV, but it is also seen in patients who do not have HIV. In most instances, they are known to be immunocompromised, especially after organ transplant, although other conditions with immune suppression can predispose to cryptococcal meningitis. The diagnosis is suspected with a subacute onset of headache, often with cognitive changes, but this diagnosis should be considered in almost any immunocompromised patient with headache and/or cognitive change.

Viral meningitis is common and is likely to be underdiagnosed. Diagnosis is suspected with headache often with nausea, fever, and malaise. Focal signs or frank encephalopathy should not be present. Diagnosis is confirmed by LP.

ENCEPHALITIS

Encephalitis means brain inflammation. The most common cause is viral, but nonviral pathogens may also cause encephalitis. Immune-mediated encephalitis is an important etiology.

Acute encephalitis typically presents with fever, headache, and mental status change. These are nonspecific symptoms, so bacterial meningitis, bacterial cerebritis, tuberculous, and fungal infections must be considered. Mild to moderate cerebrospinal fluid (CSF) pleocytosis supports the diagnosis of acute encephalitis. A markedly elevated CSF white blood cell count suggests a bacterial process. Moderate CSF pleocytosis with high protein levels and very low glucose suggests tuberculous meningitis.

Herpes Simplex Encephalitis

Identification of herpes simplex encephalitis is important because treatment with acyclovir has been shown to alter the course of the illness, although most viral encephalitides do not respond well to antiviral treatment. Patients can appear with all the symptoms of acute viral encephalitis, including headache, fever, and mental status change. In addition, patients usually have focal signs including hemiparesis, aphasia, visual field deficits, ataxia, cranial nerve palsies, and focal seizures.

There are two subtypes of herpes simplex virus, HSV-1 and HSV-2. HSV-1 causes cold sores, and HSV-2 causes genital herpes. HSV-1 is the most common cause of herpes encephalitis in adults, whereas HSV-2 is the most common cause in neonates, due to vaginal or transplacental transmission of infection.

HSV encephalitis differs in presentation from most other viral encephalitides because of the predilection for focal damage, especially in the temporal and frontal regions. HSV encephalitis in neonates, however, is global, so focal findings are often absent.

Diagnosis of HSV encephalitis is suspected when a patient with symptoms and signs of encephalitis has focal findings. Diagnosis is supported by imaging and/or electroencephalogram (EEG) showing focal abnormalities and by CSF pleocytosis. Note that the pleocytosis may be polymorphonuclear early in the course. Herpes simplex polymerase chain reaction (PCR) and antigen testing is routinely available. Brain biopsy is almost never needed; clinical suspicion with supportive laboratory findings provides enough security in the diagnosis to warrant antiviral treatment. The PCR for HSV is about 90% sensitive and 90% specific. A negative test in a patient with the appropriate clinical history should be followed by another test as there is a 50% likelihood of a false negative, if the pretest probability is high.

Arbovirus Encephalitis

Arboviruses are carried by mosquitoes and ticks. Distinction between individual arboviruses is not clinically important, although it may be important for control of the insect vector. Infection in humans presents as acute encephalitis, with fever, headache, and mental status change.

Differentiation from HSV encephalitis is important, as arbovirus encephalitis does not respond to antiviral therapy. Arbovirus encephalitis lacks the focal findings of and may be less fulminant than HSV encephalitis. Overall, the prognosis for full recovery is better with arbovirus encephalitis.

Neurologic Complications of Systemic Infections

Systemic infections often result in neurologic complications. Sometimes complications are caused by the spread of the infectious agent into the CNS, but this section refers to remote or secondary effects of the systemic infection.

Delirium in addition to the usual symptoms of urinary tract infection or pneumonia, these conditions can produce malaise and sometimes confusion; ultimately delirium can develop, especially in patients of advanced age and in patients with reduced cognitive reserve. Hospital delirium associated with medical illness is second only to stroke as the reason for neurologic consultation in most general hospitals.

Critical illness neuromuscular weakness is common in the intensive care unit (ICU) and is suspected when a patient has weakness after recovering from sedation. There are myopathic and neuropathic forms, and some patients show elements of both. Critical illness myopathy (CIM) presents with flaccid weakness; these patients are often hard to wean from ventilatory support. CIM can develop within days. Critical illness polyneuropathy (CIP) presents with sensory and motor deficits, and it tends to occur later than CIM, usually after more than a week of critical illness.

Neurologic complications of treatments are likely underdiagnosed. Some commonly used medications may predispose patients to the neuromuscular syndromes; encephalopathy and even seizures can be related to certain medications, especially if doses are not adequately adjusted for impaired clearance or if higher doses are needed. One of these is cefepime neurotoxicity. This can develop in patients with impaired renal function. Patients present with encephalopathy and ataxia, often with associated myoclonus, seizures, or even status epilepticus including nonconvulsive status epilepticus.

Tumors With Neurologic Involvement and Remote Effects of Tumors

Eli E. Zimmerman and Karl E. Misulis

Clinical Presentation of Tumors With Neurologic Involvement

Tumors of the central nervous system (CNS) have protean manifestations. Although they commonly present with focal neurologic findings, they can often be more insidious in onset, with more subtle manifestations. Intracranial tumors (benign or malignant, or supra- or infratentorial) often present with evidence of intracranial hypertension or elevated intracranial pressure. Patients have headache with nausea or vomiting and focal neurologic signs that commonly can result in accurate localization.

Tumor is suspected when a patient presents with focal neurologic findings and headache. Alternatively, a patient without headache may present with focal symptoms and signs that are progressive.

Specific Disorders

CEREBRAL TUMORS

Common Supratentorial Tumors

The most common type of CNS tumor is a metastatic lesion from a systemic source. These arise from the most common systemic tumors, including lung, breast, colon, and renal cell. These tumors often show multiplicity of lesions (although not always), with a pattern of ring enhancement.

Glioblastoma multiforme (GBM) is the highest grade of astrocytic tumors. They are infiltrative and relentlessly progressive, with very high mortality. These are often solitary, with ring enhancement. Lower grade astrocytomas (anaplastic astrocytomas, diffuse astrocytomas, oligodendrogliomas) show variable enhancement patterns by imaging and often progress to glioblastoma.

Meningiomas are tumors arising from the meninges and are often discovered either incidentally or after the development of seizures given their propensity to irritate the cortex.

Other intracranial tumors include tumors of the skull base or pituitary gland.

Common Infratentorial Tumors

Infratentorial tumors, or ones in the posterior fossa, are more common in the pediatric population. The three most typical tumors to present in children and in the posterior fossa are medulloblastomas, ependymomas, and pilocytic astrocytomas. Medulloblastomas are aggressive and typically highly cellular. Ependymomas are commonly found squeezing through skull foramina. Pilocytic astrocytomas are the most benign of the group and are often comprised of a cyst with a mural nodule.

In adults, infratentorial tumors are most commonly metastases, but astrocytoma and hemangioblastoma can occur. Schwannomas (often on the vestibular nerve) are benign histologically but can cause neurologic manifestations, including hearing loss or facial weakness without other evidence of intracranial pressure elevation.

MENINGEAL TUMORS

Meningiomas are the most common primary brain tumor. They are usually benign. Meningioma usually presents with location-specific symptoms; growth is usually so slow that headache is not the most common symptom. In fact, the most common presentation is no symptoms at all; meningioma is discovered incidentally on imaging performed for an unrelated neurologic problem or at the time of autopsy. Seizures can occur. Focal signs depend on location. Focal weakness suggests involvement of the motor pathways. Hearing loss and ataxia suggest a posterior fossa lesion, especially at the cerebellopontine angle. Visual deficit develops with some skull-based tumors and other meningiomas affecting the optic nerve pathways. Confusion and behavioral change without focal signs can occur, especially with lesions affecting the frontal lobes.

SPINAL TUMORS

Spinal cord tumors are either intramedullary, intradural extramedullary, or extradural. There are no definite indicators from history on examination that can pinpoint one location. All spinal cord tumors produce pain, which can be local in the region of the tumor or radiate down the neural distribution of the level(s) affected.

Intramedullary tumors are most commonly glioma, such as ependymoma or astrocytoma. The etiology can also be metastases, most commonly from lung cancer. Other cancers known for widespread metastases can produce intramedullary metastases, including breast cancer, melanoma, and renal cell cancer.

Intradural extramedullary tumors are primarily meningiomas, but alternatives include neurofibromas.

Extradural tumors are usually metastatic, and lung cancer and breast cancer are the most common etiologies.

TUMORS AFFECTING PERIPHERAL NERVES

Peripheral nerve tumors are uncommon, but they do occur. Most are benign; neurofibroma and schwannoma are the most common. Patients present with neuropathic findings of pain or loss of function usually in the distribution of a single nerve. The suspicion is enhanced with a detectable mass in an appropriate location.

Remote Effects of Tumors

There are a host of direct effects of tumors on the nervous system, including deficits from local cerebral, spinal, or peripheral nerve destruction to seizures or intracranial hemorrhages. There are also a host of remote effects that fall into a few categories.

As remote effects of cancer, paraneoplastic disorders are a prominent cause of neurologic dysfunction. A few of the most important are as follows:

- Cerebellar degeneration is often associated with ovarian, breast, and lung cancer, but other cancers can cause this. Patients present with appendicular and gait ataxia and often have cerebellar speech abnormalities and eye movement abnormalities.
- Limbic encephalitis is often associated with lung cancer, although testicular and other cancers cause this. Patients present with behavioral change, confusion, and sometimes seizures.

- Encephalomyelitis can be due to one of a variety of antibodies. In older patients, it is most often seen with lung cancer; in younger patients, it is often seen with testicular cancer. Patients present with symptoms and signs of brain and spine involvement and various combinations of mental status (cerebral), ataxia and tremor (brainstem), and corticospinal (brain or spinal) dysfunction.
- Encephalitis with anti-NMDA receptor antibodies is classically seen in young women with ovarian teratoma. Patients present with psychiatric and cognitive changes that can often be mistaken for primary psychiatric disorder.

Nutritional deficiency is common in patients with some cancers. Wernicke encephalopathy is classically described in patients with alcohol abuse, but it occurs in some patients with cancer.

Immune deficiency can be an effect of the cancer, but it is more often due to antineoplastic therapy. This can produce opportunistic infections of the nervous system.

Bleeding from the cancer or from antineoplastic therapy due to impaired and reduced platelet count or the use of anticoagulation medications for a cancer-related hypercoagulable state create a heightened risk of cerebral and spinal hemorrhage.

Functional Disorders

Karl E. Misulis, Martin A. Samuels, and Howard S. Kirshner

Overview of Functional Disorders

Functional disorder is a disorder of the function of the patient without a neurologic cause. The etiology is in the mind of the patient, usually subconsciously but sometimes with conscious intent.

Conversion disorder is considered to be a subconscious and neurologic manifestation as a representation of the underlying psychiatric etiology.

Malingering implies the conscious intent to deceive. There is usually some secondary gain, either in attention, medication, or compensation, but sometimes the etiology is unclear.

It is debated whether malingering can be truly distinguished from conversion reaction. One prominent neurologist, Raymond D. Adams, said that the neurologist can be sure only if the patient admits to deliberate falsification. In some patients, true symptoms are present, but the patient exaggerates them for secondary gain. For example, some patients with seizure disorder have both epileptic and psychogenic events.

Diagnosis of Select Functional Presentations

SEIZURES

Patients can present with clinical seizures that can be of various types. Because there is such a broad spectrum of clinical seizure activity and there are many individuals with atypical manifestations of seizures, it is often difficult to be certain that an event is an epileptic seizure on clinical grounds alone.

If an event looks like a seizure but on clinical and/or electroencephalogram (EEG) grounds is shown not to be a seizure, then the term paroxysmal nonepileptic seizure (PNES) has historically been used and is still used by some. However, the terminology on seizures has evolved. International standards have defined a seizure as being a manifestation of a disorder of neuronal activity in the brain. However, when what appears to be seizure is not due to abnormal activity, it is not a seizure. Hence, the former terminology of PNES is no longer preferred. The new terminology is nonepileptic event and, in this case, psychogenic nonepileptic event (PNEE).

Clues to the diagnosis of PNEE include the following:

- Responsiveness during an apparent generalized convulsive activity
- Pelvic thrusting
- Large-amplitude side-to-side head movements
- Alternating movements of the two sides, for example, bicycling
- Eyes closed during event
- Often precipitated by suggestion
- Absence of seizure discharge on EEG with clinical event

None of these symptoms are absolute, but they are of help in making the diagnosis. There are pitfalls in diagnosis. Rare patients can have responsiveness during a bilateral motor seizure (supplementary motor area seizure). There can be an absence of seizure discharge with a clinical event because some inferior frontal and medial temporal focal seizures can have behavioral manifestations, yet no discharges are seen from scalp electrodes because of the deep nature of the focus.

MOVEMENT DISORDER

Functional movement disorder is the preferred term for psychogenic movement disorders.

Types of functional movements vary. Among them are

- Tremor,
- Rigidity, and
- Gait abnormality.

As with seizures, there are clues, but none of these are definitive. Clues to functional movement disorder include the following:

- Tremor that alternates between the two sides
- Movements that are normal when gesturing as part of dialog but then abnormal during examination
- Reduced movement with distraction
- Associated signs such as give-way weakness
- Gait that does not fit within that typically seen with a corticospinal or extrapyramidal defect, such as astasia-abasia

Some organic movement disorders can appear to be so bizarre as to be psychogenic, including hemiballismus; sometimes these patients have been initially diagnosed as functional.

COMA

Psychogenic unresponsiveness can resemble coma, but examination is usually able to make the diagnosis. Psychogenic unresponsiveness is usually considered when diagnostic studies are negative, including imaging and EEG. In many circumstances, however, the diagnosis can be made clinically.

Clues to psychogenic unresponsiveness include the following:

- The patient is on a gurney with hands folded on lap, legs crossed, head straight, and mouth closed.
- The patient holds eyes closed during physical examination, especially of the eyes.
- The patient forcibly resists passive movements by activating muscles on demand.

A pitfall in diagnosing psychogenic coma includes catatonia. Although catatonia is psychiatric, it does need to be accurately diagnosed and treated.

Another pitfall is a missed diagnosis of locked-in syndrome. A bilateral brainstem infarction, usually involving the pons, results in the patient being unable to move the limbs or face, yet the patient is awake. The only movement a locked-in patient can make is to move the eyes vertically or occasionally to blink. Unless a careful examiner attempts to communicate by eye movement code, the diagnosis of locked-in syndrome can be missed. Rarely, Guillain-Barré syndrome can produce such profound weakness that the patient appears locked in.

HEMIPLEGIA

Functional hemiplegia can usually be suspected on the basis of the examination, but neurodiagnostic studies are usually needed. Clues to a functional etiology for hemiparesis include

- Absence of brisk tendon reflexes;
- Holding limbs down when examiner is attempting passive movement of the affected limb(s); and
- Absence of corticospinal tract signs, including brisk tendon reflexes, generalization of reflexes (spread to involve other muscles), and absence of pathologic reflexes (such as Babinski).

The Hoover sign is useful in diagnosing patients with functional weakness. The patient is asked to push up with one leg while pushing down with the other leg. When the patient attempts to lift the "weak" limb, the supposedly "strong" limb does not push down forcefully. When the patient lifts the "strong" limb, the "weak limb" pushes down forcefully.

A pitfall in diagnosing functional hemiparesis or hemiplegia includes seizure activity. Occasionally a patient is seen with hemiplegia with reduced tone in the absence of imaging abnormalities; the EEG shows nonconvulsive seizure. This combination is rare.

Another pitfall is complex migraine. Patients with complex migraine can develop hemiplegia with normal CTA and magnetic resonance imaging.

Aarsland D, Kurz MW. The epidemiology of dementia associated with Parkinson disease. *J Neurol Sci*. 2010;289(1–2):18–22.

Acosta LMY, Stubblefield K, Conwell T, Espaillat K, Koons H, Konrad P, et al. Protocolizing the workup for idiopathic normal pressure hydrocephalus improves outcomes. *Neurol Clin Pract*. 2021;11(4):e447–e453.

Almeida OP. Prevention of depression in older age. *Maturitas*. 2014;79(2):136–141.

Brune AJ, Gold DR. Acute visual disorders—what should the neurologist know? *Semin Neurol*. 2019;39(1):53–60.

Clark LN, Louis ED. Essential tremor. *Handb Clin Neurol*. 2018;147:229–239.

Folstein MF, Folstein SE, McHugh PR. Mini-mental state: a practical method for grading the cognitive status of patients for the clinician. *J Psychiatr Res*. 1975;12:(3):189–198. PMID: 1202204.

Ginsberg L. Acute and chronic neuropathies. *Medicine (Abingdon)*. 2020;48(9):612–618.

Harada CN, Natelson Love MC, Triebel KL. Normal cognitive aging. *Clin Geriatr Med*. 2013;29(4):737–752.

Heilman KM, Meador KJ, Loring DW. Hemispheric asymmetries of limb-kinetic apraxia: a loss of deftness. *Neurology*. 2000;55:523–526.

Helmich RC, Toni I, Deuschl G, Bloem BR. The pathophysiology of essential tremor and Parkinson's tremor. *Curr Neurol Neurosci Rep*. 2013;13(9):378.

Hermann P, Appleby B, Brandel JP, et al. Biomarkers and diagnostic guidelines for sporadic Creutzfeldt-Jakob disease. *Lancet Neurol*. 2021;20:235–246.

Hoogstraten MC, Lakke JP, Zwarts MJ. Bilateral ballism: a rare syndrome. Review of the literature and presentation of a case. *J Neurol*. 1986;233(1):25–29.

Inouye SK, Bogardus ST Jr, Charpentier PA, Leo-Summers L, Acampora D, Holford TR, et al. A multicomponent intervention to prevent delirium in hospitalized older patients. *N Engl J Med*. 1999;340:669–676.

Johnston SC, Gress DR, Browner WS, Sidney S. Short-term prognosis after emergency department diagnosis of TIA. *JAMA*. 2000;284:2901–2906.

Kernan WN, Ovbiagele B, Black HR, Bravata DM, Chimowitz MI, Ezekowitz MD, et al. American Heart Association Stroke Council, Council on Cardiovascular and Stroke Nursing, Council on Clinical Cardiology, and Council on Peripheral Vascular Disease. Guidelines for the prevention of stroke in patients with stroke and transient ischemic attack: a guideline for healthcare professionals from the American Heart Association/American Stroke Association. *Stroke*. 2014;45(7):2160–2236.

Kirshner HS. *First Exposure to Neurology*. New York: McGraw Hill; 2007.

Liepmann H. Das Krankheitsbild der apraxie ("motorischen asymbolie"). *Monatschr Psychiatr Neurol*. 1900;8:15–44:102-132, 182-197. [Translated in part in Rottenberg DA, Hochberg FA. *Neurological Classics in Modern Translation*. New York: Hafner; 1977: 155-181.]

Lipowski ZJ. Delirium (acute confusional states). *JAMA*. 1987;258:1789–1792.

Loy CT, Schofield PR, Turner AM, Kwok JB. Genetics of dementia. *Lancet*. 2014;383(9919):828–840.

Markus HS. Stroke genetics. *Hum Mol Genet*. 2011;20(R2):R124–R131.

McKee AC, Stern RA, Nowinski CJ, et al. The spectrum of disease in chronic traumatic encephalopathy. *Brain*. 2013;136:43–64.

Mendez MF. *The Mental Status Examination Handbook*. Philadelphia: Elsevier; 2022.

Naeser MA, Palumbo CL, Helm-Estabrooks N, Stiassny-Eder D, Albert ML. Role of the medial subcallosal fasciculus and other white matter pathways in recovery of spontaneous speech. *Brain*. 1989;112:1–38.

Nasreddine ZS, Phillips NA, Bédirian V, Charbonneau S, Whitehead V, Collin I, et al. The Montreal Cognitive assessment, MoCA: a brief screening tool for mild cognitive impairment. *J Am Geriatr Soc*. 2005;53(4):695–699.

Newman-Toker DE, Kerber KA, Hsieh YH, Pula JH, Omron R, Saber Tehrani AS, et al. HINTS outperforms ABCD2 to screen for stroke in acute continuous vertigo and dizziness. *Acad Emerg Med*. 2013;20(10):986–996. PMID: 24127701.

Ochipa C, Rothi LJG, Heilman KM. Ideational apraxia: a deficit in tool selection and use. *Ann Neurol*. 1989;25:190–193.

Ossenkoppele R, Jansen WJ, Rabinovici GD, et al. Prevalence of amyoid PET positivity in dementia syndromes: a meta-analysis. *JAMA*. 2015;313:1939049.

Pandharipande PP, Ely EW, Arora RC, Balas MC, Boustani MA, La Calle GH, et al. The intensive care delirium research agenda: a multinational, interprofessional perspective. *Intens Care Med*. 2017;43(9):1329–1339.

Payne LE, Gagnon DJ, Riker RR, Seder DB, Glisic EK, Morris JG, et al. Cefepime-induced neurotoxicity: a systematic review. *Crit Care*. 2017;21(1):276.

Powers WJ, Rabinstein AA, Ackerson T, Adeoye OM, Bambakidis NC, Becker K, et al. Guidelines for the Early management of patients with acute ischemic stroke: 2019 update to the 2018 guidelines for the early management of acute ischemic stroke: a guideline for healthcare professionals from the American Heart Association/American Stroke Association. *Stroke*. 2019;50(12):e344–e418.

Pozdnyakova A, Laiteerapong N, Volerman A, Feld LD, Wan W, Burnet DL, et al. Impact of medical scribes on physician and patient satisfaction in primary care. *J Gen Intern Med*. 2018;33(7):1109–1115.

Prasad S, Galetta SL. Approach to the patient with acute monocular visual loss. *Neurol Clin Pract*. 2012;2(1):14–23.

Low molecular weight heparinoid ORG 10172 (danaparoid), and outcome after acute ischemic stroke: a randomized controlled trial. The Publications Committee for the Trial of ORG 10172 in Acute Stroke Treatment (TOAST) Investigators. *JAMA*. 1998;279:1265–1272.

Qureshi AI, Tuhrim S, Broderick JP, Batjer HH, Hondo H, Hanley DF. Spontaneous intracerebral hemorrhage. *N Engl J Med*. 2001;344:1450–1460.

Rao AK, Louis ED. Ataxic gait in essential tremor: a disease-associated feature? *Tremor Other Hyperkinet Mov (N Y)*. 2019;9.

Rubin DI. Brachial and lumbosacral plexopathies: a review. *Clin Neurophysiol Pract*. 2020;5:173–193.

Sacks O. *The Man Who Mistook His Wife for a Hat and Other Clinical Tales*. New York: Summit Books; 1985: 7–21.

Safdieh JE, Govindarajan R, Gelb DJ, Odia Y, Soni M. Core curriculum guidelines for a required clinical neurology experience. *Neurology*. 2019;92(13):619–626. (Erratum in: *Neurology*. 2019;93(3):135.).

Sandercock PA, Counsell C, Tseng MC, Cecconi E. Oral antiplatelet therapy for acute ischaemic stroke. *Cochrane Database Syst Rev*. 2014;2014(3):CD000029.

Schmahmann JD. Disorders of the cerebellum: ataxia, dysmetria of thought, and the cerebellar cognitive affective syndrome. *J Neuropsychiatry Clin Neurosci*. 2004;16(3):367–378.

Schwendimann RN. Metabolic and toxic myelopathies. *Continuum (Minneap Minn)*. 2018;24(2 Spinal Cord Disorders):427–440.

Shaban A, Leira EC. Neurological complications in patients with systemic lupus erythematosus. *Curr Neurol Neurosci Rep*. 2019;19(12):97.

Vyas D, Bohra V, Karan V, Huded V. Rapid Processing of Perfusion and Diffusion for Ischemic Strokes in the Extended Time Window: An Indian Experience. *Ann Indian Acad Neurol*. 2019;Jan-Mar;22(1):96-99. PMID: 30692767.

Walker HK. The suck, snout, palmomental, and grasp reflexes. In: Walker HK, Hall WD, Hurst JW, eds. *Clinical Methods: The History, Physical, and Laboratory Examinations*. Boston: Butterworths; 1990:chap 71.

Walker K, Ben-Meir M, Dunlop W, Rosler R, West A, O'Connor G, et al. Impact of scribes on emergency medicine doctors' productivity and patient throughput: multicentre randomised trial. *BMJ*. 2019;364:l121.

INDEX

Page numbers followed by "*f*" indicate figures, "*t*" indicate tables, and "*b*" indicate boxes.